IMPORTANT PRESCRIBING INFORMATION

All doses recommended in this book are, unless stated otherwise, based on an average (70 kg) adult. Doses suggested are those typically suitable for critically ill patients. Individual patients may, however, require more or less than the doses stated to achieve the optimal therapeutic, effect depending on particular circumstances. Many drugs for example may need dose adjustment in presence of reduced creatinine clearance.

Every effort has been made to ensure the accuracy of the information contained in this book, particularly that relating to drugs and drug doses. It is, however, the responsibility of the prescribing practitioner to ensure that all drug prescriptions are correct and neither the authors nor the publishers can be held liable for any errors.

If in doubt seek advice from your pharmacist or consult the *British National Formulary* (BNF).

D1352063

Intensive Care

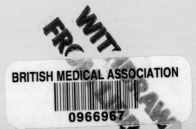

Commissioning Editor: Timothy Horne
Senior Development Editor: Ailsa Laing
Project Manager: Frances Affleck
Designer: Kirsteen Wright
Illustration Manager: Bruce Hogarth
Illustrations: Cactus

Intensive Care

Simon M Whiteley MB BS FRCA MA
Consultant, Intensive Care, St James's University
Hospital, Leeds, UK

Andrew Bodenham MB BS FRCA
Consultant, Intensive Care, The General Infirmary
at Leeds, Leeds, UK

Mark C Bellamy MA MB BS FRCA
Professor, Intensive Care, St James's University
Hospital, Leeds, UK

THIRD EDITION

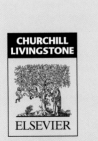

CHURCHILL
LIVINGSTONE

ELSEVIER

EDINBURGH LONDON NEW YORK OXFORD
PHILADELPHIA ST LOUIS SYDNEY TORONTO 2010

CHURCHIL LIVINGSTONE
An imprint of Elsevier Limited

First Edition © Pearson Professional Limited 1996
Second Edition © Elsevier Limited 2004
Third edition © 2010, Elsevier Limited. All rights reserved.

ISBN 978-0-443-06977-2

British Library Cataloguing in Publication Data
A catalogue record for this book is available from the British Library

Library of Congress Cataloging in Publication Data
A catalog record for this book is available from the Library of Congress

Notice
Knowledge and best practice in this field are constantly changing. As new research
and experience broaden our understanding, changes in research methods, professional
practices, or medical treatment may become necessary.

Practitioners and researchers must always rely on their own experience and knowledge
in evaluating and using any information, methods, compounds, or experiments
described herein. In using such information or methods they should be mindful of
their own safety and the safety of others, including parties for whom they have a
professional responsibility.

With respect to any drug or pharmaceutical products identified, readers are advised to
check the most current information provided (i) on procedures featured or (ii) by the
manufacturer of each product to be administered, to verify the recommended dose or
formula, the method and duration of administration, and contraindications. It is the
responsibility of practitioners, relying on their own experience and knowledge of their
patients, to make diagnoses, to determine dosages and the best treatment for each
individual patient, and to take all appropriate safety precautions.

To the fullest extent of the law, neither the Publisher nor the authors, contributors, or
editors, assume any liability for any injury and/or damage to persons or property as a
matter of products liability, negligence or otherwise, or from any use or operation of
any methods, products, instructions, or ideas contained in the material herein.

Printed in China

PREFACE

This small book follows other successful titles in the Churchill's Pocketbooks format. It is not intended to compete with the many already well-established texts in the field of intensive care, but is intended to present a distillation of sensible practice and ideas.

Every new doctor who is resident in the intensive care unit will be faced with a large variety of clinical problems to be solved. This book is therefore based on the common problems the authors are asked about on a regular basis, most of which can be easily solved by following simple rules. The aim has been to use the minimum of space by avoiding excessive detail, and no apology is made for repetition, or for what may on occasion appear a didactic approach. Information related to the specialist areas such as paediatric and cardiothoracic intensive care has been specifically excluded, although the general principles described are equally applicable in those areas. In many countries there are increasing moves to rotate trainees from different specialties, without previous intensive care experience, through intensive care. The hope is that this guide will prove timely and useful in this respect.

In the 13 years since the first edition and nine years since the second was published, there have been a number of changes in intensive care. We have incorporated these changes into this new edition. As a result, we have extensively revised the text and included a number of new or revised figures. The overall format however, remains the same. We hope that this edition will continue to provide new trainees in intensive care with safe, sensible and practical advice.

We are also aware that the book has proved popular with critical care nurses, physiotherapists and other healthcare professionals working in critical care, and hope that we have pitched the detail at the right level to also satisfy this readership

S.M.W.
A.B.
M.C.B.

CONTENTS

1. Organizational issues

Introduction 2
Definitions 2
Levels of care 3
Identification of patients at risk 4
Critical care outreach 5
Admission policies 6
Prediction of outcome 7
APACHE II severity of illness score 8
Alternative severity of illness scoring systems 12
Discharge policies 13
ICU follow-up clinics 15
National audit databases 15

2. Introduction to intensive care

Introduction 18
The multidisciplinary team 18
Daily routine 19
Infection control 19
Assessing a patient 22
Formulating an action plan 25
Medical records 26
Confidentiality 27
Talking to relatives 28
Consent to treatment in ICU 29

3. Basic principles

Care bundles 34
Sedation 34
Muscle relaxants 43
Psychological care of patients 47
Fluids and electrolytes 49
Nutrition 53
Enteral feeding 57
Parenteral nutrition 60
Stress ulcer prophylaxis 62
DVT prophylaxis 63

4. Cardiovascular system

Shock 66
Oxygen delivery and oxygen consumption 68
Cardiac output 70
Monitoring haemodynamic status 74
Optimization of haemodynamic status 78
Optimization of filling status 80
Optimization of cardiac output 82
Optimization of perfusion pressure 85
Rational use of inotropes and vasopressors 86
Hypotension 87
Hypertension 88
Disturbances of cardiac rhythm 90
Conduction defects 98
Myocardial ischaemia 100
Stable angina 100
Acute coronary syndromes 101
Cardiac failure 105
Cardiogenic shock 106
Pulmonary embolism 107
Pericardial effusion and cardiac tamponade 108
Cardiac arrest 109
Adult patient with congenital heart disease 111

5. Respiratory system

Introduction 114
Interpretation of blood gases 114

Definitions of respiratory
  failure   116
Management of respiratory
  failure   118
Continuous positive airway
  pressure (CPAP)   121
Non-invasive positive
  pressure ventilation   122
Invasive ventilation   123
Ventilation strategy and
  ventilator settings   127
Care of the ventilated
  patient   128
Common problems
  during artificial
  ventilation   131
High frequency modes of
  ventilation   133
Weaning from artificial
  ventilation   135
Airway obstruction   138
Community-acquired
  pneumonia   141
Pandemic influenza   143
Hospital-acquired
  pneumonia   143
Pneumonia in
  immunocompromised
  patients   145
Management of
  pneumonia   146
Aspiration
  pneumonitis   148
Asthma   149
Chronic obstructive
  pulmonary disease   152
Acute lung injury   154
Chest X-ray
  interpretation   158

6. Gastrointestinal system

Gastrointestinal tract in
  critical illness   168
Reduced gastrointestinal
  motility   170
Diarrhoea   170
Stress ulceration   172
Gastrointestinal
  ischaemia   172
Gastrointestinal
  bleeding   172
Intra-abdominal
  sepsis   174
Abdominal compartment
  syndrome   174
Hepatic dysfunction
  during critical
  illness   176
Hepatic failure   176
Acute pancreatitis   181

7. Renal system

Renal dysfunction in
  critical illness   184
Investigation of acute renal
  dysfunction   185
Oliguria   188
Management   188
Acute renal failure   189
Renal replacement
  therapy   190
Peritoneal dialysis   194
Outcome from acute
  renal failure in
  intensive care   195
Management of patients
  with chronic renal
  failure   195
Prescribing in renal
  failure   196
Plasma exchange   199

8. Metabolic and endocrine problems

Introduction   202
Sodium   202

Potassium   204
Calcium   207
Phosphate   209
Magnesium   210
Albumin   210
Metabolic acidosis   212
Metabolic alkalosis   215
Disturbances of blood
    glucose   215
Diabetic emergencies   217
Adrenal insufficiency   221
Phaeochromocytoma   222
Thyroid dysfunction   223
Temperature control   224

**9. Overdose, poisoning
and drug abuse**

Overdose and
    poisoning   230
Investigations   231
Measures to reduce
    absorption/increase
    elimination of
    drugs   231
Antidotes   233
Intensive care
    management   234
Paracetamol   235
Salicylates (aspirin)   236
Benzodiazepines and
    opiods   237
Antidepressants   237
Insulin overdose   238
Carbon monoxide and
    cyanide poisoning   239
Methanol and ethylene
    glycol   240
Alcohol   241
Recreational drug
    abuse   242
Problems associated
    with intravenous drug
    abuse   243

**10. Haematological
problems**

Introduction   246
Anaemia in the
    critically ill   246
Indications for blood
    transfusion   246
Blood products in
    the UK   247
Administration of blood
    products   250
Major haemorrhage   251
Risks and complications of
    blood transfusion   252
Patients who refuse
    transfusion   254
Normal haemostatic
    mechanisms   255
Coagulopathy   258
Thrombocytopenia   262
Disseminated intravascular
    coagulation   263
Purpuric disorders   264
Thrombotic disorders   264
The immunocompromised
    patient   266

**11. Brain injury,
neurological and
neuromuscular
problems**

Patterns of brain injury   272
Key concepts in brain
    injury   272
Immediate management of
    traumatic brain injury   274
Indications for CT scan   279
Indications for
    neurosurgical
    referral   280
ICU management of
    traumatic brain
    injury   281

Common problems in traumatic brain injury 284
Monitoring modalities in brain injury 288
Outcome following brain injury 290
Stroke and intracranial haemorrhage 292
Subarachnoid haemorrhage 292
Hypoxic brain injury 294
Infection 295
Seizures 296
Brainstem death 297
Neuromuscular conditions 301
Critical illness neuromyopathy 304
Neurological deficits following ICU 304

12. Trauma

Introduction 306
Primary survey 306
Exposure and secondary survey 308
Intensive care management 309
Head, face and neck injuries 310
Spinal cord injuries 311
Thoracic injuries 313
Abdominal injuries 316
Skeletal injuries 317
Fat embolism 318
Peripheral compartment syndromes 319
Rhabdomyolysis 320
Burns 320
Electrocution 322
Near drowning 323
Outcome following trauma 324

13. Infection and inflammation

Infection 326
Systemic inflammatory response syndrome (SIRS) 326
Definitions 327
Distinguishing infection 328
Sepsis care bundles 329
Septic shock 331
Investigation of unexplained sepsis 334
Empirical antibiotic therapy 336
Source control 336
Problem organisms 336
Catheter-related sepsis 340
Infective endocarditis 341
Necrotizing fasciitis 342
Meningococcal sepsis 342
Notifiable infectious diseases 345

14. Postoperative and obstetric patients

Peri-operative optimization 348
Stress response to surgery and critical illness 348
Postoperative analgesia 349
ICU management of the postoperative patient 357
Postoperative haemorrhage 359
Anaphylactoid reactions 361
Malignant hyperpyrexia 363
Obstetric patients 364

Pre-eclampsia/
  eclampsia   365
Peripartum
  haemorrhage   366
HELLP syndrome   366
Pregnancy-related heart
  failure   367

15. Practical procedures

General information   370
Arterial cannulation   372
Use of pressure
  transducers   374
Central venous
  cannulation   376
Changing and removing
  central venous
  catheters   386
Large-bore introducer
  sheaths/dialysis
  catheters   387
Pulmonary artery
  catheterization   389
Measuring PAOP   393
Measurement of
  cardiac output by
  thermodilution   394
Pericardial aspiration   395
Defibrillation and DC
  cardioversion   396
Intubation of the
  trachea   398
Extubation of the
  trachea   403
Insertion of laryngeal mask
  (supraglottic airways)   403
Percutaneous
  tracheostomy   404
Cricothyroidotomy/
  minitracheostomy   410
Fibreoptic bronchoscopy   412
Bronchoalveolar
  lavage   415

Insertion of chest drain   416
Passing a nasogastric
  tube   421
Passing a Sengstaken–
  Blakemore tube   422
Peritoneal tap/drainage of
  ascites   424
Turning a patient
  prone   425
Transport of critically ill
  patients   426

16. End of life issues

Introduction   430
Treatment limitation
  decisions   430
Managing withdrawal of
  treatment   431
Confirming death   433
Breaking bad news   434
Issuing a death
  certificate   434
Post-mortem
  examinations   435
Reporting deaths to the
  coroner   436
Brainstem death and organ
  donation   437
Non-heart beating organ
  donation   439
Cultural aspects of death
  and dying   440
Dealing with death at a
  personal level   443

Appendices

1. Drug information   445
2. Drug levels   449
3. Useful links   451

Index   453

ABBREVIATIONS

A&E accident and emergency
ACE angiotensin converting enzyme
ACN acute cortical necrosis
ACT activated clotting time
ACTH adrenocorticotrophic hormone
ADH antidiuretic hormone
AF atrial fibrillation
AIDS acquired immune deficiency syndrome
ALI acute lung injury
APTT activated partial thromboplastin time
ARDS adult respiratory distress syndrome
ARF acute renal failure
ASB assisted spontaneous breathing
AST aspartate aminotransferase
ATLS Advanced Trauma Life Support
ATN acute tubular necrosis
AV arteriovenous; atrioventricular
ANCA antineutrophil cytoplasmic antibodies
BAL bronchial alveolar lavage
BIPAP biphasic positive airways pressure
BNF British National Formulary
BSA body surface area
CCU coronary care unit
CFM cerebral function monitor
CK creatinine kinase
CMV controlled mandatory ventilation; cytomegalovirus
CO cardiac output
COPD chronic obstructive pulmonary disease

CPAP continuous positive airway pressure
CPDA citrate, phosphate, dextrose, adenosine
CPP cerebral perfusion pressure
CRP C-reactive protein
CSF cerebrospinal fluid
CT computerized tomography
CVA cerebrovascular accident
CVP central venous pressure
CVS cardiovascular system
CVVHD continuous venovenous haemodialysis
CVVHDF continuous venovenous haemodiafiltration
CVVHF continuous venovenous haemofiltration
CXR chest X-ray
DI diabetes insipidus
DIC disseminated intravascular coagulation
DKA diabetic ketoacidosis
DVT deep venous thrombosis
EBV Epstein–Barr virus
ECF extra cellular fluid
ECG electrocardiogram
ECMO extracorporeal membrane oxygenation
EDTA ethylenediamine tetra-acetic acid
EPO erythropoietin
ERCP endoscopic retrograde cholangiopancreatography
ETCO$_2$ end-tidal carbon dioxide
FBC full blood count
FDP fibrin degradation product
FFP fresh frozen plasma
FRC functional residual capacity
GCS Glasgow Coma Scale

GCSF granulocytic-colony stimulating factor
GFR glomerular filtration rate
GH growth hormone
GIT gastrointestinal tract
GTN glyceryl trinitrate
HDU high dependency unit
HELLP haemolysis, elevated liver enzymes, low platelets
HIT heparin-induced thrombocytopenia
HIV human immunodeficiency virus
HR heart rate
HUS haemolytic uraemic syndrome
ICP intracranial pressure
ICNARC Intensive Care National Audit and Research Centre
ICU intensive care unit
IHD ischaemic heart disease
INR international normalized ratio
IPPV intermittent positive pressure ventilation
ISS injury severity score
LDH lactate dehydrogenase
MAP mean arterial pressure
MH malignant hyperpyrexia
MODS multiorgan dysfunction syndrome
MRSA methicillin-resistant *Staphylococcus Aureus*
NG nasogastric
NIPPV non-invasive ventilation
NSAID non-steroidal anti-inflammatory drug
PA pulmonary artery
PACS picture archiving computer systems (digital X-rays)
PACU post-anaesthesia care unit
PAF platelet activating factor
PAFC pulmonary artery flotation catheter
PAOP pulmonary artery occlusion pressure
PCA patient-controlled analgesia
PCP *Pneumocystis carinii* pneumonia
PCR polymerase chain reaction
PE pulmonary embolism
PEA pulseless electrical activity
PEEP positive end expiratory pressure
PEG percutaneous endoscopic gastrostomy
PT prothrombin time
RAST radioallergosorbent tests
RRT renal replacement therapy
RTS revised trauma score
RV right ventricle
SAGM sodium chloride, adenosine, glucose, mannitol
SAPS Simplified Acute Physiology Score
SARS severe adult respiratory syndrome
SCID severe combined immune deficiency
SDD selective decontamination digestive tract
SIADH syndrome of inappropriate antidiuretic hormone
SIMV synchronized intermittent mandatory ventilation

SIRS systemic inflammatory response syndrome
SV stroke volume
SVR systemic vascular resistance
SVT supraventricular tachycardia
T3 tri-iodothyronine
T4 thyroxine
TEG thromboelastogram
TIA transient ischaemic attack
TIPSS transvenous intrahepatic portosystemic shunt
TISS Therapeutic Intervention Scoring System
TNF tumour necrosis factor
TO4 train of four
TPA tissue plasminogen activator
TPN total parenteral nutrition
TRALI transfusion-related acute lung injury
TSH thyroid stimulating hormone
TT thrombin time
TTP thrombotic thrombocytopenic purpura
U&E urea and electrolytes
VCJD variant Creutzfeldt–Jakob disease
VF ventricular fibrillation
VPB ventricular premature beat
VRE vancomycin-resistant enterococci
VSD ventricular septal defect
WCC white cell count

CHAPTER 1

ORGANIZATIONAL ISSUES

Introduction 2
Definitions 2
Levels of care 3
Identification of
  patients at risk 4
Critical care outreach 5
Admission policies 6
Prediction of outcome 7
APACHE II severity of
  illness score 8
Alternative severity of
  illness scoring systems 12
Discharge policies 13
ICU follow-up clinics 15
National audit
  databases 15

INTRODUCTION

Modern intensive care originated during the poliomyelitis epidemics of the 1950s, when tracheal intubation and positive pressure ventilation were applied to polio victims, resulting in a substantial improvement in survival. Patients were managed in a specific part of the hospital and received one-to-one nursing care, features that still largely define intensive care units (ICUs) to this day. From these beginnings, there was a gradual development until the ICU was a recognizable component of most general hospitals.

In the early days of intensive care, patients were often young and previously fit, with only single organ failure. If they survived, a full functional recovery could be anticipated. Today, in keeping with the changing structure of society, patients are often elderly and many have complex pre-existing medical problems, which predispose them to develop multiple organ failure during critical illness. As a consequence, the prospects for survival from critical illness are sometimes limited. This, together with the realization of the large costs involved in providing intensive care, typically approaching £2000 per day, has led to debate about how intensive care should be provided in the future. In particular, there is increasing focus on the complex ethical issues that surround admission, provision and discontinuation of intensive care therapy.

Nevertheless, intensive care medicine has become an established and fundamental part of modern health care. Critical illness may arise from a variety of disease processes, but the pathophysiological changes that result lead to common patterns of organ dysfunction. By recognizing these patterns and understanding the interactions between different organ systems, intensive care teams can improve the outcome of critically ill patients. The role of intensive care includes:

- Resuscitation and stabilization
- Physiological optimization of patients to prevent organ failure
- Facilitation of complex surgery
- Support of failing organ systems
- Recognition of futility.

DEFINITIONS

Traditional definitions of ICUs and high dependency units (HDUs) attempt to separate the functions of each.

Intensive care unit (ICU)

An area for patients admitted for the treatment of actual or impending organ failure, especially those requiring assisted ventilation. There is usually at least one nurse per patient and a doctor assigned solely to the intensive care unit throughout the 24-h period.

High dependency unit (HDU)

An area for patients who require more intensive observation or intervention than can be provided on a general ward, but who do not require assisted ventilation. Nurse-to-patient ratios are generally between those of an ICU and a general ward. There is not usually dedicated medical cover.

There are, however, difficulties with such definitions. In many smaller hospitals for example, the ICU, HDU and coronary care unit (CCU) are often combined in one area, with nursing and medical staff working flexibly as required. Post-anaesthesia care units (PACUs) or recovery rooms may be used to ventilate patients when the ICU is full. Many patients with chronic respiratory disease are now ventilated on respiratory wards, either via face / nasal masks or by long-term tracheostomy.

It is increasingly recognized, therefore, that the level of medical and nursing care received by individual patients should not be a function of their physical location, in an ICU or on the ward, but a function of their clinical condition. This has led to the classification of levels of care for critically ill patients based solely on need.

LEVELS OF CARE

Critically ill patients can be classified according to the level of medical and nursing care required (see Intensive Care Society 2002 Levels of Critical Care for Adult Patients www.ics.ac.uk/icmprof/downloads/icsstandards-levelsofca.pdf) (Table 1.1).

Patients should be nursed in an area capable of providing the appropriate level of care. While level 2 care may be provided in an HDU or ICU, true level 3 care can only be provided in a suitably equipped ICU. In reality, these levels of care are not discrete entities, but represent points on a continuum or spectrum. As their condition changes, patients may need a greater or lesser level of care, and frequently move between the defined levels.

TABLE 1.1 Levels of critical care

Level 0	Patients whose needs can be met by ward-based care in an acute hospital.
Level 1	Patients at risk of their condition deteriorating (including those recently moved from higher levels of care) whose needs can be met on a normal ward with additional advice or support from the critical care team.
Level 2	Patients requiring more advanced levels of observation or intervention than can be provided on a normal ward, including support for a single failing organ system.
Level 3	Patients requiring advanced respiratory support alone or basic respiratory support together with support for at least two organ systems.

Specialist care is recorded by attaching one of the following letters as a suffix.

N – neurosurgical, C – cardiac, T – thoracic, B – burns, S – spinal injury, R – renal, L – liver, A – other specialist care.

TABLE 1.2 Typical early warning scoring system

Score	3	2	1	0	1	2	3
Heart rate		<40	41–50	51–100	101–110	111–130	>130
BP	<70	71–80	81–100	101–199		>200	
RR		<8		9–14	15–20	21–29	>30
Temp.		<35	35.1–36.5			>38.5	
CNS				A	V	P	U

A: alert; V: responds to voice; P: responds to pain; U: unresponsive

IDENTIFICATION OF PATIENTS AT RISK

As the level of care required by an individual patient can change rapidly, it is important that those at risk of deterioration and needing increased levels of care are identified early, so that the appropriate interventions can be instituted.

A number of scoring systems have been developed to help staff detect those patients who are at risk. These are based on the principle that patients develop abnormal physiological parameters as their condition starts to deteriorate. The scoring system can be used by any member of the ward medical or nursing staff and if appropriate, the intensive care outreach team can be called (see below). An example of a typical early warning scoring system is shown in Table 1.2. The response triggered by the scoring system is shown in Table 1.3.

TABLE 1.3 Typical response to early warning scoring system		
Ward area	Score > 3	Call outreach team
High dependency area	Score > 3	Call responsible medical staff
	Score > 5	Call outreach team/ICU
Any area	Score > 10	Call outreach Team/ICU

CRITICAL CARE OUTREACH

Outreach is a relatively new concept in critical care. Traditionally, intensive care staff have tended to stay in the ICU and await the referral of patients from other areas by the attending medical staff. It is increasingly recognized, however, that the ICU staff have much to offer critically ill and potentially critically ill patients outside the ICU. This has led to the development of critical care outreach teams.

These teams commonly consist of senior members of medical, nursing and physiotherapy staff from the ICU who provide a liaison service and an immediate point of contact between the ICU and other areas of the hospital. Their roles include:

- Identification of patients at risk
- Prevention of further deterioration and the need for subsequent ICU admission
- Support for level 1 care on the wards
- Education and the promotion of critical care skills
- Identification of patients unlikely to benefit from ICU admission
- Facilitation of discharges from higher levels of care back to the ward.

Once contacted, the outreach team will usually assess a patient and may offer advice and support to ward staff. Early advice on matters such as fluid management and provision of intermediate respiratory support (e.g. physiotherapy/high flow oxygen/CPAP) may prevent further deterioration and enable the care of the patient to continue at ward level (level 1 care). Alternatively, the team may institute more advanced therapy and expedite transfer to an area capable of providing a higher level of care (level 2 or 3).

Occasionally the outreach team may, in consultation with the patient, relatives, and the parent medical team, decide that a patient is unlikely to benefit from intensive care and that admission would not be appropriate (see Limitation of treatment, p. 430).

ADMISSION POLICIES

The aim of intensive care is to support patients while they
recover. It is not to prolong life when there is no hope of recovery.
Sometimes difficult decisions have to be made about whether or
not to admit a patient to intensive care, as there is often a shortage
of intensive care beds and a requirement to use the available
resources responsibly and equitably. To aid decision making, some
units have written admission policies. A typical admission policy is
shown in Box 1.1.

The difficulty with all admission policies, however, is that it is
impossible to predict with complete accuracy which individual
patients stand to benefit from admission to intensive care.

Box 1.1 Admission policy

Requests for admission
- Patients will be admitted to ICU who in the opinion of the ICU
  consultant are likely to benefit from a period of intensive care.
  Patients in whom further treatment is considered futile will not
  normally be admitted.
- Requests for admission should be made by contacting the ICU
  consultant on call. Requests should normally come from a consultant
  who has seen the patient immediately prior to making a referral.
- In the case of elective surgery where the admission of the patient
  can be foreseen a request should be made at least 24 hours prior
  to surgery. The bed should be confirmed immediately prior to
  commencement of anaesthesia.

Bed management issues
- All problems related to availability of beds will be dealt with initially
  by the ICU consultant on call, who is in a position to make decisions
  about the potential admission and the needs of the patients already
  in the ICU.
- If there are no beds immediately available, the continued provision of
  care at an appropriate level to the patient remains the responsibility
  of the staff in attendance, supported where possible by the ICU
  outreach team.
- Where no ICU bed is available, the ICU consultant may be able to
  give advice as to the location of other available ICU beds; however,
  their prime responsibility is to patients already in the ICU.

Joint responsibility
- All patients will be admitted under the care of a named ICU
  consultant and the ICU team will assume responsibility for the
  patients care. (Responsibility may be shared jointly with the admitting
  team.)

Discharges
- Will be arranged by the ICU staff in conjunction with the responsible
  consultant. In cases of emergency, however, patients may be
  discharged by the consultant on-call for the ICU.

In practice, therefore, the decision whether or not to admit a patient to intensive care is usually based on the outcome of multidisciplinary discussion and clinical expertise.

Instantaneous judgements regarding the continuation or withdrawal of treatment from patients in the operating theatre, resuscitation room or on the wards are often difficult and increasingly, lawyers, patient advocates, independent mental capacity advocates (IMCAs) and clinical ethicists are being involved in the most difficult decisions. Senior staff should be involved early on. In many cases, unless the outlook is truly hopeless, patients will be admitted for a trial of treatment to see whether they will stabilize and improve over time.

Additionally, patients with little or no prospect of survival may occasionally be admitted to intensive care. For example, patients from the resuscitation room, or those who have suffered catastrophic complications during surgery, may be admitted even though they are likely to die. This is to facilitate more appropriate terminal care, or to allow the relatives time to visit and the bereavement process to be better managed. This is a justifiable and appropriate use of a critical care facility. Admission policies need, therefore, to be sufficiently flexible to allow the admission of what may seem, on occasion, like inappropriate cases (see Treatment limitation decisions, p. 430).

PREDICTION OF OUTCOME

The difficulties outlined above have led to a wealth of work, using scoring systems, to predict the outcome of patients treated in intensive care. This generally involves the collection of a large amount of data from many patients, stratification of the data to produce a risk score, prospective validation of the score, and its subsequent application to clinical decision making in specific cases. There are, however, major difficulties with this approach:

- There is, as yet, no satisfactory diagnostic categorization for intensive care patients. Often the problems relating to intensive care admission bear little relation to the original presenting complaint or diagnostic category.
- Although patients may survive to leave the ICU, there is a significant mortality on the wards, and later at home, after leaving intensive care. Many studies use 28-day mortality as an end point. It has been suggested that 6-month or 1-year outcomes of mortality and measures of morbidity (quality of life measures) are better end points.

- Scoring systems may accurately predict population outcomes, but are unreliable for prediction in individual cases.

The APACHE II score, for example (see below), which is arguably the best known outcome score, takes into account both acute physiological disturbance and individual pre-existing co-morbidity, and correlates well with the risk of death for the intensive care population as a whole, but does not accurately predict individual mortality.

Attempts have been made using computer modelling to improve the accuracy of outcome prediction models in individual patients. The Riyadh Intensive Care Program, for example, uses daily scores as a basis on which to predict those patients in which further treatment is futile. This approach has, however, failed to gain widespread support.

Severity of illness scoring systems therefore cannot be used to predict individual patient outcomes. Their value lies in the ability to predict accurately the overall mortality expected in a particular intensive care unit based on the local 'case mix'. The ratio of the actual mortality to the predicted case mix adjusted mortality provides a measure (standardized mortality ratio) by which individual units can be compared for audit purposes. A standardized mortality ratio (SMR) less than 1 implies better than predicted outcomes, whilst a SMR greater than 1 implies a worse than predicted outcome.

In the UK, a scoring system that predicts critical illness outcomes more accurately in a British patient population has been developed by the Intensive Care National Audit and Research Centre (ICNARC). Continuous ongoing data collection will enable the score to be further refined and improved. See National audit databases, p. 15.

APACHE II SEVERITY OF ILLNESS SCORE

The APACHE II (acute physiological and chronic health evaluation) tool is the most widely used severity of illness scoring system in intensive care. While now somewhat dated and originally related to an index population in the United States, it remains widely used because it is well known, reasonably well validated and internationally accepted as a 'case mix adjustment tool'.

A score is assigned to each patient on the basis of:

- worst physiological derangement, occurring in the first 24 h of admission (Table 1.4)
- age (Table 1.5)
- chronic health status (Box 1.2).

TABLE 1.4 APACHE II
A: Acute physiological derangement score sheet

Score	+4	+3	+2	+1	0	+1	+2	+3	+4
Core temp. (°C)	>41	39–40.9		38.5–38.9	36–38.4	34–35.9	32–33.9	30–31.9	<29
Resp. rate	>50	49–35		34–25	24–12	11–10	9–6		<5
MAP	>160	130–159	110–129		79–109		55–69	40–54	<39
Oxygen: if FiO$_2$ <0.5 use A–a gradient	>66.6	46.7–66.5	26.7–46.5		<26.7				
Oxygen: if FiO$_2$ <0.5 use PaO$_2$ (kPa)					>9.3	8.1–9.3		7.3–8.0	<7.3
Serum HCO$_3$ (mmol/L) or arterial pH	>52, >7.7	41–51.9, 7.6–7.69		32–40.9, 7.5–7.59	22–31.9, 7.33–7.49		18–21.9, 7.25–7.32	15–17.9, 7.15–7.24	<15, <7.15
Sodium (mmol/L)	>180	160–179	155–159	150–154	130–153		120–129	111–119	<110
Potassium	>7	6–6.9		5.5–5.9	3.5–5.4	3–3.4	2.5–2.9		<2.5
Creatinine mmol/L (score double in ARF)	>309	169–306	125–168		53–124		<53		
Hb g/dL	>20		16.7–19.9	166–15.4	15.3–10		9.9–6.7		<6.7
White blood count × 1000	>40		20–39.9	15–19.9	3–14.9		1–2.9		<1
Glasgow Coma Scale					Score 15 minus actual GCS				

TABLE 1.5 APACHE II
B: Age points

Score	0	+2	+3	+5	+6
Age	44	45–54	55–64	65–74	75

Box 1.2 APACHE II

C: Chronic Health Score

For patients with severe organ system insufficiency or immune compromise, assign scores as shown.

Condition must have been evident prior to this hospital admission and conform to the definitions below.

Category	Score
For non-operative or emergency postoperative patients	+5
For elective postoperative patients	+2

Definitions

CVS New York Heart Association Class IV.

Respiratory Chronic restrictive, obstructive or vascular disease resulting in severe exercise restriction, i.e. unable to climb stairs or perform household duties, or documented chronic hypoxia, hypercapnia, secondary polycythaemia, severe pulmonary hypertension or respiratory dependency.

Renal Receiving chronic dialysis.

Liver Biopsy proven cirrhosis and documented portal hypertension, episodes of past upper GI bleeding attributed to portal hypertension or prior episodes of hepatic failure/encephalopathy/coma.

Immunity Decreased resistance to infection, resulting from immunosuppressive therapy, chemotherapy, radiation, long-term or recent high-dose steroids, or has a disease that is sufficiently advanced to suppress resistance to infection, e.g. leukaemia, lymphoma, AIDS.

Notes on completing APACHE II scores

In many ICUs, APACHE data are collected by audit clerks and entered into electronic databases often as part of a much larger data set. You may, however, be expected to calculate scores on your patients and you should understand the process:

APACHE II score = acute physiology score (A) + age score (B) + chronic health score (C).

- Score the worst value for each parameter in the first 24 h.
- Where results are not available, score as zero. This does not mean that you do not have to try to find the result first!

Oxygen
$FiO_2 > 0.5$: Calculate the alveolar–arterial oxygen difference or (A–a)DO$_2$ expressed in kPa:

$$(A–a)DO_2 = \text{alveolar oxygen } (PAO_2) - \text{arterial oxygen } (PaO_2).$$

$$\text{alveolar oxygen} = FiO_2 \times (\text{atmospheric pressure} - \text{SVP water}) - PaCO_2$$

$$\text{alveolar oxygen} = FiO_2 \times (101 - 6.2) - PaCO_2$$

therefore

$$(A–a)DO_2 = (FiO_2 \times 94.8) - PaCO_2 - PaO_2.$$

The result of this gives the A–a gradient, which is then scored from the APACHE table:

Score	+4	+3	+2	+1	0
Result	>66.6	46.7–66.5	26.7–46.5		<26.7

$FiO_2 < 0.5$: simply score the PaO_2 in kPa:

Score	0	+13	+2	+3	+4
PaO_2 (kPa)	>9.3	8.1–9.3		7.3–8.0	>7.15

Serum HCO$_3$
Only use bicarbonate when there are no blood gases available. Otherwise score the arterial pH.

Glasgow Coma Scale (GCS)
A number of approaches to this are adopted in different units. Either (a) assign the assumed GCS patient would have had if not artificially sedated, or (b) as patients who are ventilated, paralysed and sedated will have a GCS of 3, score as $15 - 3 = 12$ (see below). Ask what is the usual practice in your unit.

Chronic health points
This can provide a significant loading to an APACHE score. Apply only according to the criteria on the scoring chart that imply established organ system impairment.

Problems with APACHE II
There are a number of problems with the APACHE II score:

● Patients with an APACHE II score >35 are unlikely to survive. However, the score is a statistical tool based on the population, and scores for individuals cannot be used to predict outcome. Some patients, for example those with diabetic ketoacidosis, may have marked physiological abnormalities, but generally get better quickly.

- The score is based on historical data, and as new interventions are developed, the data become obsolete.
- Lead-time bias results from the stabilization of patients in the referring hospital prior to transfer. This artificially lowers the score for the patient arriving at the referral centre.
- The GCS component is difficult to assess in patients receiving sedative or neuromuscular blocking agents. There is an important difference between a GCS 3 due to head injury and due to the effects of drugs.
- The physiological components are based on adults. They do not translate to paediatrics. For children the 'Pim' (paediatric index of mortality) or 'Prism' (paediatric risk of mortality) score is usually used instead.

ALTERNATIVE SEVERITY OF ILLNESS SCORING SYSTEMS

APACHE III score

The APACHE II score has now been superseded by an updated APACHE III score. Five new variables have been added (urine output, serum albumin, urea, bilirubin and glucose), while two variables (potassium and bicarbonate) have been removed. In addition, the Glasgow Coma Scale and acid–base balance components have been altered. A complex matrix grid scoring system is used with a maximum score of 299.

SAPS

The Simplified Acute Physiology Score is similar to APACHE, and is used more commonly in mainland Europe. It utilizes 12 physiological variables assigned a score according to the degree of derangement.

TISS

The Therapeutic Intervention Score System assigns a value to each procedure performed in the ICU. The implication is that the more procedures that are performed on a patient, the sicker they are. It is dependent on the doctor and unit, however, since different hospitals will have varying thresholds for carrying out many procedures. The score is therefore not good for comparing outcome between patients or between different units, but is useful as a general guide to the type of care and resources likely to be needed by patients on an individual unit.

SOFA score

The Sequential Organ Failure Assessment score tracks changes in the patient's condition over time. It comprises scores assigned to each of six components: respiratory, cardiovascular, hepatic, neurological, coagulation and renal. These are summed to produce an overall score. A score higher than 11, or between 8 and 11 and not improving, is generally associated with an adverse outcome.

DISCHARGE POLICIES

Discharge policies are just as hard to define as admission policies (above). Patients may be discharged in the following circumstances:

● Either: the patient's condition has improved to the extent that intensive care is no longer required.
● Or: the patient's condition is not improving and the underlying problems are such that continued intensive care is considered futile by staff on the ICU.

In the second of these situations, the patient may either die on the ICU or be transferred back to the ward in anticipation that they will not be resuscitated or readmitted to the ICU if their condition deteriorates further. It is imperative that the referring staff, the patient's family and, where possible, the patient, agree that such decisions are appropriate and that decisions are clearly documented.

For patients whose condition is improving and for whom discharge is considered, two questions should be asked, as follows.

1. When are patients fit to be discharged?

In simple terms, patients are fit for discharge from intensive care when they no longer require the specialist skills and monitoring available on the ICU. This generally means that they have no life-threatening organ failure and that their underlying disease process is stable or improving. Table 1.6 gives some guidance.

2. Where is the patient to be sent?

This will depend at least in part on the patient's underlying diagnosis, current condition, and where the patient came from in the first place. Some patients, especially elective postoperative surgical patients, may be fit enough to go straight back to a general ward. Others may, because of continuing organ dysfunction or other problems, require closer monitoring, supervision and nursing care and may go back to an HDU.

TABLE 1.6 Criteria for discharge from ICU

Airway	Adequate airway and cough to clear secretions (if inadequate, tracheostomy and suction, see below)
Breathing	Adequate respiratory effort and blood gases
	May be on oxygen (e.g. from face mask)
	Not requiring CPAP or non-invasive ventilation (unless discharged to HDU or respiratory unit), see below
Circulation	Stable, no inotropes
Neurological function	Adequate conscious level
	Adequate cough and gag reflexes (if inadequate, e.g. bulbar palsy or brain injury may need tracheostomy to make airway safe and allow suction)
Renal function	Renal function stable or improving
	Not requiring renal support unless discharged to a unit which performs dialysis
Analgesia	Adequate pain control

Increasingly patients with chronic respiratory disease or those who are slow to wean from a ventilator may be transferred to a respiratory HDU capable of providing CPAP and non-invasive forms of ventilation. Some centres are developing specific long-term weaning units for this purpose and for caring for patients with tracheostomies.

Patients who have been transferred from another ICU for specialist treatment or because of lack of beds may be discharged back to the referring hospital. In general, patients should be returned to their referring hospital as soon as possible, if only for the sake of relatives who may find travelling difficult.

Wherever possible, patients should only be discharged during normal daytime hours. Indeed, the time of day at which patients are discharged is taken as a 'quality indicator' for intensive care units in the United Kingdom. There is evidence that patients who are discharged from intensive care outside the normal working day are at greater risk of subsequent deterioration and readmission. The causes of this are probably multifactorial, but may include patients being discharged prematurely to facilitate the admission of another patient, and reduced levels of out of hours supervision on the wards.

Occasionally, patients may either self-discharge or be fit for discharge home prior to a ward bed becoming available (e.g. after overdosage of sedative drugs). In such cases the patient's family or friends may be able to attend to take them home direct from ICU.

In general, it is helpful prior to discharge to document explicit decisions regarding circumstances under which treatment should be re-escalated, whether or not readmission to intensive care is appropriate, and whether or not to attempt resuscitation in the event of acute deterioration. Such decisions should not be 'written on tablets of stone', however, and should be revisited on a regular basis, in full consultation with the patient or their advocate.

ICU FOLLOW-UP CLINICS

Traditionally, outcome studies in intensive care have focused on mortality. Recently there has been increased interest in the morbidity that may occur in survivors of intensive care, and many units now run ICU follow-up clinics. Typically, patients who have survived are seen 2 or 3 months after discharge. As well as providing an opportunity to assess a patient's physical and emotional well-being after ICU admission, it gives patients an opportunity to reflect and give feedback on their experiences. It is likely, in the future, that feedback from follow-up clinics will help inform and improve overall quality of patient care during critical illness.

NATIONAL AUDIT DATABASES

The importance of national, collaborative audit and research in intensive care is now well recognized. The Intensive Care National Audit and Research Centre for England and Wales (ICNARC) and the Scottish Intensive Care Society Audit group have large national ICU databases that record demographic details, diagnostic criteria, physiological scoring, and outcome data on the majority of adult patients admitted to intensive care in the UK.

CHAPTER 2

INTRODUCTION TO INTENSIVE CARE

Introduction   18

The multidisciplinary team   18

Daily routine   19

Infection control   19

Assessing a patient   22

Formulating an action plan   25

Medical records   26

Confidentiality   27

Talking to relatives   28

Consent to treatment in ICU   29

INTRODUCTION

Setting foot in an intensive care unit for the first time can be a daunting experience. Many patients are very sick with complex, multi-system problems. Some will die. There may be large arrays of unfamiliar monitoring and therapeutic equipment at the bedside. The following pages are intended to help you survive and keep out of trouble during your first few days on the ICU. Remember, if in doubt ask someone.

THE MULTIDISCIPLINARY TEAM

The care of patients in intensive care is increasingly complex, which precludes all care being provided by a single individual or team. The critically ill patient is cared for in an area where they receive optimum care and input from a number of different specialties. A major role for junior and senior medical staff in intensive care is the coordination of all aspects of patient care, and in particular the maintenance of good lines of communication between the different teams involved. Many nursing, paramedical and technical staff are involved in the care of patients in intensive care. It is important to remember that all these people have skills and experience that you do not. Do not be afraid to ask for advice. If you treat them as colleagues you will get more from them, and remember that the unit is likely to run best when everyone supports each other.

Nursing staff

Many nursing staff in the ICU are very experienced and very knowledgeable. You should see them as allies. Listen to and carefully consider their advice. Remember also that nurses have their own job to do, which is demanding and time consuming. They are not there to run about after you, therefore if you can get something you need, get it and clear up your own mess after you!

Physiotherapists

Physiotherapists provide therapy for clearance of chest secretions. They have an important role in helping to maintain joint and limb function in bed-bound patients, and in mobilizing patients during their recovery. Physiotherapists are also key members of most outreach teams (see below). They can often provide help with the respiratory care and management of patients on general wards who are struggling to maintain adequate respiratory function, and who might otherwise require admission to a critical care unit. Their advice on when to intervene, when to temporize and when it is safe to do nothing is invaluable.

Pharmacists

The nature of intensive care is such that patients will often be on many medications. There is therefore great potential for drug interactions and incompatibility of infusions. In addition, many drug doses need to be modified in the presence of critical illness, either because of potential adverse effects in the critically ill (pharmacodynamic effect), or because their absorption, distribution and elimination may be abnormal (pharmacokinetic effect). These changes are likely to be particularly marked in patients with hepatic or renal failure, and may be difficult to predict. The pharmacist will generally review prescriptions, and is a ready source of advice on all therapeutic matters.

Dieticians

All patients who stay more than a very short time in ICU require some form of nutrition. While basic nutritional support can be provided by standard regimens, many hospitals now have nutrition teams including dieticians, who will tailor regimens to each patient's particular requirements.

Technicians

A large number of technical staff are involved in supporting the ICU. These include laboratory technicians, renal technicians who manage haemodialysis machines, and equipment service engineers. Cultivate a good relationship with all these people. They can be an invaluable source of help.

DAILY ROUTINE

The daily routine on the ICU will vary from unit to unit. There are typically one or two main business ward rounds during the day, which members of the multidisciplinary team may attend. You may well be expected to see and assess patients prior to the ward round and then to present your findings and action plan on the round. There may also be additional ward rounds during the day as other clinicians and/or results become available (e.g. microbiology).

INFECTION CONTROL

Patients receiving intensive care are, to a greater or lesser extent, immunocompromised and are at greatly increased risk of hospital-acquired (nosocomial) infection. This may result directly from the underlying disease process, as a non-specific response to critical illness, or as a side-effect of a treatment. In addition, multiple vascular catheters and invasive tubes that penetrate mucosal surfaces effectively bypass host defence barriers, and increase the risk of systemic infection. While early appropriate antibiotic therapy is one of the key factors in improving the outcome from sepsis, prolonged use of broad spectrum antibiotics encourages development of resistant pathogens and overgrowth of other organisms.

In most intensive care units, there is a nominated microbiologist who is familiar with the local microbiological flora and resistance patterns of the unit, and who performs a daily round on the ICU to advise on results and antibiotic therapy. This may occur as part of the main multidisciplinary ward round, or form a separate 'mini round'. It is vital to maintain a close and cooperative relationship with your microbiologist to help you to treat patients with sepsis in an early and effective manner, while at the same time reducing the chances of antibiotic resistant strains of organisms developing.

While patients are most at risk from their own microbiological flora, particularly those organisms associated with the gastrointestinal tract, they are also at risk from organisms transferred from other patients (cross-infection). You must therefore be scrupulous about following infection control procedures.

Dress code

White coats, jackets and neck ties can easily become contaminated and carry microbiological flora from one patient to the next, and should not be worn. (Visiting staff should leave white coats and jackets outside the clinical area.) If you are going to stay on the ICU all day, it is a good idea to wear surgical blues to prevent problems with contamination of clothes. Most units now have a 'bare below the elbow policy', which includes removing wrist watches and jewellery. These simple measures help promote effective hand hygiene and may help reduce cross-infection.

Hand hygiene

Effective hand hygiene is the single most effective way to reduce the risk of cross-infection. Therefore, before you go near any patient in the ICU, you should:

- Ensure your hands and finger nails are socially clean. If not, wash them thoroughly with soap and water.
- Decontaminate hands with an alcohol disinfectant rub before and after *every* contact with a patient or their environment. In practical terms, this means before and after contact with the

patient, equipment, monitoring systems around the bed space, plus the patient's notes and charts.
- Follow local policies on the wearing of disposable plastic aprons and non-sterile gloves.

> ⚠ **Alcohol disinfectant rub is as effective as hand washing at reducing bacterial contamination of the hands. It is not, however, effective against some spore forming organisms such as *Clostridium difficile*, so hand washing with soap and water may still be required where these types of infection are a possibility.**

Moving between patients

Following contact with a patient, remove your plastic apron and gloves, and either wash or decontaminate your hands with alcohol disinfectant rub before leaving the bed space. Do not share equipment between patients in the ICU. For example, stethoscopes are generally provided at each bed space. You should not use your own, which might be a vehicle for cross-infection.

Barrier nursing

Some patients may be isolated because they have a serious infection or are colonized with an antibiotic-resistant organism that might be transmitted to other patients, or even on occasions to members of staff. These patients will be barrier nursed.
The basic principles are:

- Do not enter the room unnecessarily.
- Wear an apron.
- Wash your hands and put on gloves.

Other precautions such as the use of visors, masks and gowns will depend on the particular nature of the problem. Instructions for entering the room are generally displayed on the door, and the nurses will help.

- Remove protective aprons, etc. before you leave the room.
- Wash your hands before you leave the room and use alcohol rub once outside the room.

Reverse barrier nursing

Some patients are at particular risk from infection because they are immunocompromised as a result of drug therapy, radiotherapy or immune disease, including HIV infection. These patients are often barrier nursed in a side room to help protect them. The precautions are generally similar to the above. Ask nursing staff for advice if unsure.

ASSESSING A PATIENT

Each patient in the ICU needs to be seen and assessed at least twice a day. Many conventional aspects of history taking and examination are either inappropriate or impracticable. This can seem daunting to the new trainee, particularly given the large amount of information available from charts, monitors and equipment at the patient's bedside. It is best to develop a system for assimilating key information efficiently, so that you can assess the patient and work out a plan.

History

Make sure you know the patient history in detail. Although the history may often not be available from the patient, there is generally a lot of information available from the notes, from other doctors, nurses or the referring hospital. If in doubt, telephone the referring team and request old notes and records. Take time to speak to family and friends to identify pre-existing health issues and physiological reserve, and try to ascertain the patient's attitudes to resuscitation and life support. It may be helpful to telephone the patient's usual doctor (GP, long-term consultant, doctors in another hospital where appropriate) for additional details of the history.

Intensive care units are often staffed using a 'shift pattern', and it is relatively easy for misinformation and myth to be perpetuated from one hand over to the next. If the clinical course does not fit well with the supposed diagnosis, question your assumptions and be prepared to go back to the original notes, and check your facts!

Patient's chart

Looking at the patient's chart next is an extension of the history. It can be scanned for general trends in the patient's condition since arrival in intensive care, or examined more closely to give a guide to progress over the preceding 24-h. Important things to note from the chart are shown below.

● Respiratory:
type and mode of ventilation, level of respiratory support
progress made in weaning
blood gases.

- Cardiovascular:
  haemodynamic stability
  trends in pulse, blood pressure, CVP, stroke volume, cardiac
    output, inotrope requirements
  evidence of adequate organ perfusion (e.g. conscious level,
    renal output, lactate).
- Gastrointestinal:
  nasogastric losses / bowel function / evidence of gastrointestinal
    bleeding
  tolerance of enteral feed (or parenteral nutrition)
  surgical drain losses.
- Renal:
  fluid intake
  volume and quality of urine
  overall fluid balance
  plasma and urinary electrolytes.
- CNS:
  consciousness level
  seizure activity
  sedation and analgesic requirement.
- Evidence of infection:
  temperature / white cell count / C reactive protein (CRP).

Examining the patient

Once you have put together the information available from the
history and the patient's chart, you should examine the patient
carefully. Remember hand hygiene and infection control issues.
(See Hand hygiene, p. 20.)

> ⚠ **Before examining a patient, you should introduce
> yourself and explain what you are going to do, even if
> the patient appears unconscious. Remember that hearing
> may be the last sense to be lost under anaesthesia or sedation.**

Examine the patient systematically, assimilating the information
available from the monitoring into your examination findings as
you go. A typical approach might be as follows:

- Respiratory system:
  trachea central, air entry bilateral and equal, breath sounds,
    added sounds

check position and adequacy of chest drains, endotracheal
tubes, etc.

check type and adequacy of ventilation and ventilator settings

look at the chest X-ray as an extension of the physical
examination in ICU patients

it is often helpful to consider blood gases at this stage as well.

- Cardiovascular system:

pulse, blood pressure, JVP, heart sounds, CVP, stroke volume,
cardiac output

evidence of adequate perfusion

cold and 'shut down' or warm and well perfused

core–peripheral temperature gradient

peripheral oedema

venous/arterial catheter sites–evidence of infection.

- Abdomen:

soft or tender, distended

bowel sounds present

bowels open regularly/diarrhoea/melaena

enteral or parenteral feeding.

- Renal:

urine output

fluid balance

oedema fluid.

- CNS:

level of consciousness

dose and duration of sedative/analgesic drugs; consider
stopping to allow assessment of neurological status

evidence of focal neurology/seizures/weakness

does the patient make purposeful movements to verbal
command or painful stimulus?

for painful stimulus, press on nail bed or supraorbital ridge
(other sites cause bruising)

intracranial pressure and cerebral perfusion pressure.

- Limbs:

adequate perfusion (especially after injury)

presence of peripheral pulses

adequate capillary refill

evidence of swelling, tenderness, DVT or compartment
syndrome.

- Skin/wounds:

surgical wounds, and trauma sites, inspection for adequate healing

evidence of infection or discharge

surgical drains, volume and nature of drainage

pressure areas intact.

⚠️ **Do not just pull dressings down to 'peek underneath'. Ask the nurse about the state of the wound and if necessary arrange to inspect it formally, either the next time the dressings are changed or earlier if necessary. If appropriate, make sure the surgical team has reviewed the wounds.**

Special investigations

When you have examined the patient, you should go back to the patient's charts and records and check on anything that you have missed. Also review the patient's important haematology, biochemical and microbiology investigations and other investigations, including CXRs and other radiological investigations.

Prescription charts

Review the patient's drug, fluid and nutrition prescription chart. Particularly check that any routine stress ulcer prophylaxis and DVT prophylaxis is appropriately prescribed. Are current prescriptions appropriate to the patient's needs? In particular, are antibiotics still needed? Do any prescribed drugs require plasma level monitoring? Are any of the prescribed drugs likely to interact?

Finally, make sure that you have spoken to nursing staff and other people involved in the care of the patient. Ask for their assessment of problems and priorities, which may be different from your own.

FORMULATING AN ACTION PLAN

When you have finished assessing the patient, record your examination findings and any important results in the medical notes. Summarize your findings by making a brief list of the current problems, for example:

● Increased WCC and CRP. Catheter-related sepsis?
● Haemodynamically unstable. Increasing inotrope requirements. Adequately filled?
● Urine output deteriorating, rising creatinine. Needs renal referral.

Formulate an action plan

Using this approach, you can prioritize problems and formulate a plan of action. In practice, this should be done in consultation with the consultant looking after the ICU. The action plan should include the following:

- Action targeted against problems identified.
- Integrated plan for each organ system requiring support.
- Ventilation and/or weaning plan.
- Nutrition and 24-h fluid balance plans.
- Changes to drug therapy.
- Any further investigations required.

Communication

When you have finished with the patient and detailed your findings and plans in the medical notes, you should tell the nursing staff and others involved in the patient's care what is planned. In particular:

- Leave detailed instructions and parameters for the manipulation of drugs such as inotropes, which are generally titrated to response (e.g. what is the target blood pressure? Specify systolic or mean).
- Discuss any major changes in therapy or new problems with the referring consultant team.
- Keep the relatives informed of progress.
- Ensure all staff and the relatives up to date with the overall prognosis of the patient. (See Talking to relatives, p. 28.)

MEDICAL RECORDS

The nature of intensive care is such that many different individuals are involved in the care of the patient. At the same time, the patient's condition may change rapidly, requiring frequent changes in therapy. If everyone is to keep up with the patient's progress, accurate, contemporaneous note-keeping is essential. It is also worth bearing in mind that medico–legal cases frequently arise where patients have suffered trauma or complications from medical and surgical treatment, and that your record-keeping might therefore be scrutinized in the future.

In many units, the patient's charts, pathology results, X-rays and prescription charts are now kept electronically or 'on line'. Whichever system is used, you should record:

- Daily examination and progress notes.
- Interventions and procedures.
- Complications of procedures, which must be recorded accurately and honestly. Complications do occur, and providing you have followed correct procedures, they do not imply negligence. (Failure to record them or act appropriately upon them does!)

- Results of important investigations.
- The patient's chart is often used to record blood gases, biochemistry, haematology and microbiology results. This is a legal document and therefore the results do not need to be routinely copied into the medical notes. Important positive and negative findings, however, particularly those which carry either diagnostic or prognostic significance, or which directly affect management, should be transcribed.
- It is essential to record the content and outcome of discussion with the patient's relatives, so that other staff do not give conflicting advice or opinions.

 All **entries in the medical records must include date, time, name (printed) designation (i.e. ICU resident / specialist registrar) and signature.**

Occasionally, because of the pressure of work in the ICU, it may not be possible to make full notes at the time, for example when admitting and resuscitating a very unstable patient. It is crucial, however, that notes are written at the earliest opportunity, and the fact that they have been written retrospectively should be recorded.

CONFIDENTIALITY

The patient's medical condition and treatment are matters of confidentiality. While it is generally accepted in intensive care that relatives should be kept informed of what is going on, you must respect the patient's wishes and confidentiality at all times. Therefore:

- Make sure you know to whom you are talking before giving out any information.
- Avoid discussing a patient's condition on the telephone. You do not know who is on the other end of the line. The press have been known to telephone and not admit who they are. If a relative lives too far away to make it to the hospital, offer to telephone them back on a previously agreed number.
- Occasionally patients may request that information is not given to one of more of their relatives. This should be respected. If difficulties ensue, discuss with senior staff.
- Never make any comment to journalists. Refer them to your hospital press liaison officer or your consultant.

- Occasionally the police may request information about a patient or request a blood test. Remember that your first duty is to the patient, no matter what he or she is alleged to have done. If in doubt, refer them to your consultant.

TALKING TO RELATIVES

The relatives of critically ill patients may well ask to speak to a doctor about the patient's condition, or you may ask to speak to them. Discussions with relatives should generally take place in a quiet room away from the patient's bedside, unless the patient is awake enough to take an active part in such communications.

- Do not talk 'over' the patient, who may be aware of the surroundings and able to hear, but unable to communicate back. (Hearing is said to be the last sensory modality to be lost with sedative drugs.)
- Do not talk standing in the corridor; use a side room away from other families.
- Avoid talking to very large groups of relatives. Speak to key members of the family and encourage them to explain things to other relatives.
- It is always advisable to take a nurse with you so that he or she knows what has been said. The relatives will probably only retain a fraction of what has been said to them, and the nurse can reinforce what you have said later. The nurse will also offer comfort and moral support to the patient's family.
- Adjust the explanation of events to the level of understanding of the relatives, and avoid medical jargon and abbreviations.
- Be honest and not overly optimistic about the ability of intensive care to turn around desperate situations. There are inherent uncertainties about the outcome of any particular disease, and it is best to be cautious rather than attempting to quote probabilities of survival. It is often useful to explain that intensive care offers a level of support that 'buys time' for the patient's body to recover, but may do little to 'cure' the patient. Rather, recovery depends largely on the physiological and immunological reserve of the patient.
- Do not criticize other medical or nursing colleagues' management of the patient. Remember that hindsight is a wonderful thing. Difficult questions or decisions should be referred to senior colleagues or the referring teams.
- Do not let family members push you into making statements that are not true. This is particularly important concerning

prognosis. Don't agree with statements like 'He is going to be all right isn't he, Doctor' if it is not true.

- Record in the medical notes what has been said to the family. This ensures continuity and prevents misunderstandings.
- Accept that relatives will not always absorb bad news the first time they hear it. Time and repeated explanations may be required. Bear in mind that relatives may also be selective about which particular items of your information they choose to retain. Complex psychological issues come into play here, and it is important not to be judgemental. Remember also that different cultural groups respond in different ways to bad news (see Breaking bad news, p. 434).

CONSENT TO TREATMENT IN ICU

Consent is a difficult area in the ICU. Patients have often had no opportunity to discuss intensive care treatment prior to admission. They are admitted on the presumption that they would wish to undergo life-sustaining treatments, if given the choice. The validity of obtaining consent from third parties (e.g. spouses, partners, other relatives, etc.) is questionable in this context. Nevertheless, it is often still considered normal practice to do so. In England and Wales, this position has recently been formalized in the Mental Capacity Act 2005 (Explanatory Notes to Mental Capacity Act 2005 Chapter 9, accessed Feb 2009 http://www.opsi.gov. uk/acts/acts2005/en/ukpgaen_20050009_en_1).

When is consent required?

Patients in the ICU will have repeated interventions performed, for example, tracheal suction, arterial and venous line insertion, and passage of tubes into various orifices. Most units would not seek specific consent for these procedures, but you should always explain to the patient, and the relatives if present, what you are going to do. For more significant invasive procedures like returning to theatre for re-laparotomy, tracheostomy, or insertion of intracranial pressure monitoring, it is usual to seek formal consent whenever possible. If the patient is obtunded but potentially able to understand the treatment being proposed, it may be appropriate to seek consent directly from the patient. If you are in any doubt, seek senior help.

Many patients requiring intensive care are unfit to give consent, that is to say, they 'lack capacity' as defined by the Mental Capacity Act 2005. Patients without capacity have the right for major decisions concerning their well-being (and this is includes significant medical interventions) to be referred to an 'advocate'.

In most cases, the next of kin will act as the advocate, even where this relationship is somewhat remote.

You should inform them of the nature of the proposed procedure, the anticipated benefits and likely risks. Where alternatives are available, these should also be discussed. Most hospital consent forms have a section for third party assent, and it is usual practice to obtain it. If the relatives are not present, then it is courteous and avoids conflict to obtain assent over the telephone. Such discussions should always be documented in the notes. If nothing else, this ensures relatives are kept informed and provides an opportunity for an update on the patient's condition. Relatives do not respond well to news of the death of a patient in the operating theatre when they did not know that an operation was planned!

Where there is no clear next of kin, or where there is conflict between the perceived best interests of the patient and the wishes of the next of kin, UK law provides for an 'independent mental capacity advocate' (IMCA) to become involved. These are potentially complex and sensitive situations, which should be referred to your consultant who in turn may refer the matter on to the hospital medical director or other senior manager. If there is continued dispute, application may have to be made to the courts for a ruling as to the patient's best interest.

COMMON PROBLEMS RELATING TO CONSENT

Jehovah's Witnesses

Jehovah's Witnesses have religious objections to receiving transfusions of blood or blood products. Where these views are declared, it is usual practice to discuss with the patient what therapy they will and will not accept, and then to obtain a written disclaimer. The patient is then managed in the appropriate way, but without the use of blood products. The situation in intensive care is difficult if the patient is unable to express his or her view at the time; if there is sufficient evidence of the patient's religious beliefs, these should be respected. Further advice can be obtained from Jehovah's Witness liaison committees. These are formed by the Jehovah's Witness churches on a regional basis, and are extremely approachable and helpful groups. Your hospital chaplaincy should have contact details.

The situation with children is different. The child should be brought under the protection of the courts to decide whether a blood transfusion should be given.

See Blood transfusion, p. 250, and Management of Jehovah's Witnesses, p. 254.

Advance directives

An increasing number of people are writing so-called advance directives to outline what treatment they would or would not wish to receive in the future, should they be unfit to make this decision at the time. The best known scenarios for such directives come from patients who have progressive neuro-muscular disease or early onset of progressive dementia. Such directives may take the form of a request not to be admitted to intensive care for assisted ventilation in the case of severe pneumonia. In general terms, where these decisions are properly documented then they should be respected.

> ⚠ **At the current time in the UK, while it is accepted that patients have a right to decline treatment, they do not necessarily have a right to demand treatment. There is no onus on medical or nursing staff to provide treatment that they otherwise believe to be unnecessary or indeed harmful just because patients and their families demand it.**

Organ donor register

Registry with the national organ donor register and the possession of a signed organ donor card is a form of advanced directive allowing people to outline their wishes regarding potential organ donation after their death. Recent legislation has emphasized the need to follow the patient's wishes in respect to potential organ donation where this has been properly documented, regardless of the views of the next of kin (see Brainstem death and organ donation, p. 437).

HIV testing

The ethical guidelines on HIV testing are clear. Patients should not be tested for HIV infection without informed consent, which is taken to include adequate counselling both before the test and after a positive test result. The situation in intensive care is therefore difficult, as it is unlikely that informed consent can be obtained. The decision whether or not to perform an HIV test depends therefore on the precise clinical situation.

In most cases, knowledge of the patient's HIV status does not alter the management of an acute critical illness, and therefore an HIV test should not be performed until the patient is over the acute illness and able to give informed consent.

There are situations, however, where knowledge of the test result may alter immediate clinical management. For example, in the context of a central nervous system infection or cerebral abscess of unknown aetiology, knowledge of the patient's immune status leads to consideration of a very different range of pathogens and may avoid the need for invasive brain biopsy. In such circumstances it may be reasonable to perform an HIV test without consent, but this can only be justified if there is likely to be direct and immediate benefit to the patient.

The social stigma surrounding HIV infection is reducing, and the benefits of long-term prophylaxis for patients, their families and partners have become well established. As the risk–benefit ratio of testing changes, it is likely that the ethical position will also change, opening the way for a more liberal stance in relation to testing in the future. At the present time, however, HIV testing remains a contentious area. Discuss matters with your consultant and, if necessary, involve the specialists in HIV or GU medicine.

 You should not perform an HIV test for the benefit of staff who consider that they may be at risk from blood contamination. Universal precautions should be adopted for all patients, to avoid occupational risk when dealing with patients' body fluids. If you receive a needle-stick injury or are contaminated with infected blood, you should follow your local occupational health guidelines. An assessment of the risk of HIV exposure will be made and, if appropriate, post-exposure prophylaxis prescribed. Post-exposure prophylaxis is time critical, and is most effective when started within 4 h of possible exposure. (See Universal precautions, p. 19.)

Consent for post-mortem examination

Issues relating to consent for post-mortem examination and the retention of tissue from deceased patients have generated significant attention lately. These are addressed in Chapter 16. (See Consent for post-mortem examination, p. 435.)

CHAPTER 3

BASIC PRINCIPLES

Care bundles   34
Sedation   34
Muscle relaxants   43
Psychological care of patients   47
Fluids and electrolytes   49
Nutrition   53
Enteral feeding   57
Parenteral nutrition   60
Stress ulcer prophylaxis   62
DVT prophylaxis   63

CARE BUNDLES

In recent years, there has been increasing emphasis on improving the consistency of care provided across different intensive care units. One way in which this has been addressed has been by the introduction of 'care bundles'.

A care bundle is a group of interventions that are applied together in a particular given circumstance. In a sense, the care bundle resembles a checklist where all the elements are essential. There is observational evidence to suggest that intensive care units that are compliant with care bundles have a reduced overall mortality rate as compared with units who are not. (See Respiratory care bundle, p. 128 and Sepsis care bundle, p. 329.)

SEDATION

The ICU can be a very frightening place for patients. They may have little control over their surroundings and may be repeatedly subjected to invasive, often painful procedures. In order to reduce pain and distress, patients are often sedated, particularly during periods of assisted ventilation.

When administering sedation, the intention is both to ensure patient comfort, and to enable nursing and medical procedures to be performed safely. Comfort encompasses a number of areas of different importance to each patient, including:

- tolerance of endotracheal intubation, assisted ventilation, invasive catheters, etc.
- analgesia (painful wounds, limbs, viscera)
- reduced awareness of frightening or noisy environment
- amnesia for unpleasant procedures
- promotion of 'sleep'.

Sedation may also be used for therapeutic purposes, for example reducing cerebral oxygen consumption or myocardial work.

The use of sedatives does, however, have disadvantages. These may result either from the direct effects of the sedation itself (e.g. confusion or disorientation) or from side-effects of the drugs used to achieve it (e.g. hypotension, immunosuppression). The decision to use sedation is therefore a balance of the risks and benefits, and there is increasing use of sedative-free periods to prevent drug accumulation and reduce side-effects (see Over-sedation below).

The ideal sedative agent

The ideal sedative agent for use in ICU probably does not exist. All sedative agents cause some degree of cardiovascular instability

TABLE 3.1 Advantages and disadvantages of opioids and benzodiazepines for ICU sedation

	Advantages	Disadvantages
Opioids	Respiratory depression Cough suppression Some sedative effects Analgesic	Nausea and vomiting Delayed gastric emptying and ileus Potential accumulation Respiratory depression Potential cardiovascular instability Withdrawal phenomenon
Benzodiazepines	Hypnotic Anxiolytic Amnesia Anticonvulsant	No analgesic activity Unpredictable duration of action Potential cardiovascular instability Withdrawal phenomenon

in critically ill patients. Longer-acting agents can be given by bolus, but may accumulate and do not allow rapid change in response to alterations in a patient's condition. Shorter-acting agents are often preferred because they can be given by infusion, are less likely to accumulate and allow rapid change in depth, but they can be difficult to titrate.

In general single agents are not effective, either because they fail to achieve all the goals of sedation or because of unacceptable side-effects as the dose is increased. For this reason, it is more common to use a tailored combination of drugs. The principle employed is similar to that of 'balanced anaesthesia'. By combining the benefits of more than one class of agent, satisfactory levels of sedation can be achieved at much lower doses than could be achieved using either agent alone, thus allowing some of the adverse effects of individual agents to be reduced. A typical combination is that of an opioid (e.g. fentanyl) together with a benzodiazepine (e.g. midazolam). This combination provides analgesia, sedation and anxiolysis. The advantages and disadvantages of these agents are shown in Table 3.1.

Choice of agents

The choice of agents will depend on local protocols and the clinical condition of the patient. If the balance of a patient's problem is pain, then analgesia is the main requirement. Epidural anaesthesia, other regional anaesthetic techniques

and patient-controlled analgesia (PCA) may be useful.
(See Postoperative analgesia, p. 349.) If the balance of the
patient's problem is agitation, then the main requirement may be
for sedative or anxiolytic agents. Haloperidol and other major
tranquillizers are appropriate for the treatment of delirium and
psychosis and recent guidelines have placed greater emphasis
on the use of these agents (see Acute confusional states below).
Tables 3.2 and 3.3 provide a guide to commonly used analgesic
and sedative drugs.

Propofol is perhaps one of the most widely used sedative agents
in adult ICU. Bolus doses of 1–3 mg/kg are sufficient to induce
anaesthesia (e.g. prior to intubation). Smaller doses of 10–20 mg
repeated to effect may be useful for increasing the depth of
sedation, e.g. prior to suction or painful procedures.

TABLE 3.2 Commonly used analgesic agents

Drug	Dose	Notes
Morphine	2–5 mg i.v. bolus 10–50 µg/kg/h	Cheap, long acting Good analgesic, reasonable sedative Standard agent for PCAS and postoperative pain Metabolized by liver, active metabolites accumulate in renal failure
Fentanyl	2–6 µg/kg/h	Shorter acting than morphine Good analgesic less sedative Metabolized by liver No active metabolites No accumulation in renal failure
Alfentanil	20–50 µg/kg/h	Shorter acting than fentanyl Good analgesic, less sedative No active metabolites, no accumulation in renal failure Rapid termination of effects after discontinuation
Remifentanil	0.1–0.25 µg/kg/min	Ultrashort-acting analgesic, very titratable Metabolized by plasma esterases Rapid clearance even after prolonged infusion Mostly used intra-operatively or for short-term ventilation Causes significant bradycardia and hypotension; avoid boluses

TABLE 3.3 Commonly used sedative agents (doses based on 70 kg adult)

Drug	Dose	Notes
Diazepam	5–10 mg bolus i.v.	Cheap, long-acting benzodiazepine Reasonable cardiovascular stability Sedative, amnesic, anticonvulsant actions Given by intermittent boluses. Metabolized in liver. Long elimination half-life. Active drug and active metabolites can accumulate in sicker patients, therefore avoid continuous infusions
Midazolam	2–5 mg bolus i.v., 2–10 mg/h	Similar properties to diazepam but shorter acting Metabolized by the liver Can be given by continuous infusion
Etomidate	0.2 mg/kg bolus i.v.	Short acting cardiovascular stable anaesthetic induction agent Used only as single bolus dose for induction of anaesthesia, e.g. prior to intubation. Associated with significant adrenal suppression **Not to be used by infusion**
Propofol	1–3 mg/kg bolus, i.v., 2–5 mg/kg/h	Short-acting intravenous anaesthetic agent Sedative, anticonvulsant and amnesic properties Used for induction of anaesthesia and intubation May cause significant hypotension Avoid infusions in children

There have been ongoing reports of inhaled anaesthetic agents being used for sedation in critical care. These may be of value in specific circumstances. Isoflurane and other volatile agents may be useful in asthma and severe bronchospasm because of their bronchodilator properties. Specific systems for delivering volatile agents into ventilator circuits on the ICU have been developed. Nitrous oxide may be of value for changes of burns dressings, but should not be used for more than 12 h because of bone marrow suppression.

Clonidine

50–150 µg bolus i.v.

0.2–2 µg/kg/h

Clonidine is an α_2 agonist at presynaptic terminals, and has a general sedative effect. The main side-effect is hypotension and a small test dose is usually given to assess the effect on blood pressure. If tolerated, doses can be increased. It produces little respiratory depression, and can therefore be used safely in patients in whom agitation is hindering weaning from mechanical ventilation. Oral or i.v. preparations are available. There are no particular problems associated with withdrawal phenomena. The use of alpha₂ agonists as a primary sedative agent is increasing. Dexmetatomidine is a similar drug in this class that is licensed for ICU sedation in the USA and is currently undergoing further trials in the UK.

Ketamine

0.5–1 mg/kg i.v.

0.2–2 mg/kg/h infusion

Ketamine is an anaesthetic agent that is also profoundly analgesic. Unlike other sedative agents it does not cause cardiovascular or respiratory depression at normal doses. Ketamine indirectly increases sympathetic activity, which in turn leads to increases in heart rate and blood pressure and produces bronchodilatation. These properties have made it a useful agent for anaesthesia in extreme environments outside hospital (e.g. for amputation at the scene of an accident) and would make it appear attractive as an agent for use in intensive care. Historically, it has been used to provide short-term analgesia for painful procedures (e.g. burns dressings) and it is occasionally used as a sedative agent in severe asthma for its bronchodilator effects. Its general use is, however, limited by the incidence of unpleasant dreams, hallucinations and emergence phenomena.

Problems associated with over-sedation

Ideally patients should be awake, pain-free, able to move about as much as possible and be able to cooperate with physiotherapy and nursing care. Excessive sedation should be avoided. The potential problems associated with over-sedation include:

- prolonged need for IPPV/intubation
- haemodynamic instability
- gastrointestinal tract stasis
- potential immune suppression
- potential organ toxicity
- difficulty in assessing neurological state

- increased withdrawal phenomena, delirium, hallucinations and nightmares in the post-critical illness period.

To avoid excessive sedation, agents should be titrated according to the balance of the patient's needs. In practice, this can be difficult. The requirement for sedation differs markedly between patients. Younger, fitter patients generally require more sedative and analgesic drugs. Patients who abuse alcohol and other centrally acting drugs may be very difficult to sedate because of cross-tolerance between the abused substance and the prescribed sedative or analgesic agents. Relatives and patients may deny or conceal such abuse. Acute tolerance to drugs used for sedation in ICU may also occur.

In addition, the pharmacokinetics of many sedative drugs used in critical illness is poorly understood. Only limited information is available on drug metabolism and excretion in the critically ill. Drug trials performed in rats, healthy 'volunteers', ASA I patients and patients with compensated cirrhosis and uraemia are of little relevance to the critically ill ICU patient, in whom abnormalities in the distribution, metabolism and elimination of drugs are common. Regular reassessment of the need for, and level of, sedation is therefore required.

Sedation scoring

Sedation scoring systems may be useful in helping titrate levels of sedation. A typical score (performed hourly) together with appropriate responses is shown in Table 3.4.

Sedation-free periods

Where drugs are given by continuous infusion accumulation can occur and studies have consistently shown that patients tend to be over-sedated. Regular reassessment of sedation, and the use of sedation-free periods or 'sedation holds' can reduce the duration of tracheal intubation and ventilatory support. Many units now consider sedation holds on a daily basis. Typically sedation (not analgesia) is stopped once a day, to allow assessment. Ideally, sedation is held until the patient is able to follow commands.

COMMON PROBLEMS RELATED TO SEDATION

Patient who is difficult to sedate

- Check that sedative infusions are running correctly and at the prescribed dose.
- Exclude possible causes of agitation, including: full bladder, painful wounds, hypoxia, hypercarbia, and endotracheal tube touching carina.

TABLE 3.4 Sedation score

Description	Score	Comment
Agitated and restless	+3	Levels +3 to +2: inadequate sedation. Give bolus of sedative/analgesic drugs and increase infusion rates
Awake and uncomfortable	+2	
Awake but comfortable	+1	Levels +1 to 0 appropriate levels of sedation.
Roused by voice	0	Reassess regularly
Roused by touch	−1	Level −1 to −3 excessive level of sedation
Roused by painful stimuli	−2	Reduce or stop infusion of sedative/analgesic drugs
Unrousable	−3	Restart when desired level attained
Natural sleep	A	Ideal
Paralysed	P	Difficult to assess level of sedation. Consider physiological response to stimulation

- Review other drug therapy and stop where appropriate. Many drugs (for example H_2 blockers) have the potential to induce confusional states.
- Consider tracheostomy or nasal intubation. These are often better tolerated, and allow sedative and analgesic drugs to be significantly reduced.
- Consider alternative sedative/analgesic agents if appropriate (e.g. paracetamol, NSAIDs, gabapentin, tricyclics). Seek advice.
- Consider alternative analgesic techniques if appropriate (e.g. epidural or regional nerve blocks).

Eventually all patients need to be weaned off sedative agents. There is often a difficult phase during which the patient is partially sedated but unable to cooperate due to residual drug effects. Real problem patients (e.g. after head injury or suffering from withdrawal of drugs or alcohol), may be best nursed on a mattress on the floor. This reduces risk of harm should the patient fall out of bed. (See Withdrawal phenomena/acute confusional states below.)

Patient who is slow to wake up

If a patient fails to regain full consciousness after sedative and analgesic drugs have been stopped for a period of time, the question invariably arises as to 'why?' This may be due to the accumulation of drugs or their active metabolites, which resolves with time, but other causes of coma or 'apparent coma' should be excluded. Consider:

● Effects of sepsis. Encephalopathy is common (for example as part of multiple organ failure).
● Metabolic derangement/encephalopathy.
● Seizure activity.
● Structural brain damage (including CVA, hypoxic brain injury).
● Awake patients who cannot respond ('locked-in syndrome').
● Residual neuromuscular blockade (see p. 45).
● Critical illness neuromyopathy (see p. 304).

Severe muscle weakness is common following critical illness so it may not be immediately apparent that the patient is actually awake, but unable to move. A similar clinical picture may also be seen in the presence of pontine lesions (e.g. following central pontine myelinolysis or brainstem stroke). Careful clinical examination is required to ascertain the true clinical picture. An EEG and CT scan may be helpful. If no other cause of coma can be established and failure to wake up is considered to result from the accumulation of sedative agents, a trial of naloxone or flumazenil may occasionally be diagnostic (Table 3.5). This is not without risk, however, and may precipitate convulsions. Seek senior advice.

TABLE 3.5 Naloxone and flumazenil

Drug	Dose	Notes
Naloxone	0.4–2 mg bolus i.v.	Competitive antagonist of opioid receptors* Used to reverse sedation and respiratory depression caused by opioids
Flumazenil	0.2–0.5 mg bolus i.v.	Competitive antagonist of benzodiazepine receptors* Used to reverse sedation and respiratory depression caused by benzodiazepines

*Both drugs have a short half-life (approximately 20 min), leading to the risk of recurrence of respiratory depression and sedation. Side-effects include fits, hypertension, and dysrhythmias. Do not infuse over long periods of time. Ventilate the patient and await resolution as redistribution and metabolism of drugs occur!

Withdrawal phenomena / acute confusional states

When drugs used before admission, or sedative drugs given in ICU are stopped, drug withdrawal states may develop. This may result in seizures, hallucinations, delirium tremens, confusional states, agitation and aggression. Elderly patients are particularly susceptible. These phenomena are difficult to control without further heavy sedation, but usually settle over time. You should look for and treat any reversible causes of confusion (Box 3.1).

Drugs that can be useful for the control of acute confusional states, including those induced by the withdrawal of mixed sedative agents, are shown in Table 3.6. You should generally seek senior advice before resorting to these agents.

Box 3.1 Causes of acute confusional states

Side-effects of prescribed drugs
Withdrawal of alcohol or other centrally acting drugs
Effects of sepsis
Renal and hepatic encephalopathy
Electrolyte disturbance
Hypoxia / hypercarbia
Brain injury (e.g. stroke, cerebral haemorrhage)
Endocrine abnormalities (e.g. use of steroids, thyroid abnormalities)
Sleep deprivation (especially REM sleep)

TABLE 3.6 Drugs for the treatment of acute confusional states

Drug	Dose	Notes
Lorazepam	1–3 mg bolus i.v.	Long acting benzodiazepine Useful for controlling seizures and withdrawal phenomenon
Clonidine	50–150 µg bolus i.v.	α_2 agonist Useful for controlling withdrawal phenomenon See previous notes
Chlorpromazine	5–10 mg bolus i.v. Repeat as necessary	Major tranquillizer* Useful in acute confusional states
Haloperidol	5–10 mg bolus Repeat as necessary	Major tranquillizer* Useful in acute confusional states

*Large number of actions and side-effects. Particularly beware of alpha blockade and hypotension. (Numerous newer antipsychotic agents, e.g. olanzapine, are now available. Seek advice.)

MUSCLE RELAXANTS

The routine use of muscle relaxants in ICU is to be discouraged. Potential problems associated with muscle relaxants include:

- 'Awareness', when paralysed patients are inadequately sedated during unpleasant procedures. Although well described in the context of inadequate anaesthesia during surgical procedures in the operating theatre this is a real risk in the ICU. Assisted ventilation, tracheal intubation, suctioning, and other invasive procedures can all be very uncomfortable or painful and frightening for a patient. Increasing numbers of surgical procedures, such as tracheostomy, are also performed in ICU!
- Potential for rapid development of severe or fatal hypoxia following accidental unnoticed disconnection of the ventilator, because the paralysed patient cannot make any respiratory effort.
- Potential for neuromyopathy, which is common in patients with multiple organ failure and may be associated with the prolonged use of muscle relaxants.

Therefore, the use of relaxants should be restricted to the following:

- To facilitate endotracheal intubation.
- The management of patients with acute brain injury or cerebral oedema (e.g. to prevent rise in ICP on coughing).
- The management of patients with critical cardiovascular or respiratory insufficiency where the balance between oxygen delivery and oxygen consumption may be improved by preventing muscle activity.

The choice of drugs depends upon the clinical situation and the patient's general condition.

Suxamethonium

Only used by bolus injection for endotracheal intubation, 1 mg/kg i.v. bolus.

This is a short-acting depolarizing muscle relaxant, which gives good intubating conditions in less than a minute. It is useful for rapidly intubating patients in an emergency and has the advantage for the inexperienced that it has a short duration of action (2–4 min), so that if intubation is difficult, spontaneous respiratory effort is rapidly re-established. In a small number of patients, however, the effects are prolonged because of a genetic abnormality in the cholinesterase enzyme, which breaks down suxamethonium.

Side-effects associated with the use of suxamethonium include bradycardia, hypotension, and increased salivation and bronchial secretions. These can be blocked by the use of atropine. Intraocular pressure and intracranial pressure are transiently increased. All patients suffer a small increase (0.5–1 mmol/L) in serum potassium following suxamethonium. The drug should therefore be avoided in patients with hyperkalaemia. In some groups of patients, this increase in potassium may be much greater and may result in a cardiac arrest. It is also best avoided in all patients with pre-existing neuromuscular disease. Contraindications to the use of suxamethonium are shown in Box 3.2.

Box 3.2 Contraindications to suxamethonium

Absolute	*Relative*
Recent (significant) burns or crush injuries	Severe overwhelming sepsis
	Prolonged immobility
Spinal injury (after first 24 h)	Neuromyopathies (including critical illness neuropathy)
Renal failure and raised K^+	
Myasthenia gravis	
Dystrophia myotonica	
History of previous allergy	
History of malignant hyperpyrexia	

! **Many junior doctors routinely use suxamethonium, as it is one of the 'first' muscle relaxants introduced during anaesthetic training. However, while it is appropriate for use by junior trainees in anaesthetic practice because of a favourable risk–benefit ratio, this is not necessarily the case in critically ill patients. Suxamethonium should not be used 'routinely' and the risk versus benefits should be carefully considered for each individual patient.**

If it is necessary to use a muscle relaxant for intubation, as an alternative to suxamethonium, non-depolarizing muscle relaxants (see below) can be used as part of a 'modified rapid sequence induction'. Any non-depolarizing muscle relaxant could theoretically be used at relatively high dose for this purpose. Rocuronium, however, has the fastest onset of action. Moreover, a specific antagonist to rocuronium is now available, so the effects may be rapidly reversed if intubation proves difficult. (See Practical procedures, p. 398.)

NON-DEPOLARIZING MUSCLE RELAXANTS

Currently available non-depolarizing muscle relaxants are slower in onset and have a longer duration of action than suxamethonium. They can be used for intubation as an alternative to suxamethonium (when this is contraindicated), or when the risk of airway contamination with gastric contents is low. Non-depolarizing muscle relaxants can be used either by intermittent bolus or infusion, to provide continuous muscle relaxation when this is required. Table 3.7 provides a guide to commonly used agents.

Monitoring neuromuscular blockade

The use of muscle relaxants should be regularly reviewed and consideration given to stopping them intermittently to assess the adequacy of sedation. Neuromuscular blockade can be monitored if required using nerve stimulators. On the ICU this is most commonly required to exclude residual muscle paralysis, for example prior to performing brainstem death tests. An electric current is passed through a peripheral nerve and the response of the muscle supplied by that nerve observed. A common method of assessment is to produce four impulses, 0.5 s apart, known as a train of four (TO4), followed by a period of continuous tetanic stimulation at 50 Hz and then another train of four. Typical responses are shown in Figure 3.1.

Other than for intubation purposes, it is usually unnecessary to completely abolish all muscle response. When using non-depolarizing muscle relaxants by infusion, 75–90% block is usually adequate. This equates to one or two twitches present on a train of four.

Reversal of neuromuscular blocking drugs

In the majority of cases in ICU the effects of muscle relaxant drugs are allowed to wear off over time. Occasionally it may be appropriate to reverse the action of non-depolarizing drugs. This can usually be achieved with anticholinesterase drugs once there is some evidence of recovery of muscle function as demonstrated by the presence of two or three twitches on TO4.

TABLE 3.7 Commonly used non-depolarizing muscle relaxants

Drug	Dose	Notes
Atracurium	0.5 mg/kg i.v. bolus 0.5–1.0 mg/kg/h infusion	Onset 1–2 min, duration 30 min Undergoes spontaneous degradation, no accumulation in hepatorenal failure. Ideal for use by infusion Localized histamine release common May cause bronchospasm
Cisatracurium	150 µg/kg i.v. bolus 1–3 µg/kg/min infusion	Onset 1–2 min, duration 45 min Similar to atracurium, less histamine release
Vecuronium	0.1 mg/kg i.v. bolus 0.05–0.2 mg/kg/h infusion	Onset 1–2 min, duration 40 min Can be associated with bradycardia Parent drug and active metabolites can accumulate in hepatorenal failure
Rocuronium	600 µg/kg i.v. bolus 300–600 µg/kg/h infusion	Faster onset of action than vecuronium More prolonged block Similar in other aspects to vecuronium Higher frequency of allergic reactions
Pancuronium	0.1 mg/kg i.v. bolus	Onset 2 min, duration 1 h Produces tachycardia and increased blood pressure Relatively long-acting usually given by intermittent bolus Can accumulate in renal failure

A new drug, sugammadex, has recently become available that selectively binds and inactivates rocuronium and vecuronium, but not other non-steroid structure muscle relaxant drugs. This can rapidly reverse the effects of rocuronium (and to a lesser extent vecuronium and possibly pancuronium) even when only just administered.

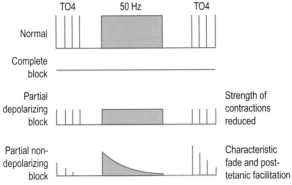

Fig. 3.1 Monitoring neuromuscular function – typical patterns. TO4 represents 'train of four' stimulation, 50 Hz represents maximal tetanic stimulation.

PSYCHOLOGICAL CARE OF PATIENTS

Despite the provision of analgesic and sedative agents to patients on intensive care, it is important to realize that they are not anaesthetized and may be aware of their surroundings during their stay. Even the sickest patients, who may be heavily sedated during critical phases of their illness, will hopefully go on to a period of convalescence, when they will be fully aware of their surroundings. This can be very stressful for patients. A number of factors may contribute to patients' distress.

Environment

The ICU is a very noisy place and often the only lighting is artificial. Patients may spend long periods in the same room with little knowledge of the outside world. The appreciation of day and night may be lost, resulting in disturbed sleep patterns. In addition, sedative drugs abolish rapid eye movement (dream) sleep and this can cause marked psychological disturbance, particularly during the convalescent stage.

Communication difficulties

Communication difficulties following tracheal intubation have not been adequately resolved. Written messages and letter boards are cumbersome, and lip reading is often difficult. Speaking aids for ventilated patients are available in the form of an artificial larynx to produce tones, but none is satisfactory for acute use as they take time and practice to work well. Speaking tracheostomy tubes or tracheostomy tube cuff deflation may be helpful in the recovery phase of illness.

Dependency

Patients in intensive care are totally dependent both on the nursing staff for their personal needs, and on machines and drugs. In addition, they may be repeatedly visited by large groups of doctors and other staff. This may be humiliating and depersonalizing.

Pain, fear and anxiety

Many patients in intensive care will have painful surgical wounds and many will also have stiff painful limbs and joints as a result of immobility and critical illness neuropathy (see p. 304). Almost all will be subjected to repeated, potentially painful, procedures. Patients may be aware how sick they are, or even that they are dying. The overall experience is very frightening.

To reduce the impact of these problems, think about the psychological care of your patients. In particular:

- Take time to get to know patients. Acknowledge their fears and anxieties. Give appropriate explanations and reassurance.
- Respect patient privacy as much as possible.
- Avoid unnecessarily large ward rounds and talking over the patient.
- Always explain procedures to patients and provide adequate analgesia or anaesthesia.
- Avoid disturbing the patient at night if possible. Encourage daytime stimulation in the form of visits from relatives and children, television and radio, all of which improve morale.

Despite every effort, many patients on ICU will suffer distressing, vivid nightmares and dreams during their stay. Some will develop apparent psychoses, which require treatment. Others (particularly long-stay patients) may become markedly depressed and withdrawn. Consideration should be given to the use of antidepressant therapy, although there are arguments against its use in 'reactive' depression. Amitriptyline (or similar agent) at night may aid nocturnal sleep and help to elevate mood and motivation, but may be associated with excessive sedation, lasting well into the following day. Fluoxetine given in the morning is an alternative. Advice may be sought from local 'liaison psychiatry' services.

One of the roles of the intensive care follow-up clinic is to facilitate better recognition and earlier, more appropriate management of the late psychological sequelae of intensive care, including post-traumatic stress disorder. (See ICU follow-up clinics, p. 15.)

FLUIDS AND ELECTROLYTES

The management of fluid and electrolyte balance in critically ill patients is fundamental to intensive care. In health, daily input and output are in balance and the figures are approximately as shown in Figure 3.2. This translates to daily water and electrolyte requirements as shown in Table 3.8.

Simplistically therefore, fluid management is a matter of selecting an appropriate fluid and volume to provide the required amount of water and electrolytes. The constituents of commonly available fluids are shown in Table 3.9.

Daily requirements could, for example therefore, be provided by 2–3 L of 4% dextrose and 0.18% saline, with 20 mmol of potassium added to each litre. For the critically ill patient on the intensive care unit, however, the situation is more complex than this, with a number of factors often simultaneously affecting fluid and electrolyte balance.

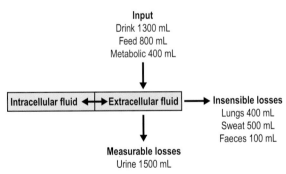

Fig. 3.2 Typical fluid balance for healthy 70 kg adult under normal environmental conditions.

TABLE 3.8 Typical daily water and electrolyte requirements	
Water	30–35 mL/kg/day
Na$^+$	1–1.5 mmol/kg/day
K$^+$	1 mmol/kg/day

TABLE 3.9 Composition of commonly available intravenous fluids

	Na^+ (mmol/L)	Cl^- (mmol/L)	K^+ (mmol/L)	Ca^{2+} (mmol/L)	HCO_3^- (mmol/L)	Dextrose (mmol/L)	Osmolality* (mosmol/kg)
Hartmanns/Ringer's lactate	131	112	5.0	2.0	29		278
0.9% saline	154	154					287
0.45% saline	77	77					144
0.18% saline 5% dextrose	31	31				222	284
5% dextrose						278	278

*Calculated osmolality. Measured osmolality may differ.

Factors potentially reducing fluid requirements

- Provision of warmed humidified respiratory gases reducing insensible losses.
- Increased activity of the renin–angiotensin–aldosterone axis results in reduced sodium excretion, and increased secretion of antidiuretic hormone (ADH) reduces secretion of free water. (See Stress response to critical illness, p. 348 and SIADH, p. 203.)
- Oliguric renal failure.

Factors potentially increasing fluid requirements

- Widespread capillary leak associated with sepsis and inflammatory conditions may result in redistribution of body water out of the vascular compartment, and the development of pulmonary, central and peripheral oedema.
- Gastrointestinal tract dysfunction, fluid sequestration and diarrhoea.
- Increased fluid losses associated with burns, skin loss, wounds and fistulae.
- Increased insensible losses due to poor humidification of inspired ventilator gases and/or pyrexia. (Fluid requirements may increase by as much as 150 mL/day for each 1°C rise in temperature.)
- Non-oliguric (high-output) renal failure, e.g. in the recovery phase of acute tubular necrosis.
- Neurogenic diabetes insipidus (e.g. accompanying brain injury) or nephrogenic diabetes insipidus (e.g. due to drugs).

Factors affecting electrolyte requirements

- At cellular level: hypoxia, acidosis, toxins and the effects of drugs can interfere with ionic pump mechanisms and lead to alterations in normal electrolyte balances and requirements.
- Fluid shifts and increased losses can be associated with altered electrolyte balance.
- Altered gastrointestinal and renal function further impair electrolyte homeostasis.

In addition, the underlying condition, repeated venesection and multiple procedures may lead to the need for repeated blood transfusions. Significant coagulopathy may require use of other blood products such as fresh frozen plasma (FFP) and platelet concentrates. There is frequently a requirement for multiple drug infusions. All these factors and additional volumes of fluid need to be taken into account when managing fluid and electrolyte balance.

Practical fluid management

The aim is to keep the patient hydrated, with an adequate circulating volume and normal electrolytes. Exact fluid regimens will depend on the patient's clinical state of hydration (look at tongue, mucous membranes, tissue turgor, urine output), cumulative fluid balance on the daily charts, and electrolyte investigations.

● Measure 24-h fluid balance accurately. The nurses will usually record the totals of all fluids, in and out, hourly. This will include all intravenous and nasogastric fluids, all drugs and all measurable losses. (It does not include unmeasurable insensible losses or shifts between intra- and extravascular spaces.)
● Measure serum electrolytes frequently. Sodium (Na^+) and potassium (K^+) at least every 4–6 h in sicker patients. Magnesium (Mg^{2+}), calcium (Ca^{2+}) and phosphate ($PO_4{}^{3-}$) daily or as required. Increasing Na^+ and urea suggest dehydration.
● Additional measurements such as plasma and urinary osmolality and urinary electrolytes are useful in difficult cases. (See Oliguria, p. 188.)

A typical fluid regimen for a 70 kg adult patient not receiving nutritional support, and with normal renal function, is shown in Table 3.10.

Despite careful fluid management patients frequently become significantly fluid-overloaded, as measured by positive fluid balance and generalized oedema. This usually reflects the severity of the underlying clinical condition and resolves as the patient's condition improves.

Measurement of patients' weight as a means to aiding fluid management has never proved to be that useful due to difficulties in accurate measurement. In addition, progressive loss of lean body mass and fat in the immobilized critically ill patient over time make baseline measurements unrepresentative of ideal weight.

TABLE 3.10 Typical fluid management in 70 kg adult with normal renal function

Maintenance	Dextrose 4% and saline 0.18% 20–60 mmol/K^+/L	80–100 mL/h
Additional losses	0.9% saline 20 mmol/K^+/L	Replace nasogastric and drain losses mL for mL
Other electrolytes	K^+, Ca^{2+}, Mg^{2+}	As required
Colloids	Gelatin /starch	As required to maintain adequate circulating volume
Blood products	Red cells/FFP/platelets	As indicated

Review the fluid balance and regimen regularly and adjust it as necessary. If in doubt, consider a fluid challenge or a trial of diuretics. A low dose of a diuretic [for example 10–20 mg furosemide (frusemide)] often produces a good diuresis in the overloaded patient, with little effect in others. This effect has been attributed to the 'overcoming' of SIADH. (See Oliguria, p. 188.)

Disturbances of fluid and electrolyte balance are discussed further in Chapter 8.

Hyperchloraemic acidosis

Many of the intravenous fluids used in critical care are not 'balanced salt solutions', i.e. their ionic composition does not mirror that of physiological fluids. Commonly, both crystalloid and colloid solutions are based on 'normal' saline, which has a chloride content equivalent to the sodium content. Administration of such fluids is associated with a progressive elevation in serum chloride, resulting in hyperchloraemic acidosis.

The typical picture is of a persistent metabolic acidosis with a low/normal anion gap (<18), high chloride and low bicarbonate. In most patients this is not physiologically significant, and will resolve as their condition improves. In those patients where the acidosis is severe (often multifactorial), or where there is a physiological or clinical effect (e.g. hyperkalaemia associated with acidosis occurring in a patient with renal dysfunction), reducing the chloride content of fluids and feeds and the use of sodium bicarbonate infusion will aid resolution. (See Metabolic acidosis, p. 212.)

Use of balanced salt solutions

The problems described above can be avoided by using balanced salt solutions, e.g. Hartmann's or Ringer's lactate solutions. Similarly, colloid solutions (both gelatins and starches), which were traditionally available suspended only in normal saline, are now available in balanced salt solutions. Although the evidence base in terms of outcomes is limited, it favours use of these over the traditional hyperchloraemic fluids. Follow local protocols or seek senior advice.

NUTRITION

During the acute phase of illness, intensive care patients are often catabolic. Muscle is broken down to provide amino acids for energy requirements and for synthesis of acute phase proteins. Nitrogen from protein breakdown is lost in the urine and patients develop a negative nitrogen balance. This may result in severe muscle wasting and weakness, greatly prolonging recovery.

TABLE 3.11 Typical daily nutritional requirements

Item	Requirement/kg/day	Typical daily requirement (70 kg adult)
Maintenance fluid	30–35 mL/kg/day	2500 mL
Na^+	1–1.5 mmol/kg/day	100 mmol
K^+	1 mmol/kg/day	60–80 mmol
Phosphate	0.5 mmol/kg/day	<50 mmol
Energy	30–40 kcal/kg/day*	2500 kcal

*Increased in critical illness. See below.

The aim of feeding patients is therefore to provide adequate amino acids and energy to minimize this process.

All critically ill patients should be assumed to have established or impending nutritional deficiency, and when examining patients in the ICU you should note their nutritional status. Muscle wasting may often be hidden by oedema fluid and it is only on recovery, when oedema subsides, that the true extent of wasting is visible. Temporal muscles and other muscles around the face may be the most obvious, due to gravity removing dependent fluid from this area.

Although there is a very large literature on nutrition in the critically ill patient, there are relatively few practice guidelines. NICE has published a set of guidelines on nutrition for patients in hospital, but these only briefly mention intensive care. A fuller set of guidelines has been produced by the Intensive Care Society, together with guidelines from the Canadian Critical Care Network and the European Society For Enteral and Parenteral Nutrition. The web sites of these organizations can be consulted for further information (Critical care nutrition http://www. criticalcarenutrition.com, National Institute for Health and Clinical Excellence (NICE) 2006 Nutrition in adults. http://www. nice.org.uk/nicemedia/pdf/CG032NICEguideline.pdf).

Nutrition can be provided by the enteral or parenteral route depending upon the circumstances, although the enteral route is preferred wherever possible (see below). Whichever route is chosen, the aim is to provide all the patient's nutritional requirements. Typical daily nutritional requirements are given in Table 3.11. (See also Fluids and electrolytes, p. 49.)

Estimation of energy requirements

Energy requirements depend on body mass and metabolic rate. They are normally 30–40 kcal/kg/day, but this may be increased in critical

TABLE 3.12 Estimated energy requirements (kcal/day)

Step 1. Estimate basal metabolic rate (kcal/day)		
Age (years)	Male	Female
15–18	BMR = 17.6 × weight (kg) + 656	BMR = 13.3 × weight (kg) + 690
18–30	BMR = 15.0 × weight (kg) + 690	BMR = 14.8 × weight (kg) + 485
30–60	BMR = 11.4 × weight (kg) + 870	BMR = 8.1 × weight (kg) + 842
>60	BMR = 11.7 × weight (kg) + 585	BMR = 9.0 × weight (kg) + 656
Step 2. Add factor for level of activity		
Bed bound/immobile		Add 10%
Bed bound mobile/sitting		Add 15–20%
Mobile		Add 25%
Step 3. Adjust for critical illness		
Burns 25–90% (1st month)		Add 20–70%
Severe sepsis/multiple trauma		Add 20–50%
Persistent increase temperature 2°C		Add 25%
Burns 10–25% (1st month) Multiple long bone fractures (1st week)		Add 10–30%
Persistent increase temperature 1°C		Add 12%
Burns 10% (1st month) Single fracture (1st week) Postoperative patient (1st 4 days) Inflammatory bowel disease Mild infection		Add 0–10%
Partial starvation (>10% loss body weight)		Subtract 0–10%

illness. In most instances when starting nutritional support it is not necessary to calculate exact energy requirements. Standard feeds can be used and the energy content can be adjusted subsequently if necessary. If required, energy requirements can be estimated using formulae such as the one in Table 3.12, or measured with a metabolic computer attached to the breathing circuit (these measure O_2 uptake and CO_2 production to derive energy consumption). Longer term requirements should be assessed by a dietician.

An alternative method of estimating energy requirements is indirect calorimetry. Metabolic computers are available which sample the patient's inspired and expired gases and, using an

> ⚠ **While adequate energy intake might prevent negative nitrogen balance (muscle breakdown) in a critically ill patient, excess feeding will not produce a positive nitrogen balance in a catabolic patient. This will only be achieved in the recovery phase of illness. Therefore avoid excessive feeding. Seek specialist advice from a dietician.**

assumed value for the respiratory quotient, can estimate total energy expenditure.

Energy requirements are generally provided as a mixture of carbohydrate and fats.

Nitrogen (protein)

To prevent muscle breakdown adequate amounts of nitrogen must be provided. This is generally of the order of 9–14 g nitrogen a day, equivalent to 1–2 g protein/kg per day. Proteins should be provided in a form that ensures that all the essential amino acids are provided. There is increasing interest in the role of individual amino acids. For example, glutamine has a specific role as a substrate for metabolism within the gastrointestinal tract where it is important in maintaining integrity and function. At the present time, there is no definitive evidence base for the benefit of such products.

Vitamins, minerals and trace elements

Vitamins, minerals and trace elements are essential for health and many have important roles in enzyme pathways. Less is known, however, about the requirements during critical illness. Both water- and fat-soluble vitamins can be provided by commercially available preparations. Folic acid and vitamin B_{12} should be prescribed separately. Trace elements and minerals, including calcium, magnesium, iron, zinc, copper, selenium, molybdenum, manganese and chromium, are available. Replacement is guided by the reference values for daily recommended intake and signs of deficiency. All patients with chronic alcohol dependency should receive vitamin B supplements (see p. 241).

Immunonutrition

There has been a lot of interest over the last 10 years in the role of several specific nutrients in modulating the immune response. Arginine, glutamine, nucleotides and omega-3 fatty acids have been studied, either alone or in combination, in a variety of patient groups. Studies have shown conflicting results, To date, there is no definitive evidence that immunonutrition improves outcome in critically ill patients.

ENTERAL FEEDING

Enteral feeding is the preferred means of nutritional support wherever possible. Advice should be sought from a dietician for exact nutritional requirements; however, ready-to-use off-the-shelf enteral feeding formulae are available and are suitable for most patients. Therefore do not wait for specialist dietetic advice before starting enteral feeding. Start empirical feeds out of hours and seek a tailored approach on the next working day. It is unnecessary in intubated patients to stop feeds for repeated surgical procedures like daily pack changes.

Indications

Unless there is a specific surgical contraindication, all patients should receive enteral feeding as soon as possible, preferably within 24 h. This provides nutrition and helps to maintain gastrointestinal tract integrity and function. Potential benefits include:

- Reduced gut atrophy.
- Reduced bacterial and endotoxin translocation.
- Reduced incidence of septic complications and SIRS.
- Reduced length of hospital stay.

(See Stress ulcer prophylaxis, p. 172 and Gastrointestinal tract, p. 166.)

Contraindications

Contraindications include paralytic ileus, intestinal obstruction and surgical conditions of the oesophagus or abdomen.

 The absence of bowel sounds alone in a ventilated patient without other evidence of ileus should not prevent attempts to commence enteral feeding.

Route of administration

The majority of patients in the ICU will already have a standard nasogastric tube in situ for gastric aspiration. This can be used for short-term feeding. In patients who require longer term feeding, fine-bore nasogastric feeding tubes are more comfortable and less likely to cause mucosal erosions. (See Practical procedures, p. 421.)

Delayed gastric emptying is a major factor limiting the success of enteral feeding. There is increasing use of feeding tubes placed through the pylorus, which deliver enteral feed directly into the duodenum or jejunum. Although it is possible to place these tubes 'blindly', more commonly placement is guided by X-ray screening, ultrasound or endoscopy. Percutaneous endoscopic gastrostomy (PEG) or gastrojejunostomy (PEGJ) is useful in patients who are likely to require long-term feeding. This can be performed on the ICU and has the advantage that it allows all nasogastric tubes to be removed, reducing the risks of nosocomial chest infections.

Typical feeding regimens

Enteral feeds are given by continuous infusion. Typically, feed is given for 20 h and then stopped for 4 h. This rest period is to allow the gastric pH to return to normal (acid) levels. This helps to prevent colonization of the stomach with gastrointestinal tract flora, which is associated with an increased incidence of nosocomial pneumonia. Many units have policies for the commencement of enteral feeding. For example:

- Commence enteral feed at 30 mL/h.
- Give feed for 4 h.
- Aspirate NG tube to assess gastric residual volume.
- If feed absorbed, increase in 25 mL increments every 4 h up to 100 mL/h.

Complications

The potential complications of enteral feeding are shown in Box 3.3.

Misplacement or dislodgement of the NG tube can result in accidental delivery and/or aspiration of feed into the lungs. The position of the tube must always be verified before feed or drugs are administered (see Passing a nasogastric tube, p. 421). Blocked NG tubes can occasionally be 'rescued' by flushing with normal saline using a syringe. Small syringes are more effective then large ones for this purpose.

Box 3.3 Complications of enteral feeding

Tube malposition or displacement

Tube occlusion

Abdominal cramps and bloating

Regurgitation and pulmonary aspiration

Diarrhoea

Increased risk of nosocomial infection associated with NG tubes

Metabolic derangement

To prevent inadvertent administration of enteral drugs/feed by the i.v. route (and vice versa) many units now use a separate colour-coded (typically purple) syringe system for enteral administration. The Luer lock on these syringes, and the enetral feeding systems to which they connect, is reversed, making them incompatible with IV ports.

COMMON PROBLEMS ASSOCIATED WITH ENTERAL FEEDING

Feed not absorbed

High gastric residual volume suggests enteral feed is not being absorbed. If after 4 h feed the gastric residual volume is more than 200 mL, return the aspirated feed to the stomach and rest for 1 h. Then reassess.

If possible, stop or reduce opioid analgesics that may delay gastric emptying. Ensure that the electrolyte balance is normal. Disturbances of potassium and magnesium in particular can contribute to gastrointestinal tract dysfunction. Consider the need for further investigation such as plain abdominal X-ray to exclude obstruction. In the absence of mechanical obstruction the use of prokinetic drugs may promote gastric emptying. Choice will depend upon local protocol. Available agents include:

- metoclopramide
- erythromycin (lower dose for kinetic use).

Unless there is a contraindication to feeding, do not stop enteral feeds purely because of 'failure to absorb'. Continue at a low rate, for example 10–20 mL/h. Consider the use of a nasoduodenal/nasojejunal tube.

Diarrhoea

Diarrhoea commonly complicates enteral feeding in the ICU. The causes of this are multifactorial. Diarrhoea is generally a nuisance rather than a serious problem; however, it may result in the need to abandon enteral feeding.

- Do not immediately stop enteral feed. Discuss, with the dietician changing the feed, reduction in the osmolality and increase in the fibre content.
- Perform a rectal examination to exclude faecal impaction (common in the elderly), which may be a cause of overflow diarrhoea. Consider suppositories or manual evacuation.

- Confirm diarrhoea is not infective in nature: send stool specimens for microscopy and culture (*Salmonella*, *Shigella* and *Campylobacter* species) and for *Clostridium difficile* toxin.
- Treat any infective process appropriately. For *Clostridium difficile* use oral or nasogastric metronidazole or vancomycin.
- Review the drug chart. Stop any prokinetic drugs such as metoclopramide. If the diarrhoea is non-infective, consider the use of loperamide.
- If the diarrhoea is bloody or if the nature is unclear, consider the need for further investigations e.g., sigmoidoscopy, colonoscopy or CT. Discuss with gastroenterology/infectious disease specialists.
- Consider the need for a faecal tube collection system and isolation in a side room

PARENTERAL NUTRITION

If enteral feeding is contraindicated or cannot be established, then total parenteral nutrition (TPN) may be required. It is generally not necessary if the patient is likely to be able to recommence enteral feeding within a few days, unless the patient is already severely wasted or malnourished. If in doubt, seek senior advice.

Practical TPN

Most units now use one or two standard mixture feeds, prepared under sterile conditions in the pharmacy or bought in from an outside supplier. The typical composition of a standard feed is shown in Table 3.13.

Some patients need regimens specifically tailored to their needs. For example, patients in renal failure, who are not on renal support, require a reduced volume and restricted nitrogen intake to avoid rises in plasma urea. For most patients, however, a standard feed can be started and advice subsequently sought from dieticians, pharmacists or a parenteral nutrition team. In practice

TABLE 3.13 Typical composition of standard TPN mixture

Volume	2.5 L
Nitrogen source (9–14 g nitrogen)	L-amino acid solution
Energy source (1500–2000 kcal)	Glucose and lipid emulsion
Additives	Electrolytes, trace elements, vitamins
Other additives	Insulin and H_2 blockers may be added if required

therefore, decide what volume of feed the patient will tolerate. Standard adult feeds are usually 2.5 L a day, but smaller volume feeds are available for fluid-restricted patients.

Parenteral feeds are hypertonic and can cause thrombophlebitis. They should normally only be given via central venous lines, although high-volume lower-osmolality feeds may be given via peripherally inserted feeding lines. When inserting multiple lumen central lines, it is a good idea to keep one lumen clean and dedicated for TPN. Parenteral nutrition mixtures make good culture mediums for bacteria, so do not break the line to give anything else. TPN is given by constant infusion over 24h and delivered by volumetric infusion pumps.

Monitoring during TPN

Advice should be sought from the nutrition team and dietician. The following should be assessed daily:

- Fluid balance.
- Urea, electrolytes, phosphate.
- Glucose. Blood sugar will often rise and require the addition of an insulin infusion. Recent evidence suggests that close control of blood sugar levels may improve outcome of critically ill patients (see p. 215).
- Adequate energy requirements. Judged by degree of catabolism clinically. Nitrogen balance can be calculated but in practice rarely is.
- Liver function tests (albumin, transferrin and enzymes) indicate adequate protein synthesis and give an early indication of TPN-related complications.
- Trace elements and micronutrient levels are typically measured weekly. Seek local advice.

Complications

The complications of TPN include all complications of central venous access (see Complications of central venous cannulation, p. 376). Metabolic derangement, particularly hyper- or hypoglycaemia, hypophosphataemia and hypercalcaemia, are common and require appropriate adjustment of the feed. Hepatobiliary dysfunction, including elevation of hepatic enzymes, jaundice and fatty infiltration of the liver, may occur. This is usually caused by a combination of the patient's underlying disease processes and overfeeding. Reduce the volume of TPN and/or energy content. If the serum becomes very lipaemic, it may be necessary to reduce the fat content.

Refeeding syndrome

This syndrome was originally described in recovering prisoners of war, but is also well recognized in patients with anorexia nervosa who have been re-established on a healthy diet. It is seen but generally under recognized in critical illness. During starvation, there is suppression of insulin secretion, resulting in progressive loss of intracellular electrolytes. When effective feeding is re-established, there is a rapid rise in blood glucose, resulting in a shift from lipid to glucose metabolism. This is characterized by a rapid shift of electrolytes into cells, and in particular by profound hypophosphataemia. These changes are accompanied by a marked elevation in metabolic rate, and can be complicated by muscle weakness, rhabdomyolysis, cardiac failure, confusion and seizures. The syndrome can be managed by gentle reintroduction of nutrition, accompanied by meticulous monitoring and correction of fluid and electrolyte abnormalities (especially hypophosphataemia). Typically, at-risk patients are started on a quarter of their predicted daily requirements of nutrients and then this is gradually increased over a number of days. Seek specialist advice.

STRESS ULCER PROPHYLAXIS

Early enteral feeding helps to maintain gastrointestinal mucosal blood flow, provides essential nutrients to the mucosa and is important in reducing the incidence of stress ulceration. (See Gastrointestinal tract, p. 168.) If enteral feeding cannot be established, patients should receive alternative prophylactic measures to prevent stress ulceration. For example:

● ranitidine 50 mg i.v. 8-hourly
● omeprazole 40 mg n.g./i.v. daily.

It was previously thought that sucralfate, which is relatively effective in preventing gastrointestinal bleeding was preferable to ranitidine for prophylaxis against gastric erosion. The rationale for this, was that while sucralfate provides an effective mucosal barrier it does not suppress gastric acid production. Agents such as ranitidine that do suppress gastric acid production are associated with increased gastric pH, which may lead to bacterial overgrowth in the stomach and the potential for an increase in nosocomial pneumonias. Recent evidence, however, suggests that ranitidine is substantially more effective at preventing gastrointestinal haemorrhage than sucralfate, and that there is little difference in the incidence of nosocomial pneumonia. On this basis, sucralfate has largely disappeared from intensive care practice in the United Kingdom.

DVT PROPHYLAXIS

Patients requiring intensive care are at risk for the development of deep venous thrombosis (DVT) and pulmonary embolism (PE). Risk factors include immobility, venous stasis, poor circulation, major surgery, malignancy and pre-existing illness. Over and above these well-known factors, intensive care itself is an independent risk factor. Upper limb venous thrombosis is more common in ITU than in other settings, usually due to thrombosis following subclavian vein catheterization. Heparin-induced thrombocytopenia (HIT) with associated venous thrombosis is probably more common than previously realized (see p. 263).

Despite all these risk factors, there has been surprisingly little research performed to document either the true incidence of DVT or PE in such a population or what constitutes the best form of prophylaxis. Guidance on prophylaxis has, however, recently been published by the Intensive Care Society (Venous thromboprophylaxis in critical care 2008, see www.ics.ac.uk). The use of compression stockings and early mobilization of patients may help to reduce the risk. Once coagulation profiles are within normal ranges prophylactic low-dose subcutaneous heparin is usually given. Low molecular weight heparins are usually preferred, for example,

● enoxaparin 20 mg s.c. daily.

Low molecular weight heparins are associated with a lower incidence of haemorrhage and HIT than unfractionated heparin. Activated partial thromboplastin time (APTT) cannot, however, be used to monitor their effect. Specific assays of factor Xa activity are required, although these are time consuming and not routinely performed. It is not considered necessary to monitor the effects of low molecular weight heparins when used prophylactically in routine clinical practice.

There are a number of newer oral and parenteral anticoagulant drugs receiving licences for DVT prophylaxis; these are likely to be increasingly used in critical care in the future.

Suspected DVT can be confirmed by ultrasound or venography. If confirmed, the patient should be fully anticoagulated either with heparin or with high-dose low molecular weight heparin. This can be followed by warfarin when conditions allow. (See Pulmonary embolism, p. 107.)

CHAPTER 4

CARDIOVASCULAR SYSTEM

Shock   66

Oxygen delivery and
  oxygen consumption   68

Cardiac output   70

Monitoring haemodynamic
  status   74

Optimization of
  haemodynamic status   78

Optimization of filling
  status   80

Optimization of cardiac
  output   82

Optimization of perfusion
  pressure   85

Rational use of inotropes
  and vasopressors   86

Hypotension   87

Hypertension   88

Disturbances of cardiac
  rhythm   90

Conduction defects   98

Myocardial ischaemia   100

Stable angina   100

Acute coronary
  syndromes   101

Cardiac failure   105

Cardiogenic shock   106

Pulmonary embolism   107

Pericardial effusion and
  cardiac tamponade   108

Cardiac arrest   109

Adult patient with
  congenital heart
  disease   111

SHOCK

The primary function of the cardiovascular system is to maintain perfusion of organs and tissues with oxygenated blood. Complex homeostatic mechanisms exist to ensure that an adequate cardiac output and blood pressure are maintained to meet the needs of the individual. When these mechanisms fail, 'shock' ensues, which uncorrected, can result in organ failure, prolonged ICU stay and death.

Definition

Shock is a syndrome of cardiovascular system failure resulting in inadequate tissue perfusion. Hypotension is a common but not universal feature. Shock is often a feature of patients suffering sepsis, pneumonia, multiple trauma or multiple organ failure. Consequently, it is commonly seen in general intensive care units.

Clinical features

The clinical features vary depending on the cause and the physiological response. Two patterns are typically recognized, although there is a continuum from one to the other:

- Hyperdynamic shock: Warm, pink, vasodilated, a tachycardia, with high cardiac output and hypotension. (typical of septic shock, see p. 33)
- Hypodynamic shock: Cold, grey, sweaty, vasoconstricted, peripherally shut down with low cardiac output, blood pressure may be relatively well maintained (typical of cardiac shock, see p. 108).

Other features of shock may include an increased or decreased core temperature, hypoventilation or hyperventilation, renal and hepatic dysfunction, disseminated intravascular coagulation, and altered mental status. (See Systemic inflammatory response syndrome, p. 326 and Multiorgan dysfunction syndrome, p. 327.) The young fit patient with an adequate cardiac reserve may well be able to initially compensate for the pathophysiological disturbances leading to shock. Consequently, shock occurring in an otherwise fit young person often represents a greater physiological disturbance or a later stage of illness as compared with the situation in an elderly patient, in whom conditions such as fixed cardiac output, peripheral and coronary artery disease and reduced organ function reduce the 'physiological reserve'.

TABLE 4.1 Typical causes of shock*

Classification	Underlying cause
Hypovolaemia	Dehydration
	Haemorrhage
	Burns
	Sepsis
	Increased capillary permeability
Cardiogenic	Myocardial infarction/ischaemia
	Valve disruption
	Myocardial rupture (e.g. VSD)
Mechanical/obstructive	Pulmonary embolism
	Cardiac tamponade
	Tension pneumothorax
Altered systemic vascular resistance	Sepsis
	Severe anaemia
	Anaphylaxis
	Addisonian crisis

*Note, more than one cause may be present in an individual patient.

Aetiology

The aetiology of shock is frequently multifactorial. Typical causes are listed in Table 4.1. Although all causes of shock are seen on the ICU, the commonest in practice is septic shock (see Septic shock, p. 331).

Management

Apart from the mechanical causes of shock, in which relief of the mechanical obstruction may take priority, the principles of managing shock states are similar in all patients regardless of aetiology. They include:

● treatment of the underlying pathology
● optimization of circulating blood volume
● optimization of cardiac output
● optimization of blood pressure
● optimization of oxygen delivery
● support for any organ failure.

You should understand the factors that influence tissue perfusion and oxygen delivery, oxygen consumption and cardiac output.

OXYGEN DELIVERY AND OXYGEN CONSUMPTION

Oxygen delivery (DO_2)

Oxygen delivery is defined as the total amount of oxygen delivered to the tissues (body) per minute. It depends on the cardiac output (CO) and the oxygen content of arterial blood, as shown:

$DO_2 = CO \times$ [arterial oxygen content]

$DO_2 = CO \times [(SaO_2 \times Hb^* \times 1.34) + (\text{dissolved oxygen})]$

$Hb^* =$ haemoglobin g/dL (divide by 100 for g/mL)

$1.34 =$ amount of oxygen (mL) bound to 1 g of fully saturated haemoglobin.

Therefore, ignoring dissolved oxygen, which is insignificant at atmospheric pressure, typical figures are:

$1000 \, mL/min = 5000 \, mL \times [(99/100 \times 15/100 \times 1.34)]$

Oxygen consumption (VO_2)

Oxygen consumption is the total amount of oxygen consumed by the tissues (body) per minute. It can be calculated from the difference in oxygen content of arterial and mixed venous blood ($S\bar{v}O_2$).

$VO_2 = CO \times$ [(arterial oxygen content) − (mixed venous oxygen content)]

$VO_2 = CO \times [(SaO_2 \times Hb \times 1.34) - (S\bar{v}O_2 \times Hb \times 1.34)]$

If cardiac index is used in the above calculations (see below), then oxygen delivery and oxygen consumption can also be expressed as an index relative to body surface area. Typical normal values are shown in Table 4.2.

TABLE 4.2 Typical adult values for oxygen delivery and oxygen consumption

Oxygen delivery	1000 mL/min
Oxygen delivery index DO_2I	550 mL/min/m²
Oxygen consumption VO_2	250 mL/min
Oxygen consumption index VO_2I	150 mL/min/m²

Oxygen extraction ratio

Under normal circumstances, oxygen consumption by the tissues is only about 25% of the oxygen delivered. This provides a large margin for safety, so that if oxygen requirements increase, for example in exercise, more oxygen can be extracted and utilized. In disease states however, while oxygen requirements may be raised, the ability of the tissues to extract and utilize oxygen may be impaired. Under these circumstances, utilization of oxygen by the tissues may be limited by the available supply. Oxygen delivery may be increased by manipulation of cardiac output, improvement in oxygen saturation and transfusion (see below). Oxygen extraction cannot be significantly influenced except by general improvement in the patient's condition.

Optimizing oxygen delivery

From the formula for oxygen delivery above, it follows that oxygen delivery can be improved by:

- Ensuring adequate arterial oxygen saturation.
- Optimizing haemoglobin (see below).
- Optimizing cardiac output (see Optimizing haemodynamic status, p. 78).

If oxygen delivery remains critical, then tracheal intubation and assisted ventilation with paralysis (muscle relaxants) may help to reduce the muscle utilization of oxygen and reduce oxygen requirements.

Optimizing haemoglobin

Since haemoglobin (Hb) carries oxygen to the tissues, one might assume that raising a patient's Hb to 15 g/dL might provide optimal oxygen delivery. However, clinical studies have not confirmed that raising the haemoglobin concentration improves outcome and indeed, the opposite is likely to be true. Evidence from the Canadian Multicentre Clinical Trials Group suggests that restrictive transfusion strategies produce the best outcome in critically ill patients and that the optimal level in most cases is a Hb of 8–10 g/dL. (See Indications for blood transfusion, p. 246.) This study excluded patients, however, with significant coronary artery and vascular disease, who may benefit from a higher Hb. If in doubt about optimal haemoglobin for an individual patient, seek senior advice.

Mixed venous oxygen saturation ($S\bar{v}O_2$)

A guide to the balance between oxygen delivery and oxygen consumption can be obtained by the measurement of mixed venous oxygen saturation. Traditionally mixed venous oxygen was measured in blood from the pulmonary artery via a pulmonary artery catheter, either intermittently (by blood gas measurement) or continuously (using an oximetric catheter.) More recently, measurement of oxygen saturation of blood from a central catheter in the superior vena cava ($S\bar{v}_cO_2$) has been shown to correlate with the true $S\bar{v}O_2$ sufficiently closely to be used almost interchangeably in clinical practice.

Resuscitation guided by $S\bar{v}O_2$ or $S\bar{v}_cO_2$ has been shown to improve outcome by reducing the severity of organ failure and the duration of intensive care. Normal $S\bar{v}O_2$ is 55–75%. Values below this imply inadequate oxygen delivery. Values above this imply either supranormal oxygen delivery or reduced oxygen consumption. Conditions that may result in impaired oxygen consumption include sepsis, metabolic poisoning and widespread cellular death.

 Despite apparently optimal oxygen delivery, guided by $S\bar{v}O_2$ or $S\bar{v}_cO_2$ differences in regional perfusion may still result in some tissues receiving inadequate perfusion and oxygen delivery. The splanchnic circulation is, for example, at particular risk of hypoperfusion.

CARDIAC OUTPUT

Assuming that oxygen saturation and haemoglobin are optimal, then the main determinant of systemic oxygen delivery is cardiac output (CO). This is defined as the volume of blood ejected by the heart per minute. It is the product of heart rate (HR) and stroke volume (SV), as shown:

cardiac output (CO) = heart rate (HR) × stroke volume (SV)

In order to take account of patient size, cardiac output is usually expressed as cardiac index (CI), which is the CO divided by the patient's body surface area (BSA). BSA can be derived from a patient's height and weight using nomograms. In practice, however, height and weight are usually entered directly into monitoring systems and all necessary calculations performed automatically. Typical values are shown in Table 4.3.

TABLE 4.3 Typical adult values for cardiac output	
Cardiac output (CO)	4–6 L/min
Cardiac index (CI)	2.5–3.5 L/min/m²

The factors that affect cardiac output are discussed below.

Heart rate

In a healthy heart there is little change in stroke volume with fluctuations in heart rate occurring within the physiological range (70–160 beats/min). Therefore, as heart rate increases, CO increases. The elderly, those with pre-existing heart disease, and critically ill patients, however tolerate a much narrower range of heart rates, and values outside 100–120 beats/min may significantly compromise CO.

At low heart rates, SV may be maintained but CO falls as a function of heart rate. At high rates, inadequate filling leads to a fall in SV and a subsequent reduction in CO. Tachycardias associated with abnormalities of cardiac rhythm (e.g. atrial fibrillation) further reduce ventricular filling and CO. Tachycardias also lead to increased myocardial oxygen consumption, while simultaneously reducing the time for diastolic perfusion of the ventricles. In patients with ischaemic heart disease, this may produce significant myocardial ischaemia, which may further compromise CO.

Stroke volume (SV)

The stroke volume is the volume of blood ejected with each heartbeat, and is the difference between the volume of the full ventricle (end diastolic volume) and the volume of the ventricle after ejection of blood is completed (end systolic volume). Traditionally, SV has been thought of as being determined by preload, contractility and afterload.

Preload

This is defined as the ventricular wall tension at the end of diastole. In simple terms preload refers to the degree of ventricular filling. According to the Frank–Starling law of the heart, the greater the degree of ventricular filling, the greater the force of myocardial contraction and thus SV. Above a certain point, however, the ventricle becomes over-stretched and further filling may result in a fall in SV. Heart failure and pulmonary oedema may then develop (see Fig. 4.1).

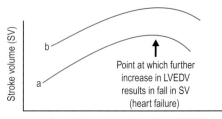

Fig. 4.1 Diagrammatic representation of Frank–Starling Curves. (a) Increasing LVEDV leads to increased SV. (b) Effect of increased contractility, e.g. as a result of inotropes.

Preload is therefore a function of the volume status of the patient. It also depends upon adequate ventricular relaxation in order to allow ventricular filling to take place. Ventricular relaxation is an active process. In critically ill patients, failure of ventricular relaxation (diastolic failure) may result in the ventricle becoming stiff and non-compliant. When this occurs, the ventricle cannot fill normally, regardless of the patient's volume status and cardiac output is reduced.

Contractility
This represents the ability of the heart to work independent of the preload and afterload. Increased contractility, as, for example produced by inotropes, results in increased SV for the same preload (see Fig. 4.1). Decreased contractility may result from intrinsic heart disease, or from the myocardial depressant effects of acidosis, hypoxia and disease processes, e.g. sepsis.

Afterload
This is defined as the ventricular wall tension at the end of systole. In simple terms this is a measure of the load against which the heart is working. It is increased by ventricular dilatation, outflow resistance (for example, aortic valve stenosis) and increases in peripheral vascular resistance.

Pressure–volume–flow loops
A more recent approach to understanding the interdependency of preload contractility and afterload and the effects thereof, on cardiac output and stroke volume, is to consider pressure–volume–flow loops of the left ventricle (see Fig. 4.2).

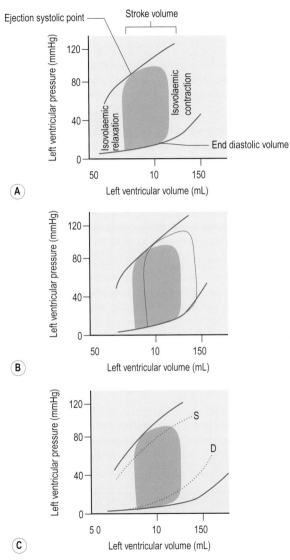

Fig. 4.2 (A) Pressure–volume loops of the left ventricle. (B) Effect of increased end diastolic volume (preload) (C) Effect of reduced contractility (S) and diastolic dysfunction (D).

End diastolic volume, which represents ventricular filling, is a function of venous return (pressure) and the diastolic compliance. Increased venous pressure leads to increased ventricular filling and this additional filling is greatest where diastolic compliance is optimal. Where diastolic dysfunction or failure occurs, the diastolic compliance is reduced (with a steeper diastolic compliance curve) and higher venous pressures are required to achieve adequate ventricular filling. Diastolic dysfunction may be seen in hypoxia, myocardial ischaemia, metabolic derangement or as a consequence of mechanical compromise such as pericardial effusion or tamponade.

The end systolic point describes the relationship between the end systolic volume (the volume of blood remaining in the ventricle at the end of systole) and the ejection systolic pressure. This point is determined by a combination of contractility and outflow resistance (afterload). The end systolic point moves upwards and to the right if the ejection systolic pressure is increased (e.g. increased afterload), and downwards to the left if the ejection systolic pressure is reduced (e.g. decreased afterload). Thus under conditions of vasodilation, (e.g. sepsis) there is reduced afterload, lower ejection systolic pressure and reduced end systolic volume. Conversely, vasoconstriction (increased afterload) leads to increased ejection systolic pressure, and increased end systolic volume.

Assuming contractility is unchanged, the ejection systolic point at the end of any heart beat will fall along a curve. Changes in contractility will shift the position of this curve (Fig. 4.2). Increased contractility for example as a result of inotropic drugs, shifts the curve upwards and to the left, so that the same ejection systolic pressure is associated with an increased ejection fraction, greater stroke volume and reduced end systolic volume. Reduced contractility, for example resulting from intrinsic heart disease, or from the myocardial depressant effects of acidosis, hypoxia or sepsis shifts the curve to the right and flattens it. The same systolic blood pressure is associated with a reduced ejection fraction and stroke volume and a much greater end systolic volume.

MONITORING HAEMODYNAMIC STATUS

Although considerable information on the cardiovascular status of a patient can be obtained from simple clinical examination (pulse, blood pressure, core peripheral temperature gradient, urine output etc.) additional information obtained from invasive monitoring is useful, particularly when assessing the response to changes in therapy.

Invasive arterial pressure monitoring

Arterial cannulation allows beat-to-beat measurement of arterial blood pressure and easy serial blood gas sampling. Significant respiratory variation in the amplitude of the arterial pressure wave ('respiratory swing') is characteristic of hypovolaemia. This pulse pressure variability (which relates to stroke volume variability caused by changes in venous return) can be formally measured by modern monitoring systems and is described as a percentage. Pulse variability less than 10% implies adequate filling and has been used as an end point for volume resuscitation. (See Arterial cannulation, p. 372.)

Central venous pressure

Central venous catheterization provides a route of delivery for drugs and fluids and enables measurement of right heart filling pressures (CVP). Central venous access can be achieved via the jugular, subclavian, brachial or femoral routes. (See Central venous cannulation, p. 376, and Optimizing filling status, p. 376.)

Pulmonary artery catheterization

Pulmonary artery (PA) catheterization has for a number of years been the gold standard cardiovascular monitoring tool in ICU. This technique enables the measurement of pulmonary artery pressure, pulmonary artery occlusion pressure (PAOP) and CO, and also allows many other haemodynamic variables to be calculated or derived. Typical values are given in Table 4.4.

The value of pulmonary artery catheters has recently been questioned and the technique has been the subject of a number of major multicentre trials leading to a critical re-evaluation of the role of PA catheterization. Recent trials failed to show benefit or harm in a mixed adult ICU population with the suggestion that it should be reserved for the more complicated case where specific questions about the dynamic variables are required to be answered. The use of PA catheterization has fallen significantly with the introduction of alternative forms of monitoring. Relatively non-invasive systems for continuous cardiac output monitoring are available based on transthoracic bioimpedance, oesophageal Doppler, pulse contour and pulse power analysis.

Pulse contour analysis

Currently, systems based on pulse contour analysis are perhaps the most likely to enter widespread use. In general terms these require venous access (peripheral or central) and an arterial line with a sensor either built in or attached. To calibrate the

TABLE 4.4 Normal values of common haemodynamic variables derived from PA catheterization

Central venous pressure (CVP)	4–10 mmHg
Pulmonary artery occlusion pressure (PAOP)	5–15 mmHg
Cardiac output (CO)	4–6 L/min
Cardiac index (CI)	2.5–3.5 L min^{-1} m^{-2}
Stroke volume (SV)	60–90 mL/beat
Stroke volume index (SVI)	33–47 mL/beat per m^2
Systemic vascular resistance (SVR)	900–1200 dyne.s/cm^5
Systemic vascular resistance index (SVRI)	1700–2400 dyne.s/cm^5 per m^2
Pulmonary vascular resistance (PVR)	<250 dyne.s/cm^5
Pulmonary vascular resistance index (PVRI)	255–285 dyne.s/cm^5 per m^2

These 'normal values' provide a guide only. They may not be achievable or appropriate for all critically ill patients (See Goal directed therapy, p. 78).

system an indicator is injected into the venous catheter and is detected by the arterial line producing a standard dilutional CO measurement. From this the systems are able to provide continuous CO, SV and systemic vascular resistance by analysis of the pulse waveform. To maintain accuracy they must be calibrated every 8–12 h or whenever there is a significant change in cardiovascular status. A popular device using this technique is the Picco system, which combines pulse contour analysis with intermittent calibration by thermodilution. The thermodilution calibration curves can also be used to estimate thermal volumes of distribution in the chest, providing a reasonably well validated measure of global end diastolic volume (a surrogate for filling) and extra vascular lung water, useful in resuscitation and the management of acute lung injury.

Pulse power analysis

A related approach is an analysis of the area under the curve of the arterial waveform. This is known as 'pulse power analysis' and has some theoretical advantages over pulse contour analysis. In particular, it does not require proximal arterial cannulation and should in theory be slightly more robust under conditions of damping. It is used commercially in the LiDCO system. This device combines pulse power analysis with calibration using lithium dilution every 12–24 h. An injection of a very low dose of lithium into a vein (not necessarily a central vein) is accompanied by measurement of a dilation curve in an artery. Blood is pumped from the arterial line across an electrode calibrated to measure monovalent cations. In theory, the only such ion whose concentration varies in the time course of the measurement is lithium. Injection of other charged substances at the same time invalidate the measurement. In practice, the only common confounding factor is recent injection of atracurium (a positively charged quaternary nitrogen compound).

Oesophageal Doppler

A Doppler ultrasound probe is placed in the oesophagus and directed to obtain a signal from the descending aorta. The signal obtained is displayed on the screen and indicates peak velocity and flow time. By making a number of assumptions about the nature of flow in the aorta, the cross-sectional area of the aorta (estimated from body surface area and age) and the percentage of CO passing down the thoracic aorta, SV and CO can be estimated. Trends in values and response to changes in therapy are more useful than absolute values. It is particularly useful for assessing response to fluid challenges but is rather operator-dependent.

> ⚠ All of these monitoring systems have advantages and disadvantages. The key to their successful utilization is in careful interpretation of the information provided. If any of these systems are in use in your unit, you should seek instruction on their use.

Echocardiography

Transthoracic echocardiography is minimally invasive and can be repeated at short intervals to assess cardiac function and response to therapy. The key information available from echocardiography is shown in Table 4.5.

There is increasing availability of bedside, transthoracic and to a lesser extent transoesophageal, echocardiography in intensive care, for use by suitably trained intensive care staff, as opposed to cardiologists or sonographers. Abbreviated training packages have been developed for this purpose, which enable individuals to undertake focused examinations (e.g. FATE). All these packages

TABLE 4.5 Key information available from echocardiography

Structure	Anatomical abnormalities (e.g. congenital heart disease)
Filling	Assessment of end diastolic volume of RA/RV/LA/LV
Function	Assessment of contractility Identification of areas of dyskinesia (suggestive of ischaemia) Presence of dilated chambers Valve function
Pericardium	Presence of pericardial effusions Evidence of tamponade

accept the limitations of examinations by non-specialists and emphasize the need for formal referral to echocardiography where there is doubt about the findings. Nevertheless it seems likely that echocardiography will increasingly become an extension of the traditional clinical examination of patients in ICU. All patients will be likely to receive a focused echocardiography examination on admission and at intervals and the findings used to guide haemodynamic therapy.

OPTIMIZATION OF HAEMODYNAMIC STATUS

Optimization of haemodynamic status is a key goal in both the critically ill patients and the high risk patient undergoing major surgery. This encompasses both optimization of cardiac output and oxygen delivery and also the maintenance of adequate organ perfusion.

Goal directed therapy

The availability of so many measured haemodynamic variables (above) led to attempts to improve the outcome of critically ill patients by manipulation of the variables to achieve 'standard goals'. Shoemaker, for example, compared measured variables in trauma survivors and non-survivors and suggested that outcome could be improved by manipulating haemodynamics to achieve supranormal values of cardiac index ($4.5 \, L/min/m^2$), oxygen delivery index ($650 \, mL/min/m^2$) and oxygen consumption index ($165 \, mL/min/m^2$). There is little evidence, however, that this approach improves outcome in the general population of critically ill patients.

The difficulty with population-based targets of this sort is that they risk over- or under-treating individual patients. The more modern approach therefore is to optimize cardiovascular performance of each individual patient by titration of fluids and vasoactive drugs to achieve the 'optimal response' for that individual.

Rational approach to optimization of haemodynamic status

Avoid aiming to achieve absolute numbers for CO and other variables. Use 'normal values' only as a guide and think in terms of achieving adequate haemodynamic performance for the individual patient. A rational approach is to optimize fluid (filling) status first and then to add an inotrope or vasoconstrictor as required. Figure 4.3 provides a simple algorithm for optimizing haemodynamic status and the management of shock regardless of the underlying cause.

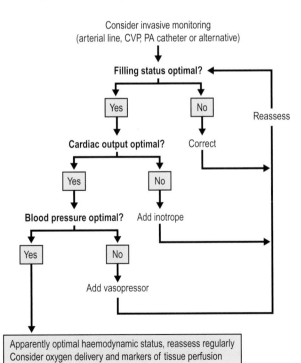

Fig. 4.3 Optimization of the haemodynamic system.

> **!** For many patients in the ICU the primary problem will be sepsis, which typically produces a high CO, low pressure state. Following the algorithm, if CO is adequate, attention moves directly to perfusion pressure. It is important, however, to assess the adequacy of cardiac output early in the management of shock to avoid missing cardiogenic causes.

TABLE 4.6 Effects of agonists on cardiovascular receptors

Receptor	Effects
α_1	Vasoconstriction
β_1	Increased myocardial contractility and heart rate
β_2	Vasodilatation (and bronchodilatation)
DA	Splanchnic and renal vasodilatation

Use of vasoactive drugs

There is a tendency to refer to all vasoactive drugs as inotropes. This is not only incorrect but can lead to confusion when deciding which agent to choose in any given circumstance. By classifying the available agents according to their receptor pharmacology and actions, a rational approach to their use can be achieved. Table 4.6 shows the effects of agonists at various receptors.

On the basis of activity at these receptors, drugs can be classified as inotropes (directly increase cardiac contractility), vasodilators, vasopressors, or a combination of these, e.g. inodilator or inopressor. Classifying agents in this way enables rational choices to be made in selecting agents for use. (See Optimizing cardiac output and Optimizing perfusion pressure below.)

OPTIMIZATION OF FILLING STATUS

The optimal filling status for a patient is that which achieves the maximal CO while at the same time avoiding any deterioration in gas exchange due to the development of pulmonary oedema. If this cannot be achieved, then assisted ventilation may be required.

Use of CVP/PAOP

The use of right atrial pressure (CVP) and to a lesser extent, left atrial pressure (PAOP) to guide fluid therapy is commonplace. Fluids are often given to achieve a predetermined CVP or PAOP. This approach should be avoided.

The relationship between filling pressure and volume status (ventricular end-diastolic volume) is complex and depends on the compliance of the ventricle. This compliance varies both between individuals and in different disease states. It may also change acutely in a single individual in response to pathophysiological changes such as myocardial ischaemia or acidosis.

Any predetermined figure for CVP/PAOP is bound, therefore, to be somewhat arbitrary and may not be optimal for an individual patient. Rather than aiming for a specific CVP or PAOP, try and determine the filling pressure which produces the best haemodynamic response from an individual patient.

- Put bed head down or lift legs as a quick way to increase venous return and assess effect.
- Give fluid to increase the CVP or PAOP in small increments and observe the increase in CO or SV
- Continue until there is no further improvement or until there is deterioration in arterial blood gases or evidence of pulmonary oedema. (Note: stroke volume index of $50\,mL/m^2$ represents a full ventricle.)
- Remember also that optimal filling may actually mean use of fluid restriction, diuretics and vasodilators to reduce preload in patients with heart failure.
- Care should also be taken in the presence of renal failure when excessive fluid is not excreted.

Volumetric haemodynamic monitoring

Increased recognition that the concept of using 'filling pressure' (CVP or PAOP) as a measure of ventricular filling status is flawed has led to the development of monitoring systems capable of directly measuring (estimating) volume status. Detailed description is beyond the scope of this book. A guide to normal values for volume indices is given in Table 4.7.

There is currently no consensus as to which of these variables is the most useful in assessing volume status. As with other haemodynamic variables, it is the trend and response to therapy which is more important than the absolute values obtained. If volumetric monitoring is available in your unit seek senior advice

TABLE 4.7 Typical values of volumetric haemodynamic variables

Right ventricular ejection fraction (RVEF)	35–45%
Right ventricular end diastolic volume (RVEDV)	100–160 mL
Right ventricular end diastolic volume index (RVEDVI)	60–100 mL/m²
Intrathoracic blood volume index (ITBVI)	850–1000 mL/m²
Extravascular lung water index (EVLWI)	3–7 mL/kg

on interpretation of the information provided. If volumetric monitoring is not available, echocardiography can also be used to provide useful information about filling status.

OPTIMIZATION OF CARDIAC OUTPUT

In all but the simplest cases of circulatory failure, where CO is inadequate consider an echocardiogram to establish diagnosis and exclude treatable mechanical causes. Transthoracic and transoesophageal echocardiography can provide useful information on structural and functional cardiac abnormalities, including pericardial collections, valvular lesions, contractility and regional wall motion abnormalities. Estimates of filling and of flows/pressures can also be made. Many critically ill patients will have small pericardial effusions without evidence of cardiac tamponade (RA and RV diastolic collapse). These do not require drainage unless CO is impaired or infection is suspected (see Pericardiocentesis, p. 395).

Inotropes
If despite optimal filling CO remains inadequate, inotropes may be added to improve cardiac performance (Fig. 4.2). The rational use of inotropes requires an understanding of the receptor pharmacology of the commonly used agents. These are summarized in Table 4.8.

Dobutamine (1–20 µg/kg/min)
Increases CO and causes a variable degree of peripheral vasodilatation. It is useful in low CO states when vasomotor tone and mean arterial pressure are reasonably well maintained.

TABLE 4.8 Actions of commonly used inotropic agents

Drug	Receptor	Actions (see notes below)	Classification
Dobutamine	$\beta_1\ \beta_2$	↑ Heart rate and stroke volume Peripheral vasodilatation	Inodilator
Dopexamine	β_2 DA	↑ Heart rate Peripheral and splanchnic vasodilatation	Inodilator
Adrenaline (epinephrine)	$\alpha_1\ \beta_1\ \beta_2$	↑ Heart rate and stroke volume Peripheral vasoconstriction	Inopressor
Dopamine	DA $\alpha_1\ \beta_1$	Actions varied depending on dose	Variable

Dopexamine (1–5 µg/kg/min)

At doses up to $1\,\mu g\,kg^{-1}\,min^{-1}$, dopexamine has little inotropic activity and increases in CO are mediated primarily by peripheral vasodilatation (reduced afterload) and reflex tachycardia. This results in improved blood flow primarily in the splanchnic and renal circulation. At doses above these, there is some intrinsic inotropic activity. Dopexamine may be useful in low CO states when there is increased peripheral vasomotor tone and mean arterial blood pressure is maintained. In addition it may be used to promote renal–splanchnic blood flow. (See Oliguria, p. 188, and GIT failure, p. 168.)

Adrenaline (epinephrine) (0.1–0.5 µg/kg/min)

At low doses the primary effect is increased CO; at higher doses there is additional potent vasoconstriction. It is useful in low output states associated with low peripheral vasomotor tone and low mean arterial pressure. Adrenaline (epinephrine) is the drug of choice in an emergency and in hypotensive states when the overall haemodynamic status is not clear. Its prolonged use is associated with impaired splanchnic perfusion, hyperglycaemia and increased serum lactate.

Dopamine (2.5–5 µg/kg/min)

Dopamine acts on α_1 and β_1 adrenoceptors and DA receptors and releases noradrenaline (norepinephrine) from adrenergic nerves. The actions of dopamine therefore vary depending on the dose. At low doses, up to 5 μg/kg/min, the primary action is said to be on DA receptors, resulting in increased splanchnic and renal perfusion. Dopamine may therefore be useful to help maintain renal blood flow and promote urine output, although the evidence for this is poor. At doses above 5 μg/kg/min vasoconstrictor and cardiac effects predominate (see Oliguria, p. 188).

Choice of inotrope

From the table and notes above, select the most appropriate inotrope for the patient's clinical condition. Generally:

- If despite low CO mean arterial blood pressure is well maintained, use dobutamine or dopexamine to increase CO, reduce afterload and improve perfusion.
- If low CO is associated with low blood pressure use adrenaline (epinephrine).
- If you are uncertain, the mixed actions of dopamine make it a reasonable choice in most settings. It is commonly used as a first-line agent in Europe; however, in the UK it has tended to be used less.

Start infusions at the lowest infusion rate possible to achieve the desired effect and continually reassess the response. Potential adverse effects include tachycardia, arrhythmias and increased myocardial oxygen consumption. Hyperglycaemia and lactic acidosis may also occur. Where the response is poor, alternative/additional agents may be used. Agents which effectively 'bypass' the β receptors may be particularly useful in heart failure, where down regulation of β receptors may occur. Two classes of drug are available (see Cardiogenic shock, p. 106).

Phosphodiesterase inhibitors

Enoximone and milrinone are examples of phosphodiesterase inhibitors. These agents act by inhibiting myocardial phosphodiesterase, thereby prolonging the action of cyclic AMP. This amplifies the effect of β-receptor stimulation, and results in increased myocardial cytosolic calcium release and hence contractility. They are very effective at increasing cardiac output, but cause profound systemic vasodilatation which can lead to hypotension. They are relatively long-acting. Introduce cautiously. Avoid loading doses. Start low dose infusions and increase gradually.

Calcium sensitizing agents

These agents have only recently become available in the United Kingdom and clinical experience is limited. The first member of this class is levosimendan. By increasing the myofibrillar response to changes in calcium concentration, this drug not only improves systolic myocardial performance but is genuinely 'lusitropic', allowing better myocardial relaxation in diastole with improved ventricular filling.

OPTIMIZATION OF PERFUSION PRESSURE

If, despite adequate filling and CO, the mean arterial pressure remains low, then vasoconstrictors should be used. The commonly available agents are shown in Table 4.9.

- Phenylephrine ($1–5\,\mu g/kg/min$).
- Noradrenaline (norepinephrine) ($0.1–0.5\,\mu g/kg/min$).

Both drugs have direct action on α_1 receptors and increase blood pressure by causing vasoconstriction. There is no appreciable direct effect on CO. They are used to generate an adequate perfusion pressure for vital organs, in particular the brain, liver and kidneys.

Excessive use of vasoconstrictors may, however, be associated with a number of adverse effects. These include increased afterload and reduced CO, reduced renal blood flow, reduced splanchnic blood flow and impaired peripheral perfusion. Vasoconstrictors should therefore be used only in the lowest possible doses required to achieve the desired effect. Consider what is a reasonable target blood pressure for your individual patient (increased with age, hypertension or peripheral vascular disease).

> ⚠ **Vasopressors should be titrated against the blood pressure and not systemic vascular resistance (SVR) or any other derived haemodynamic variable. SVR is mathmatically derived from cardiac output and blood pressure and is not a directly measured, independent variable.**

Vasopressin

There is increasing evidence that in profound shock states vasopressin or antidiuretic hormone (ADH), which is normally secreted by the posterior pituitary, becomes depleted. Replacement

TABLE 4.9 Actions of commonly used vasopressor agents

Drug	Receptor	Actions	Classification
Noradrenaline (norepinephrine)	α_1	Peripheral vasoconstriction	Vasopressor
Phenylephrine	α_1	Peripheral vasoconstriction	Vasopressor

at physiological rather than pharmacological doses, by infusion of vasopressin at 0.1–0.4 μg/kg/min, may help to restore vascular reactivity and tone. It is usually used as a second line agent in combination with other vasopressor agents. Bolus doses of terlipressin, which is a longer acting agent in this class, can also be used.

RATIONAL USE OF INOTROPES AND VASOPRESSORS

Except in emergency situations, do not start inotropes or vasopressors until adequate fluid loading has been achieved. Give only into central veins, using dedicated lumen of a central venous catheter. Be clear about the intended goal. The key is to treat the patient rather than absolute numbers or derived haemodynamic variables. If end organ perfusion is satisfactory (e.g. patient is conscious and passing urine) it may be reasonable to accept a lower cardiac output/blood pressure, rather than start inotropes/vasopressors.

Following each change in therapy you should reassess the patient's haemodynamic status. In particular, check filling status is still optimal and whether therapies have had the desired effect. When optimal haemodynamic status is apparently achieved, ensure oxygen delivery is adequate and consider markers of regional perfusion such as renal output.

No response to inotropes/vasoconstrictors
- Check that arterial and other monitoring lines are functioning correctly (check blood pressure with a cuff) and that transducers are appropriately zeroed and at the correct level.
- Ensure that filling status is optimal. Inotropes and vasoconstrictors are potentially harmful and ineffective if the circulation is empty!

- Treat any dysrhythmias. Atrial fibrillation is a common problem.
- Exclude mechanical causes of low CO and hypotension such as tension pneumothorax, pulmonary embolus and cardiac tamponade.
- Ensure that the appropriate inotrope or vasoconstrictor agent has been started at the correct dose. Check that the infusion is running at the correct rate. Note that if an infusion is started at a low rate it may take some time for the active drug to reach the end of the dead space in the infusion line.
- The myocardium responds poorly to inotropes in the presence of acidosis. Therefore, if a significant acidosis is present (pH < 7.2) consider correcting this with sodium bicarbonate. (See Metabolic acidosis, p. 212.)
- Check the ionized calcium and consider giving additional calcium. (Never give calcium and sodium bicarbonate together down the same line!)
- If there is no improvement in haemodynamic status increase the infusion rate until an appropriate response is obtained. If there is still no response, and particularly if the inotropes or vasoconstrictors have been in use for some time, consider the possibility of tachyphylaxis and receptor downregulation. Start an alternative or additional agent.
- Consider the possibility of adrenocortical failure (rare) or functional adrenal insufficiency. Consider corticosteroid replacement. (See Adrenal insufficiency, p. 221.)

Weaning inotropes and vasoconstrictors

As the patient's condition improves, inotropes and vasoconstrictor agents can be gradually reduced. Ensure optimal filling at all times and reduce drugs according to the results of haemodynamic monitoring.

HYPOTENSION

(See Optimizing haemodynamic status, p. 48.)

Assess the patient

- Is the blood pressure adequate for the patient? An MAP of 60 mmHg is generally adequate, but this will depend on the patient's normal blood pressure, which will vary with age and premorbid state.

- Is there evidence of inadequate tissue oxygenation or organ perfusion (acidosis, oliguria or altered conscious level)? If not, further treatment may not be necessary.
- Is there an obvious cause for hypotension, e.g. hypovolaemia (bleeding), myocardial failure, sepsis? This will guide specific treatment.

Optimize filling status

- Unless there is evidence of fluid overload or myocardial failure, give a fluid challenge to optimize cardiac filling, even if measured CVP is apparently adequate (e.g. 100–500 mL colloid). If there is no response (particularly if there is no rise in measured filling pressures), consider a further fluid bolus.
- If there is still no response, establish invasive monitoring CVP or pulmonary artery catheter (see Practical procedures, p. 376).

Optimize cardiac output

- Give further fluid bolus if appropriate to increase CVP/PAOP and observe the change in CO. Titrate fluids to determine CVP/PAOP that gives optimum cardiac output.
- If CO remains low, add an inotrope. The choice will depend on the clinical condition of the patient. If the peripheral resistance is low adrenaline (epinephrine) is useful as a first-line agent.

Optimize perfusion pressure

- If mean arterial blood pressure remains low despite adequate filling pressure and apparently adequate CO, add a vasoconstrictor to maintain diastolic blood pressure, e.g. noradrenaline (norepinephrine).

HYPERTENSION

Although hypotension is more of a problem in intensive care, hypertension can also occur. This may be a manifestation of pre-existing essential hypertension, but is frequently secondary to other factors. Typical causes are shown in Box 4.1.

Management

In intensive care short periods of hypertension, for example during weaning from ventilation, are not uncommon and do not generally

Box 4.1 Common causes of hypertension in ICU

Pre-existing hypertension/vascular disease

Pain and anxiety

Effects of exogenous catecholamines

Intracranial lesion

Hypervolaemia

Hypoxia

Hypercarbia

Hypothermia

result in any harm unless there is associated myocardial, cerebral or vascular disease. Therefore:

● Do not over-treat hypertension.
● If using an arterial line check the blood pressure reading using a blood pressure cuff. The readings sometimes disagree, in which case the non-invasive measurement may be the more accurate (see Arterial cannulation, p. 372).
● Ensure adequate analgesia and sedation.
● Check blood gases are acceptable.
● Ensure normal fluid status. Consider diuretics or haemodialysis/filtration if fluid overloaded.
● Correct hypothermia.
● Reduce or stop inotropes and vasoconstrictors as appropriate.

Treatment will depend upon the absolute blood pressure, age and condition of the patient. The typical hypertensive patient is the elderly postoperative arteriopath with ischaemic heart disease. Treatment is generally only required if there is sustained diastolic blood pressure >110 mmHg, systolic >200 mmHg or associated myocardial ischaemia. If treatment is required consider:

● Nifedepine 10–20 mg oral or sublingual. (Caution; sublingual nifedipine can cause a rapid fall in blood pressure.)
● Hydralazine 10 mg i.v. repeated as necessary.
● GTN infusion. Particularly if hypertensive episodes are associated with myocardial ischaemia or failure.
● Labetalol is used in small incremental boluses (5–10 mg) and by infusion.

Young hypertensive patients

The young patient with unexplained sustained hypertension, particularly if associated with end organ damage, for example

left ventricular hypertrophy, warrants further investigation.
Consider other causes such as renal artery stenosis and
phaeochromocytoma. Seek advice on appropriate treatment.
(See Phaeochromocytoma, p. 221.)

> ⚠ **Avoid the use of β-blockers as first line treatment in
> young hypertensive patients unless phaeochromcytoma
> has been excluded. Use of β-blockers can result in
> unopposed α activity, profound increases in blood pressure and
> potential death.**

DISTURBANCES OF CARDIAC RHYTHM

Disturbances in cardiac rhythm are common in the ICU, and
this highlights the need for careful monitoring of all patients.
Dysrhythmias may result from underlying heart disease, e.g.
ischaemic heart disease, cardiomyopathy or valve lesions. Other
factors which predispose to tachycardia and dysrhythmias are
listed in Box 4.2.

Initially, ensure adequate oxygenation and ventilation together
with correction of predisposing factors. Where there is no
improvement or there is haemodynamic disturbance, definitive
treatment is required.

Sinus tachycardia

This is common and generally represents an appropriate
response to a clinical stress. Management is, therefore, correction
of the underlying cause(s).

**Box 4.2 Factors predisposing to tachycardia and
dysrhythmias**

Pain and anxiety (inadequate analgesia and sedation)

Increased catecholamine levels (endogenous or from inotrope infusions)

Hypoxia

Hypercarbia

Endocrine abnormalities

Electrolyte disturbance (hypokalaemia, hyperkalaemia,
hypomagnesaemia)

Hypovolaemia

Pyrexia and myocardial effects of sepsis

Drugs

Do not give β-blockers to control sinus tachycardia. This may result in profound decompensation and even cardiac arrest. Sinus tachycardia will usually resolve when the underlying conditon improves.

Box 4.3 Causes of bradycardia

Hypoxia

Increased vagal tone (e.g response to suctioning)

Sick sinus syndrome

Conduction defects/heart block

Heart transplant (denervated heart)

Myocardial depressant drugs (including antidysrhythmics)

Brain injury

High cervical spine injury

Bradycardia

Bradycardia is arbitrarily described as a heart rate <60 bpm. As heart rate falls cardiac output becomes compromised. While younger fitter patients may tolerate heart rates below this, many older patients will not and even rates above this may be insufficient to maintain an adequate cardiac output. The key concept therefore is maintenance of an adequate heart rate for the individual.

Bradycardia frequently reflects intrinsic disease of pacemaker tissue or the conducting system. It may be precipitated by increased vagal tone, hypoxia (particularly in children) and the myocardial depressant effect of drugs. Potentially important/ reversible causes are shown in Box 4.3.

Initially, as heart rate falls, CO is maintained by increases in SV. Thereafter, as heart rate falls further, CO and blood pressure will fall. Junctional or ventricular escape rhythms may appear.

The algorithm for the management of bradycardia is shown in Fig. 4.4.

In the intensive care unit, if bradycardia occurs in association with significant hypotension, then consider adrenaline (epinephrine). Give 50–100 μg (0.5–1 mL of 1:10 000 adrenaline) boluses and titrate to effect.

Supraventricular tachycardia (SVT)

SVT encompasses all forms of tachydysrhythmia originating above the ventricles. In practice it is useful to distinguish atrial

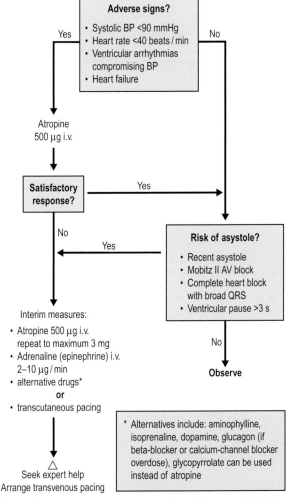

Fig. 4.4 Management of bradycardia (from Resuscitation Council UK 2005, with permission).

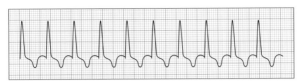

Fig. 4.5 Narrow complex tachycardia (SVT).

fibrillation and atrial flutter from other forms of SVT. In SVT the QRS complexes are always narrow (narrow complex tachycardia) unless there is an associated conduction defect (Fig. 4.5).

The management of SVT depends on the degree of haemodynamic disturbance and likely origin. As shown in Fig. 4.6, DC cardioversion is indicated if there is associated shock. Adenosine may terminate a re-entry tachycardia. Amiodarone may be the drug of choice for the treatment of persistent SVT not associated with haemodynamic compromise. Atrial fibrillation is considered separately (see below).

Atrial fibrillation (AF)

This is the commonest dysrhythmia seen in the ICU (Fig. 4.7), particularly in the elderly patient with ischaemic heart disease, intercurrent sepsis, electrolyte disturbance or inotrope dependency. AF may not settle until the patient's general condition improves. Consider the underlying causes of dysrhythmia above.

Treatment depends on the ventricular rate and the degree of associated haemodynamic disturbance as shown in Fig. 4.6. When sudden in onset, restoration of sinus rhythm (where possible) should be attempted. Synchronized DC cardioversion is indicated for sudden onset atrial fibrillation associated with rapid ventricular rate and significant haemodynamic compromise. Amiodarone is the agent of choice for most patients with lower ventricular rates and without haemodynamic compromise.

Chronic AF may be associated with ischaemic heart disease or mitral valve disease. Restoration of sinus rhythm is unlikely and control of the ventricular rate is the main aim. Digoxin remains the usual therapy, but seek cardiology advice.

● Digoxin 0.5 mg i.v. over 30 min, followed by 0.25–0.5 mg after 2 h if necessary. Once-daily dose thereafter, depending on response and levels.

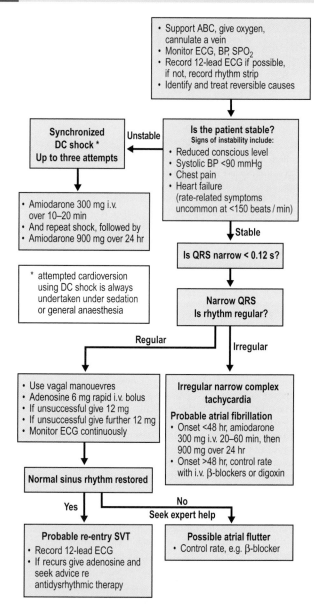

Fig. 4.6 Management of narrow complex tachycardia (from Resuscitation Council UK 2005, with permission).

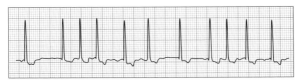

Fig. 4.7 Atrial fibrillation.

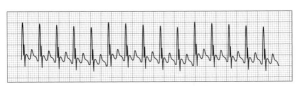

Fig. 4.8 Atrial flutter (with 2:1 block).

Atrial flutter

In atrial flutter, the atrial rate is about 300 beats per minute and the P waves have a saw tooth appearance The AV node cannot conduct all the P waves to the ventricle and there is often associated 2:1 AV block (Fig. 4.8). Suspect if the ventricular rate is 150. Use a 12-lead ECG to identify flutter waves: Treatment is synchronized DC cardioversion or control of rate with β-blockers. Seek advice.

Ventricular premature beats (VPBs)

VPBs occur normally in the general population and their significance is uncertain. They are more common in the presence of heart disease and may be increased by the effects of digoxin toxicity, catecholamines and hypokalaemia. Asymptomatic unifocal VPBs occurring fewer than five times per minute are considered to be benign. Treatment may be indicated if associated with poor haemodynamic state, if multifocal, or if occurring in runs of two or more.

- Correct hypoxia, hypercarbia, acidosis and hypokalaemia.
- Consider lidocaine (lignocaine) 1 mg/kg followed by infusion 2 mg/min.
- Consider magnesium.

Broad complex tachycardia

Broad complex tachycardia (Fig. 4.9) is usually ventricular in origin, but may occasionally be supraventricular if there

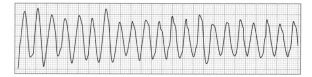

Fig. 4.9 Broad complex tachycardia.

Box 4.4 ECG features of broad complex tachycardia

VT more likely if:
- QRS very broad >0.14s
- Evidence of AV dissociation (capture beats or fusion beats)
- Dominant first R wave in VI
- Deep S wave V6
- QRS direction same all V leads

---

is an associated conduction defect, e.g. bundle branch block. Haemodynamic status is a poor guide to the underlying rhythm. An ECG may help to distinguish between the two. ECG features of ventricular tachycardia are shown in Box 4.4.

If in doubt, broad complex tachycardia should be assumed to be ventricular in origin until proved otherwise. Management of broad complex tachycardia is shown in Fig. 4.10.

Polymorphic ventricular tachycardia (torsade de pointes)

Torsade de pointes (Fig. 4.11) is a form of VT in which the complexes have a pointed shape, vary from beat to beat and the axis of the rhythm constantly changes. It is usually self-limiting, but may give rise to VF. Hypokalaemia, prolonged QT interval, bradycardia and antidysrhythmic drugs may be causes. Seek expert help.

- Give magnesium 10 mmol i.v. stat followed by 50 mmol infusion over 12 h.
- Consider β blockers.
- Consider overdrive pacing and DC cardioversion.

(See Defibrillation and DC cardioversion, p. 396.)

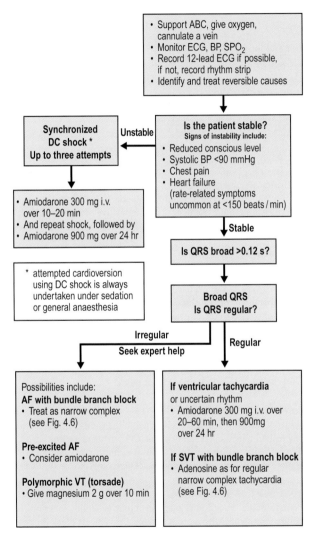

Fig. 4.10 Management of broad complex tachycardia (from Resuscitation Council UK 2005, with permission).

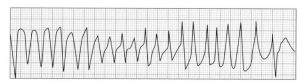

Fig. 4.11 Polymorphic ventricular tachycardia ('torsades de pointe').

CONDUCTION DEFECTS

In addition to the dysrhythmias discussed above, AV conduction defects can result in haemodynamic compromise.

1st degree heart block
PR interval >0.2 s (1 large square on standard ECG trace). This does not require treatment but is indicative of underlying heart disease, electrolyte disturbance or drug toxicity, e.g. digoxin.

2nd degree heart block
This may be of two types:

- Mobitz type 1 (Wenckebach phenomenon). There is progressive lengthening of the PR interval followed by a P wave, which is not conducted to the ventricle, and then repetition of the cycle. This is usually self-limiting.
- Mobitz type 2. The PR interval is constant but occasional P waves are not conducted to the ventricle. If high levels of block are present, e.g. 2:1 or 3:1 block, there is a significant risk that this will progress to complete heart block.

Complete heart block
No atrial electrical activity is conducted to the ventricle. This may result in ventricular standstill (no CO!) or there may be an idioventricular escape rhythm. In this case, there is no discernible relationship between visible P waves and QRS complexes on the ECG.

Treatment of heart block
Asymptomatic 1st or 2nd degree heart block generally does not require treatment. All symptomatic episodes of heart block do require treatment:

- See bradycardia algorithm above.
- Consider pacing: external or temporary pacing wire.

Indications for temporary cardiac pacing are given in Box 4.5.

Box 4.5 Indications for temporary pacing

Symptomatic bradycardia unresponsive to treatment

Mobitz type 2 heart block

Complete heart block

RBBB + left anterior or posterior hemiblock in association with prolonged PR interval (relative indication)

Pacemakers

Patients with permanent indwelling pacemakers are normally seen in pacemaker clinic regularly and should carry a card indicating the type of pacemaker that has been fitted. These are described using a coding system as shown in Table 4.10.

The commonest pacemaker is still the ventricular demand pacemaker (VVI). While the pacemaker senses normal ventricular activity, the function of the pacemaker is inhibited. If ventricular activity is not sensed the pacemaker stimulates the ventricle.

Traditional VVI pacemakers could be switched from demand to fixed rate by use of a magnet. Pacemaker technology has advanced dramatically over recent years and many pacemakers are now complicated programmable microprocessors. Automatic implanted cardiac defibrillators (AICD) are also common in patients with refractory or potentially life threatening dysrhythmias. These devices can usually be electronically interrogated to determine status and the function can be temporarily altered or suspended if necessary depending on circumstances. Do not attempt this yourself. Always seek cardiology advice regarding patients with pacemakers and AICD.

TABLE 4.10 Pacemaker coding system	
Chamber paced	V = ventricle, A = atrium, D = dual
Chamber sensed	V = ventricle, A = atrium, D = dual
Mode of response	T = triggered, I = inhibited, D = dual, O = none
Programmable functions	P = simple, M = multiple, C = communicating, O = none
Antitachydysrhythmia functions	B = bursts, N = normal rate competition, S = scanning, E = externally activated

MYOCARDIAL ISCHAEMIA

Ischaemic heart disease (IHD) is extremely common and ranges from the asymptomatic, through stable angina to crescendo angina and myocardial infarction. The understanding of acute coronary syndromes has increased in recent years (see below).

Many patients admitted to intensive care will already be on a number of cardiovascular medications and these should be reviewed in the light of the patient's condition. Where appropriate, existing drug therapy should be continued; however, many oral cardiac drugs have no parenteral preparation. In practice it is common to stop such medication in the acute phase of a critical illness and reintroduce it as the patient's condition improves. Clearly it makes no sense to be giving vasodilators and β-blockers to hypotensive patients who then require β-agonists and vasopressors to maintain a reasonable perfusion pressure.

- Oral nitrates can be replaced with GTN patches (5–10 mg every 24 h) or GTN infusion.
- Warfarin (for prosthetic valves or chronic AF) should be replaced by heparin infusion and the APTT monitored. The required level will depend upon the indication for coagulation. Low molecular weight heparins are increasingly used.
- Diuretics may be continued in equivalent doses i.v.
- Ca^{2+} channel blockers and angiotensin converting enzyme (ACE) inhibitors are usually withheld. Beta-blockers are available in parenteral form and should be titrated to effect.

STABLE ANGINA

Many patients in the ICU are unable to indicate the onset of ischaemic chest pain because of the effects of analgesia, sedation and/or ventilation. However, changes in ECG monitoring, such as ST depression, and deteriorating myocardial performance, such as reduced CO, may indicate ischaemia.

1. Give oxygen.
2. Correct precipitating factors such as tachycardia, hypertension or hypotension.
3. Administer GTN either sublingually or as oral spray. Consider GTN infusion.
4. Give analgesia if required. Usually a bolus of morphine or diamorphine i.v.

ACUTE CORONARY SYNDROMES

Acute coronary syndrome is a term used to describe onset of acute cardiac chest pain and associated signs of myocardial ischaemia (but excluding simple angina). A number of patterns of acute coronary syndrome are described based on the presence or absence of ECG changes suggestive of infarction and changes in biomarkers for heart muscle damage. Management is based on the pattern of the presenting features.

ECG changes

The following ECG changes are typical of acute myocardial infarction:

- ST segment elevation >1 mm in precordial leads or >2 mm in limb leads which persists for more than 24 h. Usually returns to normal within 2 weeks. (Persistent ST elevation at 1 month suggests development of left ventricular aneurysm.)
- Reciprocal ST segment depression in the opposite leads.
- Development of new Q waves greater than 25% of the 'R' wave and 0.04 s duration.
- T wave inversion. (This is not diagnostic by itself.)

The location of these changes on the ECG identifies the region of the infarction (Table 4.11).

Biomarkers

Biomarkers are used to indicate the extent, if any, of muscle damage sustained during an acute myocardial ischaemic event. Previously enzymes released from damaged cardiac muscles were used for this purpose but these have now been largely superseded by the use of troponin assays. Cardiac troponin (troponin I) is a protein released by damaged myocardial cells and is a sensitive

TABLE 4.11 Myocardial infarction and ECG patterns	
Area of infarction	*ECG leads*
Inferior	aVF, II and III
Anteroseptal	VI–V4
Anterior	V3–V4
Anterolateral	V3–V6
Posterior	V1

indicator of the extent of cellular damage. The measured level in fit and healthy people is normally less than 0.1 μg/L. Values above this usually indicate an acute myocardial ischaemic event or infarction.

In critically ill patients, however, myocardial damage may arise from causes other than ischaemia and minor rises in cardiac troponin may occur. The diagnostic threshold for an acute ischaemic event or myocardial infarction in intensive care patients is therefore a little higher. Levels above 0.5 μg/L are strongly suggestive of myocardial infarction.

If troponin assay is not available, creatine phosphokinase (CK) and creatinine phosphokinase isoenzyme (CK–MB) can be used. CK is released from all damaged muscle cells, whereas CK–MB is 'specific' to heart muscle. If the total CK is raised and the ratio of CK–MB to CK is greater than 6–8%, myocardial infarction is highly likely.

 Troponins and other cardiac enzymes may be raised after blunt chest trauma or cardiac compressions during resuscitation.

Patterns of acute coronary syndrome

Based on the interpretation of ECG findings and biomarkers, three principle patterns of acute coronary syndrome can be described as shown in Table 4.12.

TABLE 4.12 Patterns of acute coronary syndrome

ECG changes	Biomarkers (indicative of infarction)	Acute coronary syndrome
Ischaemic changes No ST elevation	Negative	Unstable angina
Ischaemic changes No ST elevation	Positive	Non-ST segment elevation Myocardial infarction (non-STEMI)
Ischaemic changes ST elevation	Positive	ST segment elevation Myocardial Infarction (STEMI)

The importance of understanding acute coronary syndromes in this way is the ability to stratify the risk of myocardial infarction and therefore target appropriate treatment. In reality, biomarkers such as troponin do not rise until a number of hours after muscle damage has occurred, and therefore the initial management decisions are made on the basis of ECG changes. Patients with ST segment elevation are at high risk of developing a Q-wave infarction (significant muscle damage) and should be referred to cardiology for urgent percutaneous angioplasty / stenting where available or thrombolysis where not (see below). Patients without ST elevation are at low risk of developing a Q-wave infarction and can be managed conservatively in the first instance with subsequent management guided by progress and troponin levels.

> ⚠ **All patients with acute coronary syndrome should be referred urgently to a cardiologist for advice. Patients with ST segment elevation and others at high risk may benefit from urgent percutaneous coronary interventions (angioplasty, stenting) or thrombolysis.**

Unstable angina and NSTEMI

Patients with acute coronary syndrome without ST elevation are at low risk of developing infarction and are usually managed conservatively in the first instance:

- Give aspirin 300 mg oral followed by 75 mg daily unless contraindicated.
- Consider clopidogrel 300 mg oral followed by 75 mg daily.
- Start low molecular weight heparin according to local protocol, e.g. enoxaparin 1 mg/kg s.c. twice a day.
- Consider β blocker (e.g. atenolol 25–100 mg daily, bisoprolol 12.5–5 mg twice daily) if there are no contraindications (bradycardia, hypotension, heart failure, asthma).
- Consider GTN infusion to reduce preload and reduce myocardial work. 1–2 mg/h and titrate to response.

Patients who continue to have chest pain, or who have persistent ECG changes or in whom troponin levels are raised will require coronary angiography. Seek urgent cardiology advice.

Acute myocardial infarction (STEMI)

Patients may be admitted to intensive care following a myocardial infarct or may suffer an infarction during their stay on intensive care. The diagnosis of myocardial infarction is made on the basis of a characteristic history of chest pain, ECG changes, and (subsequent) elevation of cardiac biomarkers (indicating heart muscle damage) Patients in the ICU may not be able to give a history of classic chest pain and great reliance has to be placed on the clinical picture, which may include .the sudden development of hypotension, cardiac failure (3rd or 4th heart sound), pericardial rub and pyrexia.

- Give oxygen.
- Give analgesia. e.g. morphine.
- Give aspirin 300 mg oral, followed by 75 mg daily unless contraindicated.
- Consider β-blocker unless contraindicated (bradycardia, hypotension, heart failure, asthma).
- Consider GTN infusion to reduce preload and reduce myocardial work; 1–2 mg/h. Titrate to response.

Patients with acute ST elevation are assumed to have a high risk of developing a Q wave infarction and the main goal of therapy is to restore coronary blood flow to reduce the damage to the heart muscle. Seek urgent cardiology advice regarding angiography/angioplasty or thrombolysis (see below).

Thrombolysis

The gold standard management of all ST elevation myocardial infarction is urgent restoration of the coronary blood flow to the affected area. This is best achieved by 'percutaneous coronary intervention' (PCI) comprising coronary angiography, angioplasty and stenting of the affected coronary arteries. If this is not achievable (e.g. small hospital or remote locations) or the patient is unstable thrombolysis is an alternative. Consider

- Either streptokinase 1.5×10^6 units in 100–200 mL 0.9% saline i.v. over 1 h.
- Or tissue plasminogen activator (TPA) 100 mg over 90 min (follow local protocol).

Thrombolysis is only indicated if there is irrefutable ECG evidence of acute infarction and should be started as soon as possible, preferably within 6 h of the onset of chest pain. Many

---

Box 4.6 Contraindications to thrombolysis

Recent major surgery

Intracranial pathology, e.g. previous CVA

Previous GI haemorrhage

Bleeding from any site

Allergy to streptokinase

Prolonged external cardiac massage

---

patients in intensive care will, however, have a contraindication to thrombolysis (Box 4.6). Always seek advice from a cardiologist.

CARDIAC FAILURE

Cardiac failure is common and represents an inability of the heart to maintain sufficient CO despite adequate filling. Chronic congestive heart failure leads to gross peripheral oedema, ascites, pulmonary oedema and pleural effusions. The acute picture may range from mild peripheral oedema and shortness of breath to florid pulmonary oedema and hypotension. The principles of management are the same:

- Give oxygen.
- Consider CPAP by face mask or non-invasive ventilation.
- Institute invasive monitoring as necessary. Arterial line, central venous or pulmonary artery catheter or equivalent.
- Optimize preload. Consider the use of diuretics and GTN infusion to reduce both preload and afterload.
- Add inotropes if required.
- ACE inhibitors have been shown to improve long-term survival and should be considered as soon as possible. These agents may cause profound hypotension (especially first dose) and should be introduced gradually. They should also be used cautiously in renal impairment. Seek advice.

Right heart failure and pulmonary hypertension

Both mitral valve disease and chronic pulmonary disease may result in pulmonary hypertension and subsequent right heart failure. This is a very difficult condition to manage. When pulmonary artery and right ventricular pressures are high, any fall in systemic pressure will impair perfusion of the right ventricle.

This results in worsening right ventricular performance and rapid deterioration.

- Maintain systemic arterial blood pressure. Avoid drugs that lower systemic arterial pressure. Vasoconstrictors may be necessary to maintain systemic blood pressure and right ventricular perfusion. Consider intra-aortic balloon counter pulsation pumps to maintain systemic diastolic pressure. (See Cardiogenic shock below.)
- Optimal filling of the right ventricle is vital. Use volumetric haemodynamic monitoring or right heart ejection fraction pulmonary artery catheters if available to directly estimate right ventricular end-diastolic volume.
- Consider inotropes to improve right ventricular contractility.
- Consider measures to reduce pulmonary vascular pressures and right ventricular afterload. Epoprostenol (prostacyclin) is effective but is not selective and may also reduce systemic blood pressure. Nitric oxide is more selective and may be useful although the evidence for improved outcome is limited. Seek senior advice.

CARDIOGENIC SHOCK

This is the failure to perfuse tissue adequately, as a result of poor cardiac function. It is characterized by high cardiac filling pressures, low cardiac output and increased systemic vascular resistance. This is associated with a very high mortality. The main aim is to restore oxygen delivery to tissues by increasing CO.

- Ventilate with high inspired oxygen concentration and correct any dysrhythmias (non-invasive ventilation may be appropriate).
- Establish invasive monitoring with arterial pressure and central venous or pulmonary artery catheter or equivalent.
- Optimize filling pressure. Cardiogenic shock is generally associated with increased end diastolic pressures and pulmonary oedema. Consider diuretics to remove fluid. Vasodilators such as GTN may reduce preload if the blood pressure is adequate.
- Rationalize inotropes. In the first instance adrenaline (epinephrine) infusion may be a reasonable choice. This will increase CO and maintain some degree of peripheral vasoconstriction. Once invasive monitoring is established, inodilator drugs such as dopexamine and dobutamine may be more appropriate.

- Obtain an echocardiogram to assess myocardial function and exclude surgically correctable problems such as cardiac tamponade and acute valvular dysfunction.
- If CO fails to improve, consider milrinone. This is a phosphodiesterase inhibitor (PDE-III), which acts at an intracellular level, effectively bypassing the β receptors. It is an inodilator, and causes both an increase in CO and peripheral vasodilatation. It may be associated with a marked fall in blood pressure. Do not give loading doses: start infusion at a low level and increase according to response. Hypotension may require concomitant use of a vasoconstrictor such as noradrenaline (norepinephrine) to maintain adequate diastolic pressure.
- Where there is no improvement with these measures, consider intra-aortic balloon counterpulsation. The balloon is inserted via a femoral artery and inflates in the aorta during diastole to maintain diastolic perfusion of the myocardium.
- Occasionally younger patients may be suitable for acute heart transplantation. Seek senior advice.

PULMONARY EMBOLISM

Pulmonary thromboembolism is common in immobile, critically ill, traumatized and postoperative patients. The effects range from mild discomfort and shortness of breath to sudden profound collapse and cardiac arrest. It is regularly found as an unexpected finding in post mortem studies of critically ill patients. Typical clinical features are shown in Box 4.7.

Investigations
- CXR: reduced vascular markings (oligaemia) generally unreliable.
- ECG tachycardia, right ventricular strain pattern, right axis deviation, right bundle branch block and P pulmonale.

Box 4.7 Typical clinical features of pulmonary embolism
Pleuritic chest pain
Dyspnoea
Haemoptysis
Severe hypoxia
Right ventricular failure
Cardiogenic shock/hypotension

- Evidence of dilated right heart and pulmonary hypertension on echocardiography.
- Plasma D-dimer raised.
- Traditional V/Q scans (ventilation/perfusion scans) are often not practical in ICU patients and may be difficult to interpret if there is a significant pre-existing lung problem.
- Spiral CT scans may demonstrate blood clot in the proximal pulmonary artery and are usually the most useful investigation for ICU patients. Later segmental infarcts may be seen.

Management

- Give high inspired oxygen; intubate/ventilate as necessary.
- Optimize cardiovascular status.
- For major embolism consider thrombolysis, e.g. streptokinase 0.5×10^6 units over 30 min followed by 0.1×10^6 units per h over 24 h. Then anticoagulate. Seek senior advice.
- For smaller embolism consider anticoagulation, either heparin infusion, e.g. 20–40 000 units/24 h (monitor APTT and aim to keep 2–3 × normal) or therapeutic dose low molecular weight heparin.
- Occasional patients with recurrent embolism or those considered as particularly high risk may benefit from a temporary or permanent IVC filter

PERICARDIAL EFFUSION AND CARDIAC TAMPONADE

Pericardial effusions may be caused by a variety of medical conditions. In the ICU small pericardial effusions are common in patients with widespread capillary leak and generalized tissue oedema. Significant effusions are less common but should be considered in patients with haemodynamic compromise or who fail to respond to resuscitation, particularly if there is evidence of recent chest trauma, cardiothoracic surgery or central venous access procedures. Occasional patients may develop infected collections.

The haemodynamic consequences of a pericardial effusion depend on the size and speed of accumulation. Large, rapidly formed collections typically compress the right atrium and ventricle, preventing filling and impairing CO. The clinical signs include tachycardia, elevated central venous pressures, hypotension, pulsus paradoxus, and muffled heart sounds. This may progress to profound collapse and PEA (pulseless electrical activity) arrest.

None of these signs is specific. Except in emergency circumstances a confirmatory 'echo' should be obtained before attempting pericardial drainage. The typical findings in cardiac tamponade are a large pericardial effusion with right atrial and right ventricular diastolic collapse. Urgent pericardiocentesis is required. Seek senior help. (See Pericardial aspiration, p. 395.)

CARDIAC ARREST

Most deaths in the ICU are expected. Sudden unexpected cardiac arrest is actually infrequent. If patients suffer a cardiac arrest, despite optimal intensive care management, then unless the problem is one of transient ventricular dysrhythmia or another reversible pathology, it is unlikely that the outcome will be favourable. Most well staffed units do not call the hospital cardiac arrest team unless medical staff are busy elsewhere in the hospital. Follow the advanced life support algorithm for the management of cardiac arrest in adults (Fig. 4.12).

Ventricular fibrillation
The chances of a successful outcome from VF are thought to be best if defibrillation is achieved within 90 s of onset and decrease with time thereafter. In a witnessed arrest a single precordial thump may terminate fibrillation, after which the application of defibrillating DC shock should not be delayed.

Asystole
The chances of recovery from asystolic arrest are poor. Check that the ECG leads are correctly attached and that the gain on the monitor is maximal. If VF cannot be excluded, then management commences as for VF. Severe hypoxaemia is one cause for a terminal bradycardia progressing to asystole.

Pulseless electrical activity (PEA)
Previously referred to as electromechanical dissociation. This term is used to describe the situation where electrical activity is present on the ECG but there is no discernable cardiac output. Hypovolaemia and mechanical obstruction of the cardiac output (e.g. tension pneumothorax and cardiac tamponade) should be excluded.

Management of patients following cardiac arrest
Patients who are resuscitated from cardiac arrest outside the ICU frequently require admission to intensive care. This may be because of failure to regain adequate conscious level, or inadequate

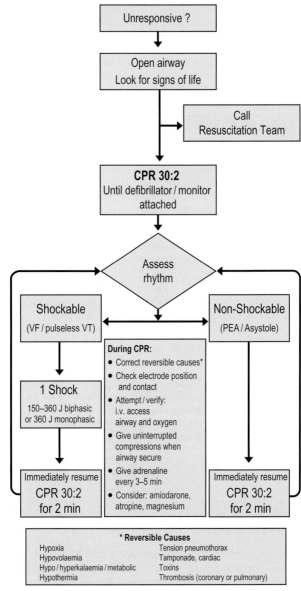

Fig. 4.12 Adult advanced life support guidelines (from Resuscitation Council UK 2005, with permission).

cardiac, respiratory or renal function. The management of these patients depends upon the underlying clinical condition, the type of arrest and the timing and adequacy of the initial resuscitation measures [see the Intensive Care Society's Standards for the management of patients after cardiac arrest 2008 (www.ics.ac.uk) and Resuscitation council UK's guidelines 2005 (www.resus.org.uk)].

The commonest problem posed by these patients is difficulty determining the extent and nature of neurological injury resulting from the period of hypoxia. It is very difficult to make any assessment of this in the first 24–48 h and most patients, therefore, will require a period of stabilization and assessment:

- Institute positive pressure ventilation according to arterial blood gases.
- Optimize haemodynamic status.
- Correct acidosis and electrolyte abnormalities.
- Correct hyperglycaemia.
- Treat any underlying conditions appropriately.
- If required, use short-acting drugs for sedation.

If the patient's neurological condition fails to improve over 48 h, then the outcome is likely to be poor. Seek advice. (See Hypoxic brain injury, p. 294.)

Hypothermia after cardiac arrest

There is some evidence that cooling patients after (VF) cardiac arrest for 24 h post-resuscitation improves neurological outcome and this is now practised in many centres. The techniques used to achieve cooling, the optimum target temperature, the optimum duration of cooling, and the benefit in other forms of cardiac arrest have not yet been fully defined. Typically patients are cooled using exposure, cold air blankets and infusion of cold fluids, to a temperature of 33–34°C for a period of 24 h and then passively rewarmed. Seek local advice and protocols.

ADULT PATIENT WITH CONGENITAL HEART DISEASE

Increasing numbers of patients are surviving into adult life with corrected/uncorrected congenital heart disease. They may present with complications of their structural heart problems like endocarditis, cardiac failure, Eisenmenger's syndrome or with unrelated problems. The cardiac physiology in these patients is often complex and the ability to resuscitate stabilize and or manipulate the haemodynamic status requires understanding of the anatomy, any corrective procedures and the consequences thereof. Always seek advice from a cardiologist, cardiothoracic surgeon or anaesthetist with an interest in this area as the effects of drugs and other interventions may be very different from the normal population.

Introduction   114

Interpretation of blood
  gases   114

Definitions of respiratory
  failure   116

Management of respiratory
  failure   118

Continuous positive airway
  pressure (CPAP)   121

Non-invasive positive pressure
  ventilation   122

Invasive ventilation   123

Ventilation strategy and
  ventilator settings   127

Care of the ventilated
  patient   128

Common problems during
  artificial ventilation   131

High frequency modes of
  ventilation   133

Weaning from artificial
  ventilation   135

Airway obstruction   138

Community-acquired
  pneumonia   141

Pandemic influenza   143

Hospital-acquired
  pneumonia   143

Pneumonia in immunocompromised patients   145

Management of
  pneumonia   146

Aspiration pneumonitis   148

Asthma   149

Chronic obstructive pulmonary
  disease   152

Acute lung injury   154

Chest X-ray interpretation   158

INTRODUCTION

Respiratory failure is one of the commonest reasons for which patients are admitted to the intensive care unit. It may be the primary reason for admission to intensive care (for example, in a patient suffering an exacerbation of chronic obstructive pulmonary disease or acute pneumonia). Alternatively, it may be a feature of a non-respiratory pathological process, for example severe sepsis from an intra-abdominal source, though it is often the respiratory failure rather than the intra-abdominal sepsis which triggers intensive care admission. Respiratory failure is conventionally classified either as 'type 1' or 'type 2' based on blood gas findings.

INTERPRETATION OF BLOOD GASES

The interpretation of blood gases is fundamental to the management of patients requiring intensive care, not just those with respiratory failure. When drawing an arterial blood sample into a heparinized syringe, ensure that any liquid heparin is completely expelled from the syringe before use, as this will contaminate the sample and influence the results. Arterial blood is obtained either by direct puncture of an artery or from an indwelling arterial line. (See Practical procedures: Arterial cannulation, p. 372.)

Most ICUs now have a blood gas analyser for 'point of care testing' (POCT). These are expensive to maintain and repair. You will be unpopular if you damage it by, for example, blocking the sample channels with clotted blood. If you do not know how to use it, ask for help. Normal blood gas values are as shown in Table 5.1.

Interpreting blood gas results will eventually become second nature. To begin with, it is helpful to follow a system, for example:

- Look at the PaO_2. Is the patient hypoxaemic?
- Note the inspired oxygen concentration (FiO_2). The higher the FiO_2 required to achieve any given PaO_2 the more significant the problem (see below).

TABLE 5.1 'Normal' blood gas values

pH	7.35–7.45
PaO_2	13 kPa
$PaCO_2$	5.3 kPa
HCO_3	22–25 mmol/L
Base deficit or excess	−2 to +2 mmol/L

- Look at the $PaCO_2$. Is it low, normal or high?
- Look at the pH. Is the patient acidotic (pH < 7.34) or alkalotic (pH > 7.45)?

If the patient has a disturbance of acid–base balance, then it is necessary to examine the blood gas further to determine the cause.

- Look again at the $PaCO_2$. Is the $PaCO_2$ consistent with the change in pH, i.e. if the patient is acidotic, is the $PaCO_2$ raised? If the patient is alkalotic, is the $PaCO_2$ low? If so the primary abnormality is likely to be respiratory.
- If the $PaCO_2$ is normal or does not explain the abnormality in pH, look at the base deficit/base excess.

The base deficit/base excess is a calculation of how much base (e.g. bicarbonate) would need to be added to or taken away (by titration) to normalize the pH of the sample. For example, in a metabolic acidosis, bicarbonate would need to be added to correct the pH because there is insufficient buffering capacity present, i.e. there is a base deficit. In metabolic alkalosis, bicarbonate would need to be taken away to correct the pH, because there is too much base (or insufficient hydrogen ions) present, i.e. there is a base excess.

- If the base deficit/base excess is consistent with the abnormality in pH then the primary abnormality is metabolic.
- If both the $PaCO_2$ and the base excess/base deficit are both altered in a way that is consistent with the abnormality in pH then a mixed picture is present.
- If the $PaCO_2$ and base excess/deficit are both altered in such a way that one is consistent with the change in pH and the other is not, then it is likely that a compensated acidosis/alkalosis is present (see descriptions below).

This simple scheme for the interpretation of blood gases is practical and will suffice for most situations. More complex systems, such as that described by Stewart, which take account of other plasma constituents, are beyond the scope of this book, but for which good up-to-date reviews are readily available. If in doubt always seek senior help.

A number of patterns of disturbance of acid–base balance are recognized.

Respiratory acidosis

Hypoventilation from any cause results in accumulation of CO_2 and respiratory acidosis. Over time, the bicarbonate concentration may rise (base excess) in an attempt to balance this and a compensated respiratory acidosis may develop, in which the pH is nearly normal.

Respiratory alkalosis

Hyperventilation from any cause results in a lowering of the $PaCO_2$ and a respiratory alkalosis. Bicarbonate concentration may fall (base deficit) in an attempt to compensate.

Metabolic acidosis

There are a number of causes of metabolic acidosis resulting from the accumulation of organic acids or the loss of bicarbonate buffer. Bicarbonate concentration is low (base deficit). If the patient is breathing spontaneously, compensatory hyperventilation may result in a low $PaCO_2$ (see Metabolic acidosis, p. 212).

Metabolic alkalosis

This is relatively uncommon and may result from the loss of acid, for example from excessive vomiting or nasogastric drainage, or from excessive administration of alkali. Other causes include hypokalaemia, diuretics and liver failure. The bicarbonate concentration is raised (base excess) and the patient may hypoventilate in an attempt to compensate, resulting in a raised $PaCO_2$ (see Metabolic alkalosis, p. 215).

 When looking at a compensated acid/base disturbance remember that the compensatory mechanisms are never sufficient to completely return the pH to normal. Therefore if the pH is acidotic (<7.4) the underlying problem is acidosis, if the pH is alkalotic (>7.4) the underlying problem is alkalosis.

DEFINITIONS OF RESPIRATORY FAILURE

Respiratory failure occurs when pulmonary gas exchange becomes impaired such that normal arterial blood gas tensions are no longer maintained, and hypoxaemia is present with or without hypercapnia. Two patterns are described: types 1 and 2.

Type 1 (hypoxic) respiratory failure

$PaO_2 < 8\,kPa$ with normal or low $PaCO_2$
(breathing air at sea level)

Type 1 respiratory failure is caused by disease processes that directly impair alveolar function, e.g. pneumonia, pulmonary oedema, adult respiratory distress syndrome (ARDS) and fibrosing alveolitis. Progressive hypoxaemia is accompanied initially by hyperventilation. The physiological benefit of hyperventilation is that it lowers alveolar carbon dioxide tension and allows for a modest increase in alveolar oxygen concentration, as can be demonstrated from the alveolar gas equation:

$$\text{alveolar oxygen } (PaO_2) = \text{inspired oxygen } (PiO_2) - \text{alveolar carbon dioxide } (PaCO_2)/\text{Respiratory quotient (R)}$$

Sick patients, however, cannot maintain aggressive hyperventilation indefinitely. Eventually, the added work of breathing has an oxygen cost that is greater than the improvement in oxygenation gained. Exhaustion ensues, and decompensation may be rapid. Carbon dioxide partial pressure in the blood and alveolae rise rapidly. Without intervention, a 'respiratory arrest' soon follows.

Type 2 (hypercapnic) respiratory failure

$PaO_2 < 8\,kPa$ and $PaCO_2 > 8\,kPa$
(in absence of metabolic acidosis)

Type 2 respiratory failure is caused by a failure of alveolar ventilation. It occurs most commonly in association with chronic obstructive pulmonary disease (COPD), but may be caused by reduced respiratory drive, airway obstruction, neuromuscular conditions and chest wall deformity.

The primary problem is carbon dioxide retention, although this is usually accompanied by hypoxaemia. This situation typically occurs in patients with chronic obstructive pulmonary disease who retain carbon dioxide. These patients have reduced sensitivity to carbon dioxide, such that increases in the partial pressure of carbon dioxide produce only a minimal increase in ventilation. Consequently, in severe disease, a progressive elevation of carbon dioxide partial pressure can occur, resulting potentially in carbon dioxide narcosis and respiratory arrest. A small number of these patients have such a severely blunted carbon dioxide sensitivity that they rely predominantly or entirely on hypoxic respiratory drive (see Chronic obstructive pulmonary disease (COPD), p. 152).

Quantifying the degree of hypoxia

The definitions above relate to patients breathing air at normal atmospheric pressure. When interpreting blood gases the inspired oxygen concentration (FiO_2) must be known. Clearly a patient who is already receiving significant oxygen therapy and still has poor PaO_2 is considerably worse than a patient with the same PaO_2 on air. For this reason, PaO_2/FiO_2 ratio, alveolar–arterial

TABLE 5.2 Measures of hypoxia in respiratory failure		
	Normal	Severe hypoxia
PaO_2/FiO_2 ratio	>40 kPa	<27 kPa
A–a gradient*	<26 kPa	>45 kPa
Shunt fraction	0–8%	>30%
*Calculation of A–a gradient, See p. 11.		

(A–a) gradient, and shunt fraction (see below) have all been used to describe the severity of hypoxia.

Normal and abnormal values for PaO_2/FiO_2 ratio, A–a gradient and shunt fraction are shown in Table 5.2.

Shunt and shunt fraction

Ventilation–perfusion mismatch can be thought of as comprising two elements. Dead space ventilation describes those areas of the lung that are ventilated but not perfused. Shunt describes those areas of the lung that are perfused but not ventilated.

Shunt occurs when blood from the right ventricle reaches the left-sided circulation without being exposed to a functioning (oxygenating) alveolar unit. Shunt may be anatomical (e.g. bronchial venous drainage, ventricular septal defect) or 'physiological' (e.g. atelectasis). Shunt fraction is an estimate of how much mixed venous blood would need to be reaching the left side of the heart without oxygenation to produce the observed arterial PaO_2.

MANAGEMENT OF RESPIRATORY FAILURE

Common causes of respiratory failure are listed in Table 5.3.

Blood gases are only one indicator of respiratory function. The primary assessment of a patient with respiratory failure is clinical:

- Look at the patient.
- Is the patient conscious? Is he or she able to talk and is lucid?
- Is the patient using accessory muscles of respiration and making adequate respiratory effort, or exhausted with minimal respiratory effort? Is there an adequate cough?
- If possible, take a history. If the patient is too short of breath to talk, the history may be obtained from the notes, staff or relatives. Try to obtain some idea of the patient's normal

TABLE 5.3 Common causes of respiratory failure	
Loss of respiratory drive	CVA/brain injury
	Metabolic encephalopathy
	Effects of drugs
Neuropathy and neuromuscular conditions	Critical illness neuropathy
	Spinal cord injury
	Phrenic nerve injury
	Guillain–Barré syndrome
	Myasthenia gravis
Chest wall abnormality	Trauma
	Scoliosis
Airway obstruction	Foreign body
	Tumour
	Infection
	Sleep apnoea
Lung pathology	Asthma
	Pneumonia
	COPD
	Acute and chronic fibrosing conditions
	ALI/ARDS

respiratory reserve. How far can the patient walk? Are they oxygen dependent? Can they leave the house?
● Examine the patient, particularly the cardiovascular and respiratory systems, bearing in mind the causes of respiratory failure. Note:
Pulse, BP, JVP, heart sounds, peripheral oedema. Is there any evidence of cardiac failure or of dehydration?
Increased or decreased respiratory rate, tracheal shift, percussion, bilateral air entry. Presence of crackles or wheeze. Is there any evidence of obstruction (stridor), collapse or consolidation, bronchospasm, pleural effusion?
● If there is wheeze, peak flow measurement may help to document severity but is often unrecordable in the critically ill.
● Look at the CXR, blood gases and other available investigations.

Management is based around correction of hypoxia, ventilatory support if required, and treatment of the underlying condition.

Hypoxaemia

Hypoxaemia is the primary concern and should be corrected:

- If there is evidence of chronic CO_2 retention, (raised bicarbonate on blood gas) give controlled oxygen therapy 24–28%, via a Venturi system. While it may be appropriate to give higher oxygen concentrations this should only be done in a controlled environment where advanced respiratory support and close observation are available (see COPD, p. 152).
- In all other cases, give high flow oxygen via a face mask, preferably via a humidified system. Higher inspired oxygen can be achieved with a reservoir mask (plastic bag attached to mask acts as an oxygen reservoir)
- Consider facial CPAP or non-invasive ventilation (see Non-invasive ventilation, p. 122).

Hypercapnia

Exhausted patients with minimal respiratory effort will require immediate intubation and ventilation. In those patients that are not in extremis, non-invasive ventilation together with treatment of the underlying condition may lead to improvement (see Non-invasive ventilation, p. 122).

Oxygen, antibiotics, nebulizers, physiotherapy and non-invasive ventilation may prove highly effective. Continually reassess the response to treatment.

Treatment of the underlying condition

- Bronchodilators. If there is wheeze, nebulized salbutamol may help. In more severe cases consider intravenous bronchodilators and steroids (see Asthma, p. 149).
- Physiotherapy may help clear secretions and re-expand areas of collapse. If possible sit patients upright or in a chair.
- Antibiotic therapy is best directed on the basis of Gram stains of sputum and on subsequent culture results. Seek microbiological advice. In the first instance broad-spectrum cover, e.g. with a cephalosporin is reasonable. A macrolide antibiotic such as clarithromycin should be added if there is a possibility of an atypical chest infection (see Pneumonia, p. 141).
- Diuretics. If there is evidence of congestive cardiac failure and pulmonary oedema, then diuretics may help. Frusemide (furosemide) 40 mg or bumetanide 1–2 mg i.v.
- Intravenous or nebulized steroids, nebulized adrenaline and helium oxygen mix may be of value in upper airway obstruction.

Box 5.1 Indications for ventilatory support in respiratory failure

Reduced conscious level

Exhaustion

Tachycardia/bradycardia

Hypotension

Increasing respiratory rate

Falling PaO_2 despite oxygen therapy

Rising $PaCO_2$ despite therapy

Worsening acidosis

Continually reassess response to treatment. If there is no improvement or if the patient's condition worsens, tracheal intubation and assisted ventilation may become necessary. Possible indications for intervention are shown in Box 5.1.

CONTINUOUS POSITIVE AIRWAY PRESSURE (CPAP)

Continuous positive airway pressure (CPAP) is a system for spontaneously breathing patients which is analogous to PEEP in ventilated patients (see p. 126). It may be provided either through a tight-fitting face mask or via connection to an endotracheal/tracheostomy tube. Newly developed full hood systems are useful for the claustrophobic/confused patient. A high gas flow (which must be greater than the patient's peak inspiratory flow rate) is generated in the breathing system. A valve on the expiratory port ensures that pressure in the system, and the patient's airways, never falls below the set level. This is usually $+5$ to $+10\,cm\,H_2O$ (Fig. 5.1).

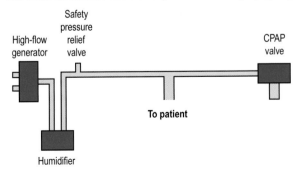

Fig. 5.1 Typical CPAP system.

The application of CPAP has a number of effects:

- Airways are splinted open, reducing alveolar collapse.
- Alveolar recruitment leads to improved oxygenation.
- Increased functional residual capacity (FRC) allows the lung to function on a more favourable part of the compliance curve and may therefore reduce the work of breathing.

CPAP is well tolerated by most patients even via a tight fitting face mask, although where it is required for a prolonged period there is a risk of skin necrosis over the bridge of the nose and this may be another indication for the use of a CPAP 'hood' rather than a face mask. Relative disadvantages of CPAP include noise, difficulties with humidification, distension of the stomach and increased risks of reflux and aspiration.

NON-INVASIVE POSITIVE PRESSURE VENTILATION

Over recent years, there has been increased use of non-invasive ventilation to manage acute respiratory failure. It may avoid the need for endotracheal intubation and conventional ventilation, so avoiding many of the associated complications. Patients with acute exacerbations of COPD have been demonstrated to have a better outcome where non-invasive positive pressure ventilation (NIPPV) has been used in place of conventional ventilation. Non-invasive ventilation techniques are also increasingly being used in the management of pulmonary oedema in congestive cardiac failure and to aid weaning from conventional ventilation (see COPD, p. 152, and Weaning from artificial ventilation, p. 135).

Biphasic positive airways pressure (BIPAP)

The most commonly used form of NIPPV is biphasic positive airway pressure (BIPAP). A high flow of gas is delivered to the airway via a tight fitting face or nasal mask, to create a positive pressure (see CPAP above). The ventilator alternates between higher inspiratory and lower expiratory pressures. The higher inspiratory pressure augments the patient's own respiratory effort and increases tidal volume, while the lower expiratory pressure is analogous to CPAP/PEEP. Typical initial settings are shown in Table 5.4.

Once established, the inspiratory pressure and inspiratory time can be adjusted to create the optimal ventilatory pattern for the patient.

TABLE 5.4 Typical initial settings for BIPAP non-invasive ventilation	
Inspiratory pressure (IPAP)	10–12 cm H_2O
Expiratory pressure (EPAP)	4–5 cm H_2O
Inspiratory time (It)	1–2 s
FiO_2	As required to maintain oxygen saturation

BIPAP is generally well tolerated by patients. The face or nasal mask can be removed intermittently for short periods to enable eating and drinking and oral medication. Regular arterial blood gas measurement should be performed to assess response to treatment. If the patient's condition deteriorates, owing to inadequate oxygenation, progressive hypercapnia or general exhaustion then conventional ventilation may still be required.

INVASIVE VENTILATION

Most intensive care ventilators are now highly sophisticated, computer-controlled machines with complicated interfaces, a large number of different ventilatory modes, and inbuilt monitoring and alarm systems. Detailed descriptions and discussion are beyond the scope of this book.

One problem is that there is no uniformly agreed terminology in relation to ventilator modes and different manufacturers use different terms for similar functions. The following terms and modes are in common use but are by no means universal. Before using a ventilator you should familiarize yourself with it. If you have any difficulties seek advice.

Volume controlled ventilation

The simplest form of volume controlled ventilation is controlled mandatory ventilation (CMV) (Fig. 5.2).

The patient is ventilated at a preset tidal volume and rate (for example, tidal volume 500 mL and rate 12 breaths/min). The tidal volume delivered is therefore predetermined and the peak pressure required to deliver this volume varies depending upon other ventilator settings and the patient's pulmonary compliance. One disadvantage, therefore, of volume controlled modes of ventilation

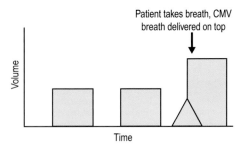

Fig. 5.2 Controlled mandatory ventilation.

is that high peak airway pressures may result and this can lead to lung damage or barotrauma.

This is suitable for patients who are heavily sedated and/or paralysed and who are making no respiratory effort. It is not suitable for patients who are attempting spontaneous breaths. There is no pressure support for spontaneous breaths and ventilator valves may be closed during attempted inspiration or expiration. The ventilator may also deliver a breath immediately after the patient's own inspiration, or as the patient tries to breathe out. This is uncomfortable and distressing, and may result in trauma to the lungs (see below).

Pressure controlled ventilation

To overcome some of the disadvantages of volume controlled ventilation, pressure controlled modes of ventilation are preferred in patients with poor pulmonary compliance. Instead of setting a predetermined tidal volume, a peak inspiratory pressure is set. The tidal volume delivered is a function of the peak pressure, the inspiratory time and the patient's compliance. By using lower peak pressures and slightly longer inspiratory times the risks of barotrauma can be reduced. As the patient's condition improves and lung compliance increases, the tidal volume achieved for the same settings will increase and the inspiratory pressure can therefore be reduced (see Acute lung injury p. 154).

It is important when using pressure controlled ventilation to understand the relationship between rate, inspiratory time and the I:E ratio (ratio of inspiratory time to expiratory time). Rate determines the total time period for each breath (60s divided by rate = duration in seconds for each breath). The I:E ratio then determines how this time is apportioned between inspiration and expiration.

For example:

If respiratory rate is 10/min, total time for breath 60/10 s = 6 s.
If I:E ratio 1:2, then inspiratory time = 2 s and expiratory time = 4 s.

If the rate is reduced while the I:E ratio is fixed, inspiratory time becomes progressively longer, effectively holding the patient in sustained inspiration. To avoid this, the inspiratory time should be fixed whenever pressure controlled ventilation is used (e.g. 1.5–2 s), so that, as the respiratory rate is changed, it is only the length of expiration that alters.

Synchronized intermittent mandatory ventilation (SIMV)

Although historically a volume controlled mode of ventilation, the equivalent of SIMV is now available in both volume controlled and pressure controlled modes (Fig. 5.3). Immediately before each breath there is a small time window during which the ventilator can recognize a spontaneous breath and respond by delivering the set (SIMV) breath early.

SIMV modes improve patient synchrony with the ventilator and reduce the problems described with CMV above. SIMV modes are therefore potentially more comfortable for the patient.

Pressure support / assisted spontaneous breathing (ASB)

Breathing through a ventilator can be difficult because respiratory muscles may be weak and ventilator circuits and tracheal tubes provide significant resistance to breathing. These problems can

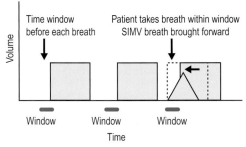

Fig. 5.3 Synchronized intermittent mandatory ventilation.

be minimized by the provision of pressure support. The ventilator senses a spontaneous breath and augments it by addition of positive pressure. This reduces the patient's work of breathing and helps to augment the tidal volume. Pressure support modes are available on all modern ventilators and can be used in conjunction with both volume and pressure controlled modes of ventilation.

Pressure support is usually set at 15–20 cm H_2O in the first instance and can be reduced as the patient's condition improves. It is best not to remove pressure support completely, however, because of the resistance of the ventilator. (See Weaning from artificial ventilation, p. 135.)

Positive end expiratory pressure (PEEP)

Intubation, artificial ventilation and the effects of lung disease leads to a reduction in the functional residual capacity (FRC) of the lung. This results in the collapse of small airways, particularly in dependent lung zones, increasing ventilation–perfusion mismatch and worsening blood gases. To prevent this +5 to +10 cm H_2O of PEEP can be used to help maintain FRC and alveolar recruitment. Disadvantages of PEEP include reduced venous return to the heart and a subsequent reduction in CO and blood pressure. Unnecessarily high levels of PEEP are therefore best avoided.

Patients with severe expiratory airflow limitation, e.g. due to asthma or obstruction, may develop high levels of intrinsic PEEP, with the risk of progressive air trapping. Most modern ventilators include functions for displaying dynamic compliance curves and calculating intrinsic PEEP. If you are unsure how to use or interpret these functions, seek advice.

If a patient has high levels of intrinsic PEEP, evidence suggests that applying external PEEP up to, but not exceeding, the level of intrinsic PEEP, causes little cardiovascular compromise, does not increase air trapping and may improve gas exchange by facilitating recruitment in non-flow limited parts of the lung. Increasing external PEEP above the level of intrinsic PEEP may worsen hyperinflation and should be avoided. Seek advice.

PEEP is relatively contraindicated in asthmatics and in chronic emphysema. Although some patients benefit, there are also risks: seek senior help.

Triggering

Both SIMV and pressure support modes of ventilation require the ventilator to be able to detect the patient's own respiratory effort in order to trigger the appropriate ventilator response. Historically triggering was achieved by detection of pressure changes in the circuit. There was no gas flow in the breathing circuit between ventilator delivered breaths and the patient's inspiratory effort was detected as a drop in pressure in the breathing circuit. This was an inefficient method of triggering which was uncomfortable and exhausting for patients. Modern ventilators rely on flow triggering. There is a constant low level of gas flow in the circuit at all times. Flow sensors detect small changes in flow in the circuit in response to spontaneous respiratory effort by the patient, triggering the appropriate ventilator response. This is a more efficient and comfortable method of triggering.

VENTILATION STRATEGY AND VENTILATOR SETTINGS

Ventilation strategy

Over the past few years the role that mechanical ventilation plays in producing lung damage has been increasingly recognized and there is evidence that the ventilation strategy used can adversely affect outcome (see Complications of IPPV below). Current trends in ventilation strategy are therefore based on the following:

- Limiting peak pressure to 35 cm H_2O.
- Limiting tidal volume to 6 mL/kg.
- Acceptance of higher than normal $PaCO_2$ levels (6–8 kPa), so-called 'permissive hypercapnia'.
- Acceptance of PaO_2 7–8 kPa, $SaO_2 \geq 90\%$.
- Use of higher levels of PEEP to improve alveolar recruitment.
- Use of longer inspiratory times.
- Use of ventilation modes which allow and support spontaneous respiratory effort.

In most patients an SIMV volume controlled mode of ventilation with added pressure support will be adequate. Typical initial ventilator settings for an adult are as shown in Table 5.5.

Pressure controlled ventilation can be used for all patients, although it is frequently reserved for those with poor pulmonary compliance (see ALI, p. 154). Typical initial settings are as shown in Table 5.6.

TABLE 5.5 Typical ventilator settings (SIMV, volume control and pressure support)

Tidal volume	6–10 mL/kg
Rate	8–14 breaths/min
I:E ratio	1:2
PEEP	5–10 cm H_2O
Pressure support	15–20 cm H_2O
FiO_2	As required to maintain oxygenation

TABLE 5.6 Typical ventilator settings (SIMV, pressure control and pressure support)

Peak inspiratory pressure	20–35 cm H_2O
Rate	8–14 breaths/min
Inspiratory time	1.5–2 s
PEEP	5–10 cm H_2O
Pressure support	15–20 cm H_2O
FiO_2	As required to maintain oxygenation

CARE OF THE VENTILATED PATIENT

Ventilator care bundles

The ventilator care bundle is designed to reduce the incidence of ventilator associated pneumonia and other complications with their attendant prolongation of intensive care unit stay and increased mortality (NICE National patient safety agency. Technical patient safety solutions for ventilator-associated pneumonia in adults 2008. www.nice.org.uk/guidelines). The elements of the ventilator care bundle are:

● Elevation of the head of the bed.
● Daily 'sedation holds' and assessment of potential extubation.
● Stress ulcer prophylaxis.
● Deep venous thrombosis prophylaxis.

In addition, a number of other factors are important in the ventilated patient.

Humidification

Some form of humidification is essential in every case. Adequate humidification prevents drying and thickening of secretions that can accumulate in the airways and endotracheal tube. Humidification is generally provided by a heated 'water bath' on the inspiratory limb of the ventilator circuit.

Physiotherapy and tracheal suction

The presence of an endotracheal tube and the effects of analgesia and sedation impair the ability to cough and clear secretions. Regular physiotherapy and suction of the airway is essential to prevent accumulation of secretions.

Monitoring

In addition to regular clinical assessment, all ventilated patients should have continuous SaO_2 and end tidal carbon dioxide, $ETCO_2$ monitoring and regular blood gases measurement.

The $ETCO_2$ approximates to arterial carbon dioxide tension $PaCO_2$. In a healthy patient the difference between $ETCO_2$ and $PaCO_2$ is usually less than 0.5 KPa. In the critically ill patient the difference may be significantly greater. Therefore, do not rely solely on $ETCO_2$ and always take blood gases for comparison. The value of continuous $ETCO_2$ monitoring is in the early detection of changes in ventilation, obstruction of endotracheal tubes and ventilator disconnection.

 Sudden loss of $ETCO_2$ indicates either failure of ventilation (e.g. obstruction of the endotracheal tube / disconnection of the breathing circuit) or loss of cardiac output.

Ventilator function should be continuously monitored. Modern intensive care ventilators have a large number of built-in monitors and alarms which do this, although you may have to set values or limits for some of these. In particular you should note:

- Inspired oxygen concentration.
- Tidal volume and minute volume delivered and expired. A discrepancy between the two indicates a leak in the circuit.
- Peak airway pressure. If the peak airway pressure does not reach a predetermined value, the breathing circuit may have become disconnected. If the peak pressure is too high this may indicate obstruction of the airway or breathing

circuit, or poor compliance. The patient may be at risk of barotrauma.
● Spontaneous effort. Many ventilators are able to record and measure any spontaneous contribution the patient makes to the minute volume.

Complications of ventilation

There are many complications of artificial ventilation. These include the following:

● Risks associated with endotracheal intubation, including inability to intubate and dislodgement or blockage of the endotracheal tube, for example with secretions.
● Prolonged tracheal intubation may be associated with damage to the larynx (particularly the vocal cords) and trachea. Traditionally tracheostomy was performed at about 14 days but many units now perform percutaneous tracheostomy earlier. There is limited evidence for enhanced recovery with early tracheostomy in some patient groups (see Tracheostomy, p. 34).
● The drying effect of gases and impaired cough lead to retention of secretions and increases the likelihood of ventilator associated pneumonia.
● Problems associated with the need for anaesthesia and/or sedation. These include the cardiovascular depressant effects of drugs, delayed gastric emptying, reduced mobility and delayed recovery. (See Sedation and analgesia, p. 34.)
● Haemodynamic effects of IPPV and PEEP include reduced venous return, reduced CO and reduced blood pressure. In turn, this reduces gut/renal blood flow and function.
● Barotrauma. The effects of high pressures applied to the airway can result in damage to the delicate tissues of the lung. This may be manifest as pneumothorax, pneumopericardium, subcutaneous surgical emphysema, interstitial emphysema and even air embolism. Where possible peak pressure should not be allowed to exceed 35–40 cm H_2O. If pressures above this are required, consider the underlying cause and the need for pressure controlled ventilation and 'permissive hypercapnia' (see ALI, p. 154).
● Volume trauma. Even at low pressures excessively large tidal volumes or unequal distribution of the tidal volume through the lung, so that some segments become overdistended, can result in volume trauma. The clinical manifestations of this are similar to barotrauma above, and include air leaks and cystic and emphysematous changes in the lung parenchyma.

COMMON PROBLEMS DURING ARTIFICIAL VENTILATION

Poor oxygenation

Gradual deterioration in oxygenation may represent continuing development of the pathophysiological process, while more sudden deterioration may represent the onset of a new problem or complication.

- Consider disconnecting the patient from the ventilator and 'hand bagging'. This effectively excludes a ventilator problem and provides 100% oxygen (see note below).
- Are both sides of the chest being ventilated equally? Check the position of the endotracheal tube. Is the tube too long or the tip abutting the carina on CXR?
- Is there any evidence of new collapse, pulmonary oedema, effusions or pneumothorax? Obtain a CXR (effusions/pneumothoraces may be better demonstrated on erect or semi-erect films). Treat any findings as appropriate.
- Increase FiO_2. Consider increasing PEEP, tidal volume and altering the I:E ratio (increase the inspiratory time). Consider pressure control ventilation, and alveolar recruitment manoeuvres.
- Ensure optimal cardiac output and haemodynamic status.
- Consider permissive hypoxaemia where aggressive ventilation is more likely to result in harm than poor oxygenation. PaO_2 above 8 kPa and SaO_2 above 90% are considered safe.
- Consider use of prone positioning and alternative modes of ventilation.
- Consider the need for extracorporeal membrane oxygenation (ECMO) if ventilated for less than 5–7 days.

(See Ventilation strategy, p. 127, ALI, p. 154 and ECMO p. 158.)

Hypercapnia

Hypercapnia generally results from inadequate ventilator settings and is simple to resolve. It may be associated with complications of ventilation which result in reduced compliance, particularly pneumothorax. Occasionally it may result from hypermetabolic states in which there is increased CO_2 production.

- Check ventilator settings, tidal volume and rate. Ensure that dead space in the ventilator circuit is minimal.
- Check the endotracheal tube. Is there any evidence of obstruction (e.g. tube kinked or blocked with secretions)? Are both sides of the chest being ventilated equally? Are there any new clinical

signs? Particularly, evidence of pneumothorax? Obtain a CXR if there is any doubt. Treat findings as appropriate.

- Is there any evidencve of bronchospasm? Consider bronchodilators or in extreme cases volatile anaesthetic agents.
- Increase tidal volume and/or rate.

> ⚠ **Endotracheal tube problems are more common than acute severe bronchospasm, and do not respond to bronchodilators. A blocked, kinked, malpositioned or obstructed endotracheal tube can be rapidly fatal. There is a great wisdom in the old saying 'If in doubt, take it out'.**

- Consider permissive hypercapnia: sometimes an elevated $PaCO_2$ is acceptable, either because lung pathophysiology makes reduction difficult/hazardous, or because the patient's habitual $PaCO_2$ is elevated.
- If permissive hypercapnia is not acceptable (e.g. head-injured patients and those at risk of raised intracranial pressure) consider extracorporeal CO_2 removal. There are bedside proprietary devices available (e.g. Novalung), the use of which has been described in this setting. Seek advice.

Increased airway pressures

Increases in airway pressure generally indicate a significant problem and should be dealt with promptly, both to resolve the underlying cause and to prevent injury from barotrauma. Common causes of increased airway pressure are shown in Table 5.7.

You should have a logical way of approaching this problem, such as:

- Disconnect the patient from the ventilator and attempt to ventilate with 100% oxygen via a bag and mask.
- Check the patient. Is there partial or complete obstruction of the endotracheal tube or major airway? Suction may clear this. Consider bronchoscopy to clear major airways.
- If there is any doubt about the patency of the endotracheal or tracheostomy tube, remove/change it. Use a bougie or airway exchange catheter if difficulty in reintubation is anticipated.
- Are there any new clinical signs? Is there evidence of bronchospasm or pneumothorax? Treat any findings as appropriate. This may require physiotherapy and suction, improved humidification, nebulized bronchodilators.

TABLE 5.7 Common causes of increased airway pressure

Endotracheal or tracheostomy tube	Kinked
	Patient biting endotracheal tube
	Obstructed with blood, secretions, etc.
	Too long (endobronchial)
	Misplaced outside trachea
Major airway	Obstructed with blood, secretions, etc.
Reduced compliance	Pulmonary collapse/ consolidation/ALI
	Pneumothorax
	Pleural effusion
	Bronchospasm
Poor synchrony with ventilator	Inadequate sedation
	Inappropriate ventilator settings

- Check ventilator settings. Are tidal volume, I:E ratio and inspiratory flow rate appropriate?
- If there is no evidence of an acute problem and airway pressures are rising due to reduced lung compliance or underlying pathophysiology, consider pressure control or alternative modes of ventilation.

> **In any of the above scenarios it may be helpful to disconnect the ventilator and ventilate the patient by hand in order to exclude ventilator problems, improve oxygenation or assess compliance. The principle advantage is application of 100% oxygen and increased mean airway pressure. The disadvantage is even short periods of disconnection can lead to atelectasis/collapse (loss of PEEP). Only disconnect the patient if really necessary.**

HIGH FREQUENCY MODES OF VENTILATION

In patients with low pulmonary compliance, conventional IPPV can result in high airway pressures, barotrauma and haemodynamic disturbance. High frequency ventilation has been tried as a means of reducing transpulmonary pressure, while providing adequate gas exchange. In most cases the tidal volume generated is less than anatomical dead space, and the exact mechanisms by which gas exchange is maintained are poorly understood. If you are considering these alternative modes of ventilation seek senior advice.

High frequency oscillation

A piston oscillates a diaphragm across the open airway resulting in a sinusoidal flow pattern with I:E ratio 1:1 (variable). This is unique in that both inspiration and expiration are active. Airway pressure oscillates around a slightly increased mean but the peak airway pressure is reduced. Increasing the mean airway pressure recruits more alveoli and improves oxygenation. CO_2 clearance is controlled by altering the rate and amplitude of oscillation. Clearance of secretions is improved. This type of ventilation is well established in neonatal and paediatric intensive care. Oscillators capable of use in adults have recently become available and are becoming more established in adult practice. A typical approach to establishing high frequency oscillation is shown in Table 5.8. Always seek senior advice.

Once established, HFOV is highly effective in alveolar recruitment leading to improved oxygenation. As recruitment continues lung compliance improves and the lung can become overdistended with potential for volume trauma. Perform regular chest X-rays and reduce mean airway pressure as the patient's condition improves.

High frequency jet ventilation

This appears at present to be an increasingly obsolete mode of ventilation in critical care units. Pulses of gas are delivered at high pressure either through an attachment to the endotracheal

---

TABLE 5.8 Approach to establishing high frequency oscillation ventilation

Mean airway pressure	3–5 cm H_2O above mean airway pressure on conventional ventilation
Amplitude	Increase sufficiently to generate visible and effective chest 'wobble'
Frequency	6–8 Hz
Inspiratory time	33%
FiO_2	1.0

TABLE 5.9 Typical settings for jet ventilator

Driving pressure	1.5–2.5 atmospheres (150–250 kPa)
Frequency	60–200/min
I:E ratio	1:1–1:1.5

tube or via a special endotracheal tube. The driving pressure and frequency can be varied. The jet of gas produced entrains air/oxygen from an open circuit (e.g. T-piece) and the tidal volume generated is generally of the order of 70–170 mL. Expiration is passive. Gas trapping may occur. The technique can be noisy and cumbersome. Humidification can be problematic. Typical settings are shown in Table 5.9.

There are two possible roles for jet ventilation:

- Management of bronchopleural fistula. During conventional ventilation most of the tidal volume may be lost through the fistula, making effective ventilation of the patient impossible. Jet ventilation has been claimed to reduce transpulmonary pressures, thus reducing the leak. The evidence for this, however, is not strong; the main determinant seems to be the mean airway pressure, regardless of ventilator used.
- As an aid to weaning. Patients can comfortably breathe over jet ventilation. As the patient's condition improves, driving pressure is reduced and frequency increased. The use of non-invasive ventilation as an aid to weaning has reduced the use of jet ventilation for this indication.

WEANING FROM ARTIFICIAL VENTILATION

As the patient's condition improves, artificial ventilation can gradually be reduced until the patient is able to breathe unassisted. The decision to start weaning is largely one of clinical judgement, based on improving respiratory function and resolving underlying pathology. Studies have shown, however, that weaning is often delayed unnecessarily and there is evidence that the use of weaning protocols may reduce the time to extubation and reduce ICU stay. Typical criteria for successful weaning are shown in Table 5.10.

Some patients, particularly postoperative elective surgical cases, will tolerate weaning well and can be rapidly extubated. Others, particularly those who have been ventilated for some time, or who have significant lung damage or muscle wasting, may take longer and benefit from tracheostomy. There is no widely agreed

TABLE 5.10 Typical criteria for successful weaning

Neuromuscular	Awake and co-operative Good muscle tone and function Intact bulbar function
Haemodynamic	No dysrhythmias Minimal inotrope requirements Optimal fluid balance
Respiratory	$FiO_2 < 0.5$ $(A–a) DO_2 < 40\,kPa$ Vital capacity $> 10\,mL/kg$ Tidal volume $> 5\,mL/kg$ Can generate negative inspiratory pressure $> 20\,cm\,H_2O$ Good cough
Metabolic	Normal pH Normal electrolyte balance Adequate nutritional status Normal CO_2 production Normal oxygen demands

policy on the best way to wean patients from ventilation. A typical approach is described below:

● Ensure the patient's general condition is optimal.
● Reduce/stop sedative drugs.
● Ensure adequate but not excessive analgesia for surgical wounds, etc.
● Where possible, sit the patient up or out in a chair, and mobilize as much as possible.
● Gradually reduce the ventilator rate to allow the patient to take more breaths. Ensure adequate pressure support and PEEP to reduce the work of breathing.
● When the patient is taking an adequate number of breaths with a good and sustained respiratory pattern, switch to CPAP with pressure support.
● If the patient manages well, gradually reduce the level of pressure support further. When the pressure support is down to $10\,cm\,H_2O$ do not reduce it any further.
● Either extubate directly from CPAP and pressure support if the patient is likely to manage or switch to separate flow generator CPAP system and extubate later when it is anticipated that the patient will manage without any support (see Extubation, p. 403).

Different patients will progress through weaning at different rates depending on their underlying problems. Some patients may be so agitated that there is no choice but to rapidly wean and extubate. Others may manage only brief periods of CPAP and pressure support before getting tired, as indicated by sweating, increasing pulse and respiratory rate (rapid shallow breaths). These patients will need rest periods on the ventilator between periods of CPAP and pressure support and weaning is often protracted.

Following weaning some patients will extubate without difficulty, others will rapidly deteriorate. This is often due to inability to clear secretions. These patients will require reintubation, ventilation and another period of optimization. Consider tracheostomy to aid clearance of secretions and weaning. (See Percutaneous tracheostomy, p. 404.)

Role of 'non-invasive' ventilation in weaning

There has been increasing recognition over the past few years of the role of 'non-invasive' ventilation techniques as an aid to weaning. Patients with difficulty weaning from conventional ventilation can, for example, be extubated and managed on BIPAP delivered via face mask. This is more comfortable for the patient than prolonged intubation, may avoid the need for tracheostomy and, as the patient's condition improves, can be removed intermittently to allow eating and drinking. Patients who have required a tracheostomy can also be weaned using similar ventilators (via the tracheostomy).

Step-down tracheostomy care

Not all general wards are appropriately staffed or possess the necessary training and expertise to care for patients recently stepped down from an intensive care unit with a tracheostomy. This is particularly likely to be the case when the patient still requires frequent suctioning of secretions. In many centres, therefore, the appropriate 'step-down' location for patients who have been weaned from ventilation using a tracheostomy on which they are still dependent, is a high dependency unit or a respiratory care unit. Precise arrangements vary greatly from hospital to hospital.

Weaning centres

There is interest in the concept of centralized weaning centres, where patients who no longer require full intensive care support, but still need respiratory support, might be managed with lower nursing and medical input. This model has been successfully adopted in several European countries. Patients are gradually weaned over time, either to full independence from ventilation or to partial independence (nocturnal ventilation). Some patients, typically those with severe chronic lung disease, chronic neuromuscular conditions and high cervical spine injuries, may require long-term ventilation.

AIRWAY OBSTRUCTION

Airway obstruction is common in the immediate postoperative period while patients are in the recovery room and the effects of anaesthetic drugs wear off. Occasionally airway obstruction may persist or may be a potential risk following a particular surgical procedure. These patients will frequently be admitted to the ICU. (See Postoperative complications, p. 355.) Causes of airway obstruction are shown in Box 5.2.

It is crucial to recognize actual or impending airway obstruction before the patient suffers a hypoxic episode. In the spontaneously breathing patient, airway obstruction produces obvious respiratory distress. Use of accessory muscles of respiration, tracheal tug, intercostal recession (mostly in children) and paradoxical respiratory movements all suggest significant obstruction. Stridor is typical, but indicates at least some airflow; the silent patient may be in much greater danger.

Management
The management of any patient with airway obstruction is essentially the same, i.e. secure the airway by endotracheal intubation or tracheostomy as soon and as safely as possible.

Box 5.2 Causes of airway obstruction

Facial trauma

Soft-tissue obstruction in upper airway

Bleeding/swelling/tumour/foreign body in upper airway

Vocal cord paralysis following damage to laryngeal nerve/hypocalcaemia

Bleeding/swelling/tumour/foreign body in lower airway

External compression of trachea, e.g. from bleeding/swelling in the neck

Collapse of trachea, e.g. tracheomalacia

Allergic reactions e.g. ACE inhibitors, anaphylaxis, angioneurotic oedema

There are, however, a few points to bear in mind, depending on the situation and your own experience:

- Do not leave the patient unattended.
- Do not delay management of the problem by sending the patient for investigations.
- Give high flow oxygen by face mask.

 Helium–oxygen mix is less dense than air and may reduce the work of breathing in patients with airway obstruction. Heliox® is a commercially available mixture containing 79% helium / 21% oxygen. The low fractional inspired oxygen limits its usefulness.

- Nebulized adrenaline may reduce obstruction caused by airway oedema
- Support ventilation with a bag and mask if necessary and practicable.
- Simple manoeuvres such as extending the neck, jaw thrust and suctioning of the airway may improve the situation particularly in the obtunded patient.
- Seek help from senior anaesthetist and ENT surgeon as appropriate. In these circumstances intubation / reintubation can often be difficult.

 Seek urgent senior help. Do not delay getting help because of apparently good oxygenation. Hypoxia on the pulse oximeter / arterial blood gases is likely to be a very late sign.

The definitive management is to secure the airway by tracheal intubation or tracheostomy. If time allows, this should be performed in theatre with surgeons scrubbed and prepared for emergency tracheostomy. Awake fibreoptic intubation, awake tracheostomy or gaseous anaesthetic induction with the patient breathing spontaneously may be appropriate, depending on the circumstances. It is beyond the scope of this text to cover these in detail. The usual problem at intubation is gross swelling and distortion of the tissues, which makes the laryngeal inlet difficult to visualize. Often the endotracheal tube has to be passed blindly through swollen tissues into the larynx. Occasionally obstruction proves to be lower down the airway and ventilation may be impossible even when the trachea is intubated.

Once the airway is secured the management is that of the underlying condition. Allow time for swelling to subside. Steroids may be of value. Elevate the head of the bed, and reassess over time.

Airway obstruction in the intubated patient

This is common in the ICU and may be due to kinking of the endotracheal or tracheostomy tube or the effects of thick secretions, blood clot or even occasionally a foreign body. Adequate humidification, regular suctioning and careful fixation of endotracheal tubes avoid most problems, but these may still arise, particularly in children where the endotracheal tube is smaller in diameter and blocks more easily.

It is important to recognize and act on these problems immediately. Typical clues are increased airway pressure, inability to inflate the chest manually with a bag, falling SaO_2 and absent $ETCO_2$ trace.

- Ventilate with 100% oxygen if possible. If not, remove the endotracheal tube and manually ventilate the patient with a bag and mask before reintubation.
- If able to ventilate satisfactorily, suction the endotracheal tube. Use 10–20 mL saline instilled down the endotracheal tube to loosen secretions.
- Bronchoscopy may be helpful.

In 'ball valve' obstruction the chest can be inflated but exhaled gas is trapped by a plug of mucus or blood impinging on the end of the tracheal tube. Apply suction directly to the endotracheal or tracheostomy tube. If the obstructing plug does not come up the tube, remove the tube while maintaining suction hopefully dragging the plug out at the same time. (A similar effect can be achieved by pulling plugs out on the end of a bronchoscope.) Ventilate the patient by bag and mask before reintubation.

Post-extubation stridor

Airway obstruction and stridor may occur following extubation. This may be as a result of underlying pathology but frequently results from laryngeal oedema, particularly in children whose airways are narrower. This may occasionally require reintubation. Two or three doses of dexamethasone (4 mg) given prior to extubation may reduce laryngeal swelling. Nebulized adrenaline and use of CPAP may be helpful. Where these measures prove ineffective, reintubation should not be delayed. A range of (small) endotracheal tubes and other emergency airway adjunct should be available. Seek senior help.

COMMUNITY-ACQUIRED PNEUMONIA

Pneumonia is defined as infection occurring in terminal respiratory airways. The pattern of illness and pathogens responsible depend on whether the infection was acquired in the community or in hospital, and on the patient's immune status. Community acquired pneumonias can be divided into those of 'typical' and 'atypical' presentation.

Typical pneumonia

The features of a 'typical' pneumonia include the following:

- sudden onset of fever with rigors
- cough productive of mucopurulent sputum
- shortness of breath
- pleuritic chest pain.

Chest X-rays show the appearances of consolidation, which may affect a single lobe, a whole lung or both lungs. The diagnosis is confirmed by raised WCC (predominantly neutrophils) and CRP, and by results of sputum and blood culture. The common causative organisms are shown in Table 5.11.

Atypical pneumonia

Atypical pneumonias are so called because their mode of presentation is different from that seen in classic pneumonia. In particular the following presentations occur:

- Present over a few days, compared to the 24–36 h of classic pneumonia.
- Non-respiratory symptoms may predominate. Fever, malaise, myalgia and arthralgia are common. Some may be associated with severe systemic illness.
- Cough may only appear after a few days and is often non-productive. Sputum that is produced is clear and often negative on Gram stain and culture.

TABLE 5.11 Common causes of typical community-acquired pneumonia

Lobar pneumonia	*Streptococcus pneumoniae*
Bronchopneumonia	*Strep. pneumoniae* *Haemophilus influenzae* *Staphylococcus aureus* Enterobacteria (less common unless risk factors/comorbidity)

Cont'd

TABLE 5.12 Cont'd	
Viral	Influenza A, B Parainfluenza Respiratory syncytial virus
Bacterial	*Legionella pneumophila* *Coxiella burnetii* *Mycobacterium tuberculosis*
Chlamydia	*Chlamydia psittaci*
Mycoplasma	*Mycoplasma pneumoniae*

- There may be disparity between the clinical signs on chest examination and the CXR with minimal signs on examination of the chest, whereas CXR shows widespread patchy consolidation with interstitial and alveolar infiltrates.
- WCC may be normal or mildly elevated.

Causes of atypical community-acquired pneumonia are shown in Table 5.12.

While the list of causes is not exhaustive it gives an indication of the range of pathogens that may be responsible. The difficulty is often in making the diagnosis. You should seek advice from local microbiologists regarding investigations and treatment. The features of some atypical pneumonias are described below.

Mycoplasma pneumonia

Mycoplasma pneumoniae is a community-acquired infection that tends to affect young adults. It may progress to a multisystem disease with the following features:

- haemolytic anaemia, thrombocytopenia
- pericarditis, myocarditis, rarely endocarditis
- meningitis, encephalitis, peripheral and central nerve palsies
- vomiting and diarrhoea, hepatitis
- rashes, myalgia and arthralgia.

The diagnosis is confirmed by rising antibody titre. Cold agglutinins occur in up to 50% of patients, although this is non-specific and can occur in other atypical pneumonias, notably *Legionella*.

Legionella pneumonia

Legionella pneumoniae infection may occur in outbreaks associated with infected showers and water-cooling systems, but also occurs sporadically, particularly among older patients. Typical features are:

- prodromal flu-like illness
- dry cough
- fever up to 40°C associated with rigors
- mental confusion
- nausea, vomiting, diarrhoea, abdominal pain, and jaundice
- haematuria and renal failure may develop
- multi-lobar shadowing and small pleural effusions on CXR.

The diagnosis is confirmed by rising antibody titre. *Legionella* may be identified by immunofluorescence on sputum, bronchial washings and urine.

PANDEMIC INFLUENZA

There is ongoing concern regarding the potential for future pandemic influenza affecting large subsets of the population with the risk of acute medical services becoming rapidly overwhelmed with patients in respiratory and multiple organ failure. There are national and local contingency plans for dealing with this (and other contagious outbreaks). See DOH guidance and local policies.

HOSPITAL-ACQUIRED PNEUMONIA

Hospital-acquired pneumonias are a common cause of morbidity in hospitalized patients. Up to 20% of all mechanically ventilated patients develop ventilator-associated pneumonia and the incidence is higher in the immunocompromised patient. Gram-negative organisms and *Staphylococcus aureus* are particularly common. A number of factors may increase the risk of pneumonia in critically ill patients, by impairing host defence mechanisms and increasing colonization of the upper airway. These are summarized in Table 5.13.

Since little can be done to improve host defence mechanisms in the critically ill ventilated patient, the best approach to reducing the incidence of nosocomial infection is to prevent contamination of the airway with pathogenic bacteria, in particular by reducing the incidence of colonization of the upper airway.

Hygiene measures

Ensure adequate hygiene procedures and aseptic technique at all times. Suction the oropharynx regularly to prevent secretions pooling above the larynx and nurse patients in a semi-recumbent position to reduce the risk of passive aspiration. Ensure adequate

TABLE 5.13 Factors predisposing to nosocomial pneumonia

Critical illness	Impaired host defences and immune systems
Sedation	Impaired mucus transport and cough mechanisms
Endotracheal and tracheostomy tubes	Bypass normal host defence mechanisms Increased colonization of upper airways Laryngeal incompetence increases risk of aspiration
Antacids	Reduce gastric acidity, allow increased colonization of stomach with lower GI flora
Nasogastric tubes	Provide route for increased colonization of upper airway with lower GI flora from stomach
Broad-spectrum antibiotics	Destroy normal commensal flora and promote colonization with pathogenic microorganisms

humidification of inspired gases and regular physiotherapy and tracheal suction. Use closed suction devices or wear sterile gloves when suctioning the airway. The use of chlorhexidine mouthwashes has been advocated.

Maintenance of gastric acidity

The maintenance of a normal gastric pH is a major barrier to the colonization of the upper airway with gut flora, occurring via nasogastric tubes or the reflux of gastric contents. Therefore although the use of H_2 blockers, such as ranitidine, to reduce gastric acidity and prevent stress ulceration has been shown to improve outcome, there are some potentially undesirable effects. H_2 blockers can often be stopped once enteral feeding is established. Therefore, establish enteral feeding early but stop feed periodically (typically 4 h per day) to allow gastric acidity to return to normal. (See Stress ulcer prophylaxis, p. 172, and Enteral feeding, p. 57.)

Selective decontamination of the digestive tract (SDD)

SDD is a method of reducing colonization of the upper airways by using oral, non-absorbable antibiotics in an attempt to reduce the bacterial load in the GI tract. There is some evidence that this is effective at reducing nosocomial infection; however, at the current time SDD is not in widespread use in the UK because of concerns that it may drive the emergence of multi-drug resistant bacteria and promote MRSA infection. Further studies are ongoing.

PNEUMONIA IN IMMUNOCOMPROMISED PATIENTS

(See also The immunocompromised patient, p. 226.)

Patients who are immunocompromised for any reason may present with pneumonia. In addition to the typical and atypical conditions already described, a number of other opportunistic pathogens typically infect these patients. These are shown in Box 5.3.

Pneumocystis carinii pneumonia (PCP)
Typical features are:

● fever
● dry cough
● breathlessness and severe hypoxaemia
● bilateral diffuse alveolar and interstitial shadowing.

Eighty per cent of PCP can be detected by immunofluorescence on bronchoalveolar lavage fluid (BAL). PCR tests are now also available. Occasionally transbronchial biopsy may be necessary.

Fungal pneumonia
Colonization of the pharynx, GIT, perineum, wounds and skin folds is common and rarely requires treatment. Significant fungal infections may occur after prolonged treatment with antibiotics and particularly in immunocompromised patients. Infection is suggested by significant growth in sputum, tracheal aspirates, BAL fluids and blood cultures. In addition there may be rising serum antibody titres to *Candida* or the presence of *Aspergillus* antigens. Fungal infection, particularly fungal septicaemia, is associated with a high mortality.

Box 5.3 Common opportunistic infections

Pneumocystis carinii
Cytomegalovirus (CMV)
Herpes virus (simplex and zoster)
Candida sp.
Aspergillus sp.

Cytomegalovirus (CMV)

CMV pneumonitis in immunocompromised patients is generally part of a disseminated infection in which there may be encephalitis, retinitis and involvement of the gastrointestinal tract. Cytology (BAL washings or biopsy) may show characteristic inclusion bodies. Diagnosis may be made by polymerase chain reaction (PCR), fluorescent antibody tests and tissue culture.

MANAGEMENT OF PNEUMONIA

All patients with pneumonia requiring admission to intensive care should have full blood count, urea and electrolytes, liver function tests, C-reactive protein (CRP) and CXR performed. Possible microbiological investigations are summarized in Table 5.14. Not all patients require the full spectrum of investigations: these should be guided by severity, risk factors and response to treatment.

The treatment of any pneumonia is twofold:

● Supportive therapy including humidified oxygen and ventilation as necessary. Regular physiotherapy and tracheal suction to aid clearance of secretions.

TABLE 5.14 Microbiological investigations for pneumonia

Sample	Investigation
Sputum/tracheal aspirate	Microscopy, culture and sensitivity
BAL	M,C & S (including AAFB) *Legionella* immunofluorescence Viruses Fungi Pneumocystis
Nasopharyngeal aspirate/ pernasal swab	Viruses
Blood	Blood culture Serology (acute and convalescent samples) Viral titres Complement fixation (*Mycoplasma*, *Chlamydia*)
Urine	*Legionella* immunofluorescence
Pleural fluid	M,C & S

● Antibiotic therapy. Choice will depend upon the clinical picture and the nature of the infecting organism. Wherever possible, microbiological specimens should be obtained prior to the commencement of antibiotics.

Flexible bronchoscopy may be helpful for obtaining specimens and removal of tenacious secretions. Where this is not available, blind (non-directed) bronchoalveolar lavage has been shown to be a very effective diagnostic aid (see BAL, p. 415).

Recommended empirical antibiotic therapy for severe community-acquired pneumonia is either a second-generation cephalosporin (e.g. cefuroxime) or a broad-spectrum lactamase stable antibiotic (e.g. coamoxiclav), plus a macrolide antibiotic (e.g. clarithromycin) to cover the common atypical agents. Where specific infective agents are identified or suspected, treatment should be based on microbiological advice.

The presence of effusion should be looked for on chest X-ray or ultrasound. Effusions can be tapped for diagnostic purposes. If the effusion is large, drainage increases lung volume and improves lung compliance. Empyema requires physical drainage to remove the source of infection. Occasional surgical intervention may be required, particularly in the case of complex multi-loculated collections. Surgical drainage and decortication by video-assisted thoracoscopic surgery may be the only solution in some cases.

Lung abscess are suggested by the presence of fluid levels and progressive cystic changes in the lungs. Abscesses may complicate a number of bacterial and other infections. The management is largely supported with postural drainage and appropriate antibiotics and other support. There is little place for thoracic surgical intervention in this context.

Hospital-acquired pneumonia

The management of hospital acquired pneumonia is similar to the management of any other pneumonia (see above). Ideally antibiotics should be used only for microbiologically proven infection. If, however, the patient's condition dictates blind antibiotic therapy, ensure microbiological specimens are obtained before commencing treatment. Antibiotic therapy needs to be guided by the likely source of the pathogens and by the local pattern of microbial antibiotic resistance. Seek microbiological advice. (See Empirical antibiotic therapy, p. 336, MRSA, p. 336 and VRE, p. 336.)

Pneumonia in immunocompromised patients

This group of patients provides a great clinical challenge, as there may be diagnostic difficulty distinguishing the radiological and clinical features of pneumonia from those of some other interstitial process. For example, lymphomatous infiltrates in the lung may resemble the picture of an immunocompromised infective pneumonia. Diagnosis can be assisted by bronchoalveolar lavage, bronchial brushings and if necessary, biopsy. Serological tests may also help support the diagnosis. The management of pneumonia in immunocompromised individuals is essentially the same as in the non-immunocompromised, although the range of potential infective agents is greater. Always seek advice on the likely pathogens, appropriate investigations and initial treatment. Common first-line agents are as follows:

- *Pneumocystis* pneumonia. High-dose co-trimoxazole (Septrin) and steroids to reduce the inflammatory response.
- Fungal pneumonia. High-dose fluconazole or (liposomal) amphotericin.
- Cytomegalovirus (CMV). Ganciclovir. Beware of nephrotoxicity and bone marrow suppression.

Tuberculosis

Most tuberculosis infections are treated with triple or even quadruple therapy. Isoniazid, rifampicin, ethambutal, streptomycin and other agents are frequently used in combination. Many strains of tuberculosis are multi-drug resistant; seek advice from your microbiologist and local infectious diseases consultant.

ASPIRATION PNEUMONITIS

Patients with impaired conscious level, cough or gag reflexes are at risk of aspiration of gastric contents into the airway. Aspiration may present with acute airway obstruction if the aspirated matter is solid. More commonly it presents as gradual onset of respiratory distress and respiratory failure, either due to bacterial infection of the lungs or due to the inflammatory effects of acid aspiration. Some patients will develop ALI following aspiration (see ALI, p. 154).

If a patient is known to have aspirated gastric contents, e.g. during an anaesthetic, management is as follows:

- Suction the trachea to remove debris. If possible suction should be applied before any form of positive pressure ventilation.

- Consider bronchoscopy and lavage if available.
- Monitor clinical condition and oxygen saturation. Give humidified oxygen as required.
- Avoid antibiotics unless there is evidence of infection. If necessary, antibiotic therapy should cover the normal respiratory pathogens plus Gram-negatives and anaerobes. A combination of broad-spectrum cephalosporin and metronidazole is appropriate initially. Further treatment should be guided by the results of microbiological investigation.
- There is no role for routine prophylactic steroids.
- Treat bronchospasm appropriately. If wheeze persists, consider possible foreign body aspiration and the need for rigid bronchoscopy.
- If the patient's condition deteriorates, ventilatory support may be necessary.

ASTHMA

Asthma occurs principally in young people and the incidence of this potentially life-threatening condition is increasing. Asthma involves increased airway reactivity, often triggered by an environmental stimulus, or following infection. An inflammatory process results in narrowing of small airways, mucus plugging, expiratory wheeze and air trapping. Severe asthma is a medical emergency. It may be rapidly progressive and clinical signs may be misleading. The clinical signs of severe asthma are shown in Box 5.4.

Box 5.4 Clinical signs of severe asthma	
Severe asthma	Life-threatening asthma
Inability to talk in sentences	Exhaustion, confusion, reduced conscious level
Peak flow $< 50\%$ predicted/best	Peak flow $< 33\%$ predicted/best
Respiratory rate > 25/min	Feeble respiratory effort or 'silent' chest
Pulse rate > 110/min; pulsus paradoxus	Bradycardia or hypotension: $SaO_2 < 92\%$ $PaO_2 < 8\,kPa$ $PaCO_2 > 5\,kPa$ pH < 7.3

Management

- Give high flow humidified oxygen and monitor oxygen saturation continually.
- Give nebulized β-agonists (salbutamol 2.5–5 mg neb.) and anticholinergics (ipratropium bromide 0.5 mg neb.). Repeat as frequently as required. Ensure nebulizers are given in oxygen not air.
- Give i.v. corticosteroids to suppress the inflammatory response. Hydrocortisone 200 mg bolus then 100 mg 6-hourly.
- There is no role for antibiotics unless there is clear evidence of a precipitating bacterial infection.
- Commence i.v. fluid, to correct dehydration.
- If there is no improvement, commence i.v. β-agonist, either salbutamol 4 μg/kg loading dose over 10 min followed by infusion 5 μg/min or aminophylline 5 mg/kg loading dose over 10 min followed by infusion 0.5 mg kg h.
- Consider a single bolus dose of magnesium sulphate 1.2–2 g i.v. over 20 min.
- If there is no improvement or the patient's condition is life-threatening, consider need for ventilation. Indications for ventilation are shown in Box 5.5.

Asthma is unlike other forms of respiratory failure in that the problem is not immediately solved by intubation and ventilation. Airway obstruction may be initially worsened by tracheal intubation and attending staff are faced with a paralysed intubated patient who cannot be ventilated!

Patients with severe life-threatening asthma are often dehydrated and have high levels of endogenous catecholamines. When anaesthesia is induced to facilitate intubation, the cardiovascular depressant effects of the drugs, the reduction in endogenous catecholamines and the effects of dehydration and acidosis can lead to profound cardiovascular collapse.

Following intubation ensure adequate analgesia and sedation. The presence of an endotracheal tube in the larynx of an

---

Box 5.5 Indications for ventilation in asthma

Exhaustion
$PaO_2 < 8$ kPa
$PaCO_2 > 6.5$ kPa
pH < 7.3
Cardio-respiratory arrest

inadequately sedated asthmatic is a potent source of irritation and continued bronchoconstriction. Standard sedative regimens are generally sufficient. There may be a role for ketamine infusion both as a sedative agent and as a bronchodilator in refractory bronchospasm. Muscle relaxation may be required initially in severe cases. Avoid agents likely to release histamine, such as atracurium or mivacurium. Cisatracurium, vecuronium or pancuronium are less likely to cause direct release histamine.

During ventilation, severe bronchoconstriction may result in air trapping and hyperinflation. This may lead to difficulty in ventilating the patient adequately using conventional ventilator settings. High airway pressure may be required, with the risk of barotrauma and development of a pneumothorax.

To minimize these problems, ventilator settings should be adjusted to allow adequate time for expiration. The optimal combination of ventilation settings in any individual patient is best determined by trial. In general, set a slow rate and prolonged expiratory time (I:E, 1:3–1:4) to allow adequate time for full expiration. The short inspiratory time may result in higher peak airway pressure. This is partly offset by the slower rate. In severe cases it may be necessary to accept a higher $PaCO_2$ rather than increase inspiratory pressures.

The role of PEEP in asthma is controversial. In theory, adding PEEP increases FRC and may worsen air trapping in patients who are hyperinflated. Judicious levels of PEEP have, however, been used to recruit airways and improve ventilation. In practice, try adding PEEP cautiously and observe the response (see PEEP, p. 126).

If severe hyperinflation becomes a problem it may be necessary to disconnect the patient from the ventilator and manually ventilate with a long expiratory time. Manual compression of the chest wall has been used to expel trapped air and improve respiratory mechanics. Volatile anaesthetic agents may be useful in severe bronchospasm. These can be either given through an anaesthetic machine but the attached ventilators are often incapable of ventilating such patients. There are specialized pumped injector delivery systems for volatile agents into ICU ventilator circuits. Occasional patients can be managed with ECMO or related technology, though this is likely to require transfer to a specialist centre, which may be problematic or impossible in the patient with severe acute bronchospasm. Simple systems for extracorporeal CO_2 removal are available (e.g. Novalung®) that can be used outside specialist centres to reduce a high $PaCO_2$.

CHRONIC OBSTRUCTIVE PULMONARY DISEASE

Chronic obstructive pulmonary disease (COPD) is a broad
'description' applied to patients with chronic bronchitis and
emphysema. These conditions frequently coexist, and in severe
cases may result in respiratory failure, which may be precipitated
by intercurrent viral or bacterial respiratory infection.

Acute exacerbation

Patients with so-called acute exacerbations of COPD are generally
managed in A&E and on medical wards with a combination of
antibiotics, bronchodilators, controlled oxygen therapy (usually
24–35% oxygen by a fixed performance, Venturi system) and non-
invasive ventilation. Pathophysiologically, there is some overlap
between chronic obstructive pulmonary disease and asthma,
with features of airway reactivity occurring in both diseases.
Some patients may genuinely suffer both conditions. There
are increasing numbers of respiratory units that provide high
dependency care to this group of patients, who are, therefore, only
likely to be admitted to an ICU when these measures have failed
and tracheal intubation and full ventilatory support is required.
(See Non-invasive ventilation, p. 122.)

Management

- Due to the effects of long-term compensatory mechanisms,
  these patients often tolerate markedly deranged blood gases
  (hypoxia and hypercapnia) very well. Therefore, it is the clinical
  condition of the patient rather than blood gases that determines
  the need for ventilatory support. Assess the patient clinically. If
  able to talk, and not distressed, the patient is unlikely to need
  immediate ventilation, regardless of the blood gas picture.
- Correct hypoxia by incremental increase in FiO_2. Aim to
  achieve PaO_2 7–8 kPa, $SaO_2 \geq 90\%$ or that which is normal for
  the patient.
- In some patients with COPD and type 2 respiratory failure,
  chronic hypercapnia results in loss of the normal ventilatory
  responsiveness to CO_2. In these patients hypoxia is the main
  stimulus to respiration. High concentrations of inspired
  oxygen can result in the loss of the stimulus to respiration
  and precipitate respiratory arrest. Look at the bicarbonate
  concentration on the blood gas. If this is normal, or only
  slightly raised (<30 mmol/L), chronic CO_2 retention is unlikely
  to exist and the patient should not be dependent on hypoxic
  drive. Increase the inspired oxygen concentration as necessary

and repeat the blood gases after 30 min. In cases where the patient is dependent on hypoxic drive, the $PaCO_2$ may rise and the need for assisted ventilation may be precipitated earlier.

- Avoid respiratory stimulants such as doxapram. These generally do not help and can result in patients becoming exhausted and requiring ventilation. Consider use of CPAP or non-invasive ventilation.
- Give nebulized β-agonists (salbutamol 2.5–5 mg neb.) and anticholinergics (ipratropium bromide 0.5 mg neb.). Repeat as frequently as required. Ensure nebulizers are given in oxygen not air.
- Give i.v. corticosteroids (hydrocortisone 200 mg bolus then 100 mg 6-hourly) to suppress the inflammatory response.
- There is no role for antibiotics unless there is clear evidence of a precipitating infection.
- Commence i.v. fluid, to correct dehydration.
- If there is no improvement, commence i.v. β-agonist, either salbutamol 4 μg/kg loading dose over 10 min followed by infusion 5 μg/min or aminophylline 5 mg/kg loading dose over 10 min followed by infusion 0.5 mg/kg/h.
- If the patient remains severely hypoxic, becomes increasingly hypercapnic, acidotic or clinically exhausted, urgent ventilation is likely to be necessary.

Most patients with acute exacerbations of COPD who require a short period of ventilation do well and leave hospital. Patients in end-stage respiratory failure, however, particularly those that have been ventilated before and who have been difficult to wean from ventilators, may not be suitable for further admission to intensive care. This decision should be taken by a senior doctor in consultation, where possible, with the patient and/or the next of kin. Seek senior advice.

Intensive care management

These patients are typically very distressed and have a high level of sympathetic catecholamine activity. Anaesthetic drugs used to intubate may abolish this and unmask relative hypovolaemia, with subsequent cardiovascular collapse. In addition, there are frequently coexisting medical problems such as ischaemic heart disease. Therefore:

- Where possible transfer the patient directly to the ICU for intubation and ventilation rather than attempting this on the ward.

- If the patient's condition allows, site an arterial line and institute arterial pressure monitoring before induction.
- Consider giving a fluid bolus (e.g. 500 mL of colloid) prior to induction. Have adrenaline (epinephrine) available for resuscitation.
- After securing the airway, institute IPPV. SIMV mode is usually adequate. Avoid hyperventilation. Rapid lowering of the $PaCO_2$ may further reduce sympathetic drive and lower the blood pressure.
- Continue antibiotic therapy according to local protocol. (See Pneumonia, p. 141, and Empirical antibiotic therapy, p. 336.)
- Give nebulized bronchodilators. Salbutamol 2.5 mg and ipratropium bromide 0.5 mg.
- Consider intravenous bronchodilator therapy. Aminophylline 5 mg/kg loading dose (if not on long-term theophylline and not already loaded) followed by infusion aminophylline 0.5 mg/kg/h. Check levels.
- Corticosteroids. Hydrocortisone 200 mg initially then 100 mg 6-hourly.

Many of these patients require a relatively short period of ventilation and wean easily from the ventilator. Weaning can often be facilitated by the use of non-invasive ventilation techniques such as BIPAP. Some patients, however, particularly those with type 2 respiratory failure, may be more difficult to wean and early tracheostomy may be considered to facilitate tracheal toilet and improve patient comfort while allowing a reduction in sedative drugs. Once stable, patients on BIPAP via mask or tracheostomy may be transferred to medical wards or weaning units for further weaning (see Weaning from artificial ventilation p. 135).

ACUTE LUNG INJURY

The clinical signs of acute lung injury (ALI) and acute respiratory distress syndrome (ARDS) are those of increasing respiratory distress, with associated tachycardia, tachypnoea and onset of cyanosis. Blood gases indicate severe hypoxaemia. The CXR shows acute bilateral interstitial and alveolar shadowing. The non-cardiogenic nature of the alveolar oedema can be confirmed by pulmonary artery catheterization (PAOP < 18 mmHg, CI > 2 L/min/m^3) or echocardiography and infective processes excluded by BAL.

TABLE 5.15 Criteria for diagnosis of ALI and ARDS

	Timing	Oxygenation (PaO_2/FiO_2)	Chest X-ray	PAOP
ALI	Acute onset	< 40 kPa (regardless of PEEP)	Bilateral infiltrates	<18 mmHg or no evidence of left atrial hypertension
ARDS	Acute onset	< 27 kPa (regardless of PEEP)	Bilateral infiltrates	<18 mmHg or no evidence of left atrial hypertension

The principal diagnostic criterion used to distinguish ALI and ARDS is the degree of hypoxaemia, as shown in Table 5.15.

Pathophysiology

A large number of conditions have been associated with the onset of ALI/ARDS, as indicated in Box 5.6.

It is clear that an ALI can develop in response to a wide range of insults. The exact processes by which this occurs are not fully understood. It is characterized by proliferation of inflammatory cells, increased permeability of the alveolar capillaries and leak of proteinaceous fluid into the alveoli (so-called 'non-cardiogenic pulmonary oedema'). This protein-rich material precipitates, forming hyaline membranes. In survivors, the acute inflammatory process gradually subsides and healing occurs. This may result in widespread interstitial lung fibrosis. Not all patients who have ALI go on to develop severe ARDS. There is a spectrum of disease ranging from mild to severe.

Box 5.6 Common conditions associated with ALI/ARDS

Physical	Infective	Inflammatory/immune
Trauma	Pneumonia	Blood transfusion
Acid aspiration	Septicaemia	Cardiopulmonary bypass
Fat embolism	Pancreatitis	Anaphylaxis
Smoke inhalation		

TABLE 5.16 Scoring system for acute lung injury

Component	Assign value
Chest X-ray appearance	
No alveolar consolidation	0
Alveolar consolidation in 1 quadrant	1
Alveolar consolidation in 2 quadrants	2
Alveolar consolidation in 3 quadrants	3
Alveolar consolidation all 4 quadrants	4
Hypoxaemia score (PaO_2/FiO_2 mmHg)*	
>300	0
225–299	1
175–224	2
100–174	3
<100	4
Compliance (mL/cmH$_2$O)	
>80	0
>60	1
>40	2
>20	3
<20	4
PEEP (cmH$_2$O)	
<5	0
6–8	1
9–11	2
12–14	3
>15	4

Score generated by dividing sum of component values by number of components used

Score = 0	No lung injury
Score < 2.5	Mild to moderate lung injury
Score > 2.5	Severe lung injury (ARDS)

Source: Murray JF, Matthay MA, Luce JM, Flick MR 1989 *American Review of Respiratory Disease* **139**: 1065.
* for kPa divide by 7.5

Although used primarily as a research tool, a scoring system for grading the severity of ALI/ARDS has been devised. This is shown in Table 5.16.

Management
Severe ARDS is associated with a high mortality ranging from approximately 25 to 80% in different series. The best outcomes

have been reported from centres using strict protocols for management. In general:

- Treat the underlying cause, as appropriate.
- Institute invasive cardiovascular monitoring (arterial line, CVP, pulmonary artery catheter or equivalent) and use inotropes/vasopressors as appropriate to optimize CO, perfusion pressure and oxygen delivery.
- Artificial ventilation is usually necessary. Reduced pulmonary compliance results in high inflation pressures, which are associated with increased risks of barotrauma. Current ventilatory strategies are intended to limit ventilator-associated lung damage while providing for alveolar recruitment. Pressure control ventilation, with longer inspiratory times (reversed I:E ratio) may be used to limit peak airway pressure. Tidal volumes should not exceed 6 mL/kg. Increased levels of PEEP are used to promote alveolar recruitment and improve oxygenation (see Ventilation strategy, p. 127).
- The FiO_2 should be kept to the minimum necessary to maintain acceptable oxygenation (PaO_2 7–8 kPa, $SaO_2 \geq 90\%$) in order to reduce lung damage associated with oxygen toxicity. Moderate levels of hypercapnia may be tolerated (permissive hypercapnia) if excessive ventilatory pressures would otherwise be required.
- BAL should be performed to identify infection, and, if appropriate, antibiotics started.
- Although in ARDS pulmonary oedema is classically thought of as non-cardiogenic, these patients often have multiple organ failure. It is estimated that 25% may develop myocardial failure, and fluid overload is common. Diuretics may be given to 'dry' the patient and may help to reduce the extent of pulmonary oedema.

Nitric oxide

Nitric oxide is a naturally occurring vasodilator produced by the endothelium of blood vessels. If added to the inspiratory gases in concentrations of 5–20 v.p.m., it results in pulmonary vasodilatation in those areas of the lung that are well ventilated. Blood is diverted away from poorly ventilated areas. Ventilation–perfusion mismatch is reduced and there is an improvement in oxygenation. At the same time pulmonary hypertension and the risk of right heart failure is reduced. Nitric oxide has a short half-life when inhaled and is generally safe for the patient. It is, however, a toxic gas, and should only be used according to the protocols established in your unit. Although nitric oxide may produce an improvement in oxygenation and therefore allow reduced FiO_2 and airway pressures, there is little evidence that it improves outcome.

Prone positioning

Turning the patient prone may improve V/Q mismatch and blood gases. The response in individual patients is unpredictable. The benefit tends to be temporary (24–48 h) and patients may need to be turned alternately prone and supine. The risks of turning large patients include injury to staff and the patient, accidental tracheal extubation, and loss of venous access, chest drains, etc. There is little evidence to show improved outcome. (See Practical procedures, p. 425.)

ECMO

Extracorporeal membrane oxygenation is a technique that allows oxygenation to be maintained while the lungs recover. The benefits are well recognized in neonatal and paediatric practice, but are less well established in adult practice, although a recent study in adults has reported favourable results [Conventional ventilation or ECMO for Severe Adult Respiratory Failure (CESAR) Trial. www.cesar-trial.org]. In the UK, ECMO is only provided in a limited number of centres and the transfer of patients with severe hypoxaemia is hazardous. Evidence suggests that to be of benefit it should be started within 5–7 days of artificial ventilation being commenced.

Steroids in ARDS

The traditional view was that therapeutic doses of steroids were of no benefit in ARDS. Despite a resurgence of interest in the use of steroids in ARDS, there is currently little evidence for any outcome advantage from therapeutic (high) dose steroids either in the acute or convalescent phase of illness.

Outcome from ALI/ARDS

Mortality in patients with ARDS is high; however, many of these patients die from the effects of multiple organ failure rather than directly from hypoxaemia. Lung function in survivors of ALI/ARDS often slowly improves over weeks or months but in severe cases lasting lung damage may persist.

CHEST X-RAY INTERPRETATION

The combination of tracheal intubation or tracheostomy and IPPV makes interpretation of classic respiratory signs in the noisy environment of the ICU very difficult. The CXR therefore assumes additional importance when evaluating the patient's condition.

You must be able to recognize the typical abnormal appearances seen in intensive care, particularly those that relate to complications of procedures. It is best, therefore, to have a standard system for evaluating the chest X-ray:

- Check name, date and orientation of film. The normal CXR orientation is posteroanterior (PA). That is, the X-rays are passed through the patient from behind towards the film, which is in front. Films taken in intensive care are generally anteroposterior (AP). This alters the magnification of structures.
- Check penetration and rotation of film.
- Check mediastinal structures, including cardiac shadow, lung hilum and pulmonary vessels.
- Check lung fields. Note position of diaphragms.
- Check bones and soft tissues.

All tracheal tubes, central venous and pulmonary artery catheters, nasogastric tubes and any drains visible by CXR should be checked for both correct placement and evidence of complications. In particular, note the following:

- Endotracheal tube, correct position above the carina, not endobronchial.
- Central venous catheters. Check intrathoracic placement with the tip positioned in a site consistent with the superior vena cava, above the pericardial reflection (see p. 376).
- Pulmonary artery catheter. Check tip lying in the pulmonary artery, preferably on the right side and not too distal (within 2 cm of edge of the spinal column).
- Nasogastric tube in the stomach.

A number of CXR patterns are common in intensive care.

Consolidation and collapse

These terms are often used incorrectly and even interchangeably. The X-ray appearances of consolidation and collapse are, however, quite distinct (Fig. 5.4).

Typical features of consolidation are:

- opacification of a lobe or segment (may be patchy)
- no loss of lung volume
- mediastinal and diaphragmatic borders partially preserved
- air bronchograms may be present.

Typical features of collapse include:

- loss of volume on side of collapse
- compensatory hyperinflation of remaining lobes

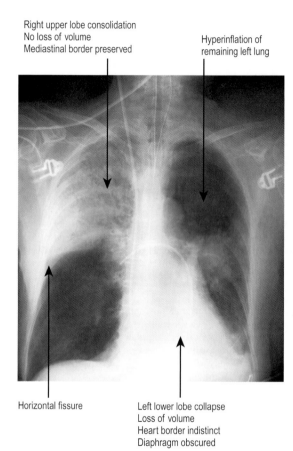

Right upper lobe consolidation
No loss of volume
Mediastinal border preserved

Hyperinflation of
remaining left lung

Horizontal fissure

Left lower lobe collapse
Loss of volume
Heart border indistinct
Diaphragm obscured

Fig. 5.4 Chest X-ray features of collapse and consolidation.

- shift of mediastinal structures towards side of collapse
- cardiac and diaphragmatic boarders obscured.

Collapse of a lung

An extreme example of collapse is collapse of an entire lung. In intubated and ventilated patients this may occur as a result of obstruction of the bronchus (e.g. by mucus plugging) or following endobronchial intubation. The anatomy of the bronchial tree is such that endotracheal tubes are more likely to pass down

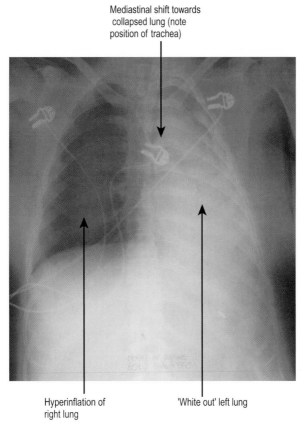

Mediastinal shift towards
collapsed lung (note
position of trachea)

Hyperinflation of
right lung

'White out' left lung

Fig. 5.5 Collapse of left lung.

the right main bronchus than the left. This commonly leads to collapse of the left lung, the typical appearances of which are shown in Fig. 5.5.

Pleural effusion / haemothorax

The classic feature of a pleural effusion in an upright patient is that of uniform opacification in the pleural space, typically obscuring the costodiaphragmatic recess, with an obvious meniscus or fluid level. In critically ill patients, CXRs are generally taken with the patient supine, often in the presence of positive

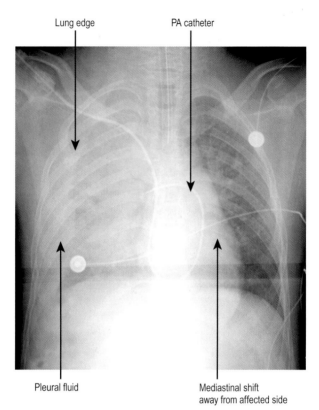

Lung edge   PA catheter

Pleural fluid

Mediastinal shift
away from affected side

Fig. 5.6 Chest X-ray appearances of pleural effusion.

pressure ventilation or CPAP. Therefore the classic appearance of pleural effusion may be missed. The only evidence of a small or moderate pleural effusion may be a general white haze to the whole lung field (imagine the fluid lying posteriorly in the pleural space). Larger effusions may have classic features or may present with a 'white-out' of that side, with shift of mediastinal structures towards the other side (Fig. 5.6).

Pneumothorax

Pneumothorax should be suspected in any patient who deteriorates while on a ventilator, particularly if there is associated trauma or

Air in pleural space

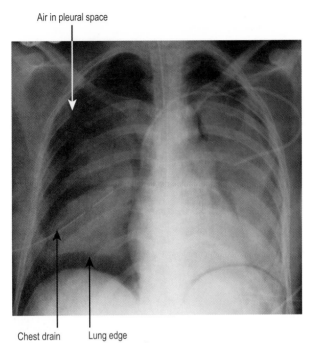

Chest drain   Lung edge

Fig. 5.7 Chest X-ray showing bilateral pneumothorax with lung edge. Right lung has not expanded despite chest drain. Check drain not blocked or kinked (presence of respiratory swing). Consider low suction. Similar changes on left but less marked.

recent insertion of a tracheostomy, central line or other practical procedure in the chest or neck. The typical appearances are that of a visible lung edge and translucent free air in the pleural space, as shown in Fig. 5.7.

The appearance may not, however, always be so obvious. In the critically ill supine patient with a small pneumothorax, free air may lie anteriorly over the lung and there may be no visible lung edge on CXR. (This is analogous to small pleural effusions lying posteriorly.) The only evidence may be that of an increased translucency (blackness) anteriorly, as shown in Fig. 5.8. If in doubt a lateral CXR or CT scan may help.

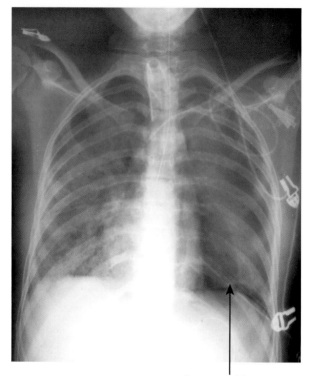

Appearance of free
air anteriorly in
pleural space

Fig. 5.8 Chest X-ray appearance of anterior pneumothorax.

Surgical emphysema and mediastinal air

Air may leak outside the pleural cavity, presenting as surgical emphysema and/or as mediastinal air on CXR. Surgical emphysema typically develops in the face, neck, mediastinum, pericardium, abdomen and scrotum and has a 'tissue paper' feel on palpation. It is visible on X-ray as black air shadows in the soft tissues of the upper body and chest wall, often outlining the pectoral muscles. Mediastinal air is visible on CXR as black translucent areas usually outlining the mediastinal shadows.

Pulmonary oedema

Pulmonary oedema is common on the intensive care unit and may indicate heart failure, fluid overload or evidence of acute lung injury. There is a spectrum from mild interstitial oedema to gross alveolar shadowing. Features include:

- interstitial shadowing (Kerley B lines)
- perihilar shadowing
- alveolar shadowing
- fluid in fissures (particularly horizontal fissure)
- Pleural effusions.

ALI / ARDS

The CXR appearances of ALI and ARDS are not specific. The common response to lung injury is leaking of capillaries, accumulation of alveolar fluid and subsequent development of areas of collapse and consolidation. The features are therefore a combination of those described above. A typical example is shown in Fig. 5.9.

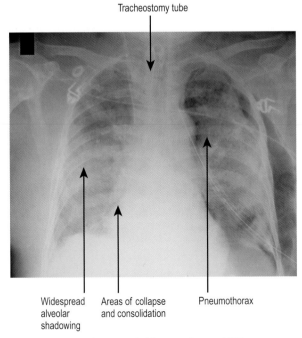

Tracheostomy tube

Widespread alveolar shadowing

Areas of collapse and consolidation

Pneumothorax

Fig. 5.9 Chest X-ray showing typical features of severe ARDS.

CHAPTER 6

GASTROINTESTINAL SYSTEM

Gastrointestinal tract in
  critical illness   168

Reduced gastrointestinal
  motility   170

Diarrhoea   170

Stress ulceration   172

Gastrointestinal
  ischaemia   172

Gastrointestinal
  bleeding   172

Intra-abdominal
  sepsis   174

Abdominal compartment
  syndrome   174

Hepatic dysfunction during
  critical illness   176

Hepatic failure   176

Acute pancreatitis   181

GASTROINTESTINAL TRACT IN CRITICAL ILLNESS

The gastrointestinal tract plays a major role in the pathophysiology of critical illness. In addition, to being a common site for surgical intervention and a common source of intra-abdominal sepsis, the gut is pivotal during critical illness in a number of ways:

- As a large 'third space' for fluid loss within the lumen of the gut.
- As a bed for altered blood flow (AV shunting) during shock states.
- As a reservoir for bacteria and endotoxins, which may translocate into the portal, lymphatic and systemic circulations, producing systemic inflammatory response syndrome, sepsis and multiorgan failure, particularly during periods of altered blood flow. (See Sepsis, p. 326).
- As a reservoir for bacteria which may colonize/infect the respiratory tract. (See Ventilator associated pneumonia, p. 143)
- As a site of secondary nosocomial infections e.g. *Clostridium difficile*.
- The maintenance of gastrointestinal integrity and function is therefore of major importance during critical illness.

Maintenance of gastrointestinal tract integrity

The pathophysiology of gastrointestinal integrity is complex. Maintenance of adequate splanchnic blood flow is thought to play a key part. In this respect, early aggressive resuscitation in shock states is crucial. Several studies have shown that both volume resuscitation and the maintenance of adequate perfusion pressure using vasopressor agents are independently important. In the 'Rivers study', early effective resuscitation, as guided by optimization of mixed venous oxygen saturation (a good surrogate for adequacy of tissue oxygen supply), was shown to reduce the patient's stay in the intensive care unit, reduce the number of organ failures and reduce eventual mortality in patients undergoing early resuscitation in sepsis. Importantly, resuscitation goals had to be achieved early (i.e. within the first 6 h). In those patients who are adequately resuscitated, early enteral nutrition may also be of value in helping to preserve mucosal integrity and gastrointestinal function.

Manifestations of gastrointestinal tract failure

Failure of the gastrointestinal tract during critical illness may present in a number of ways. These are listed in Box 6.1.

The principle aim of investigation of gastrointestinal dysfunction in the critically ill patients is to exclude serious, remediable,

---

Box 6.1 Clinical features of gastrointestinal tract failure

Delayed gastric emptying

Failure to absorb feed

Ileus, pseudo-obstruction

Diarrhoea

Stress ulceration

Gastrointestinal tract haemorrhage

Gastrointestinal ischaemia

Acalculous cholecystitis

Liver dysfunction

Systemic inflammatory response syndrome

---

intra-abdominal pathology. In some cases, the combination of history, clinical examination and blood results in the context of the overall clinical picture will suffice. In many cases however, intra-abdominal imaging will be required. Occasionally laparotomy or laparoscopy may be necessary to exclude serious pathology.

Plain abdominal X-rays

This is a first-line investigation in most cases. Check the position of the nasogastric tube and any other intra-abdominal drains. Look for gastric air and normally distributed gas pattern throughout the large bowel. Check for distended loops of thickened bowel walls and for any air bubbles visible in the gut walls (implies ischaemic gut). Check outline of major viscera and psoas shadow. Look for free air, suggesting perforation of a viscus, and air in the biliary tree, suggestive of biliary tract sepsis.

Ultrasound

This is a valuable imaging technique, which can be performed at the bedside. It is particularly useful for imaging around the liver, biliary tract, kidneys, spleen and pelvic organs and can be used to identify intra-abdominal collections of fluid for drainage. It may be difficult to obtain good images because of obesity or the presence of excessive gas in the bowel.

CT scan

This is the definitive investigation for most acute intra-abdominal problems. CT generally requires oral and intravenous contrast. Its value may be limited in the very unstable patient by the need to transport the patient to the CT scanner. Images require expert interpretation.

REDUCED GASTROINTESTINAL MOTILITY

Delayed gastric emptying and persistent ileus

Failure of gut motility is common in the critically ill. It is usually manifest as a simple ileus, with large nasogastric losses and failure to absorb feed. It will usually improve spontaneously as the patient's condition improves. Ensure that the patient's electrolyte balance is normal. Disturbances of potassium and magnesium in particular can contribute to gastrointestinal tract dysfunction. Prokinetic agents such as metoclopramide and low dose erythromycin may promote motility

Rarely, cholinergic agents such as neostigmine may be required, either as a low dose bolus (up to 1 mg) or by infusion. Neostigmine has potentially alarming cardiovascular and systemic side-effects, including abdominal pain, salivation and bradycardia. Do not embark upon this treatment lightly, and only if you are certain that there is no mechanical gut obstruction. Seek advice from your consultant.

(See Common problem: Feed not absorbed, p. 59.)

Pseudo-obstruction

Occasionally ileus will progress to marked intra-abdominal distension, with obvious signs of gut obstruction in the absence of any apparent mechanical cause. This is called pseudo-obstruction. The diagnosis is supported by plain abdominal X-ray or CT, which shows widely dilated loops of bowel.

If the colon is distended to greater than 10–12 cm in cross-section, there is a risk of colonic rupture. The use of prokinetic agents in this setting may be hazardous, and mechanical decompression is usually necessary to prevent colonic rupture. This may be achieved by flexible sigmoidoscopy, or may require surgical intervention. Seek surgical opinion.

DIARRHOEA

Diarrhoea is a common manifestation of gastrointestinal tract failure in the intensive care unit and may arise in a number of ways

- As a manifestation of multisystem disorder. For example, generalized tissue hypoxia, tissue oedema and vascular endothelial failure affect the function of all tissues. The gut is no exception to this. These pathological abnormalities are associated with a failure in cellular function and metabolic pathways, which may persist for some time. Consequently, gut failure (either diarrhoea or constipation) is often a characteristic feature of the patient in the intensive care unit.

- As a result of the osmotic load placed on the gut. This may reflect overfeeding, or feeding with a diet whose electrolyte composition is unsuitable for a particular patient.
- As a consequence of more sinister conditions, such as ischaemic colitis.
- As a consequence of infection with a gut pathogen. This is a particular problem in intensive care patients, as the widespread use of broad-spectrum antibiotics suppresses the normal gut flora and allows the emergence and predominance of potentially pathogenic organisms such as *Clostridium difficile.*

Clostridium difficile

Clostridium difficile is a spore forming organism that produces an enterotoxin. *Clostridium difficile* infection is a serious problem, as in addition to torrential diarrhoea, it gives rise to an inflammatory condition in the gut which results in pseudomembranous colitis, and potentially toxic megacolon and gut perforation. The diagnosis can be made on clinical grounds, by stool culture or by detection of the *Clostridium difficile* toxin. Additionally, pseudomembranes may be visible on sigmoidoscopy, or gut dilatation on X-ray (toxic megacolon).

   Clostridium difficile is readily transmitted from patient to patient. It is transmitted by contact, for example on the hands of health care workers. Unfortunately, because it is a spore forming organism, it is resistant to decontamination by alcohol hand rub. Rigorous hand washing using soap and water is much more effective. Patients suffering from *Clostridium difficile* diarrhoea, should be barrier nursed while in the critical care unit.

   The specific treatment of *Clostridium difficile* relies on appropriate antibiotics. You should seek guidance from your unit microbiologist, as local infection control policies are an important element in limiting the spread of this pernicious infection. Antibiotics that are most commonly effective (usually enterally) include metronidazole and vancomycin. Occasional patients may require a colectomy.

Management of diarrhoea

Supportive measures include:

- Fluid resuscitation if evidence of hypovolaemia.
- Replacement of on-going losses with an appropriate electrolyte solution usually 0.9% or 0.45% saline.
- Sending of stool samples for culture and *Clostridium difficile* toxin.

In mild cases enteral feed can be continued. Seek advice from a dietician as to the most appropriate feed. In severe cases consideration should be given to 'resting the gut' by stopping enteral feeds and instituting parenteral nutrition.

STRESS ULCERATION

Stress ulceration may occur anywhere in the gastrointestinal tract but, is most common in the duodenum and stomach. Bleeding from ulceration is common and may present as obvious haematemesis or as an unexplained fall in haemoglobin. Perforation needs to be considered in any patient with abdominal signs who deteriorates, and is suggested by the presence of free air on a plain abdominal X-ray or CT.

Stress ulceration is thought to be primarily due to inadequacy of mucosal blood flow, although concurrent use of non-steroidal anti-inflammatory drugs is a risk factor. General resuscitation measures including adequate fluid loading and maintenance of adequate perfusion pressures, together with early feeding, are more important than prophylactic measures.

(See Stress ulcer prophylaxis, p. 62.)

GASTROINTESTINAL ISCHAEMIA

This should be considered as a possible cause of deterioration, particularly in the elderly patient with pre-existing vascular disease or vasculitis. Systemic inflammatory response, oliguria, persistent acidosis, raised amylase and bloody diarrhoea may all occur but none is specific. Thickened loops of bowel with gas present in the wall may be seen on plain abdominal X-ray. CT scan may be helpful, but the diagnosis is usually made at laparotomy. Treatment requires resection of the ischaemic bowel. Difficulty at laparotomy in determining the demarcation between viable and non-viable bowel often necessitates a 'second look' laparotomy at 24–48 h. Extensive infarction is often fatal.

GASTROINTESTINAL BLEEDING

Slow bleeding from the gastrointestinal tract may occur, and is a common cause of reduced haemoglobin in the critically ill. Less commonly, but of greater immediate concern is acute massive GIT haemorrhage, which may be life threatening. The source is usually the upper GIT. Common causes are listed in Box 6.2.

> **Box 6.2 Causes of upper gastrointestinal tract haemorrhage**
>
> Duodenal ulceration
> Gastric erosion and ulceration
> Oesophageal varices
> Portal gastropathy/gastric varices
> Aortoenteric fistulae
> AV malformations
> Other small bowel lesions

Bleeding of this sort can result in haematemesis, melaena or even frank rectal blood loss. Lower GIT bleeding is less common, but may still be life threatening.

Clinical features

The history may be suggestive of the underlying diagnosis; predisposing factors include previous peptic ulceration, non-steroidal anti-inflammatory drugs (NSAIDs), corticosteroids, anticoagulants, liver disease, portal hypertension and critical illness. Brisk GI bleeding is complicated by hypovolaemic shock and oliguria. Myocardial ischaemia may occur. Patients with liver disease develop worsening encephalopathy. Patients with reduced conscious level are at risk of aspiration pneumonia.

Investigations

Full blood count and cross-match are followed by regular monitoring of haemodynamic status, urine output, haemoglobin, coagulation and electrolytes. The site of the bleeding may be identified by endoscopy or arteriography.

Management

- Large-bore vascular access is obtained and resuscitation of hypovolaemia commenced. In massive bleeds full haemodynamic monitoring, including arterial line, CVP or some other measure of volume status, are valuable.
- Coagulopathy should be corrected.
- Analgesics and anxiolytics are used judiciously in conscious patients. Massive bleeds, however, frequently necessitate intubation and ventilation.
- Endoscopy allows injection of bleeding ulcers and banding or sclerotherapy of varices. The co-administration of a proton

pump inhibitor (e.g. omeprazole 40 mg once or twice daily) is frequently all that is required to prevent recurrence.

- Persistent uncontrollable GI bleeding may necessitate surgery. Radiological embolization of actively bleeding vessels may occasionally be useful.

Variceal bleeding

Persistent variceal bleeding carries a high mortality (up to 50% from a first presentation). In addition to the above, management includes:

- Use of a Linton or Sengstaken – Blakemore tube to compress varices in the gastric fundus.
- The administration of vasopressin (up to 20 units by s.c. injection or slow i.v. infusion: beware vasopressor effects) and octreotide to reduce portal hypertension.
- Endoscopy and variceal banding once bleeding is controlled.

If these measures are ineffective, portosystemic shunting will be required. Transhepatic intravenous portosystemic shunt (TIPSS) is a radiological procedure that has a lower mortality than surgical shunt procedures, but is not considered definitive. Surgical options include splenorenal shunting, mesocaval shunting, oesophageal transection and liver transplantation. These interventions carry a high mortality.

(See Practical procedures: Sengstaken–Blakemore tube, p. 422.)

INTRA-ABDOMINAL SEPSIS

Subphrenic, pelvic and other intra-abdominal collections are an ever-present threat in critically ill patients, particularly following any intra-abdominal surgery. The clinical signs and symptoms may be vague. Persistent ileus, with failure to absorb feeds, 'grumbling sepsis' and altered liver function tests, should raise suspicion. Wound infections, urinary tract infections and genital tract infection should all be considered.

Assessment is by clinical examination followed by ultrasound or CT imaging. Management depends on the clinical condition of the patient. Options include radiologically guided drainage or open surgical drainage.

ABDOMINAL COMPARTMENT SYNDROME

The presence of blood, free fluid or gas in the abdominal cavity, splanchnic and tissue oedema and organomegally can lead to a progressive increase in the intra-abdominal pressure and to decreased splanchnic perfusion. This may result in gut, renal and liver hypoperfusion with associated clinical features. If suspected, intra-abdominal pressure can be measured via an indwelling urinary catheter (Fig. 6.1).

Normal intra-abdominal pressure is less than 15–20 mmHg. Intra-abdominal pressures above 20 mmHg with evidence of end organ dysfunction are suggestive of abdominal compartment syndrome. Decompression of the abdomen may be required. Seek surgical advice. Once opened, it may be impossible to close the abdomen at first laparotomy. The abdomen may be left 'open' under sterile plastic coverings for later closure when the swelling has subsided.

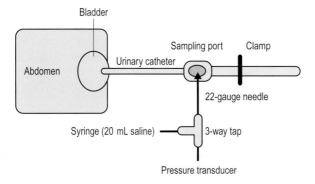

Technique
1 Clamp urinary catheter distal to sampling port.
2 Insert needle through sampling port and inject 20 mL of saline to distend the bladder and provide a continuous column of fluid between bladder and sampling point (bladder distends without increases in pressure).
3 Turn 3-way tap to connect pressure transducer. Allow pressure reading to settle and record pressure (note convention transducer zeroed to mid-axillary line).
   Bladder acts as a manometer, reflecting intra-abdominal pressure.
4 Aspirate 20 mL from the bladder, remove needle and release clamp.

Fig. 6.1 Measurement of intra-abdominal pressure via urinary catheter.

HEPATIC DYSFUNCTION DURING CRITICAL ILLNESS

Liver dysfunction (as opposed to liver failure) is common during critical illness, particularly in association with severe shock states in which there is relative splanchnic and liver hypoperfusion. It is characterized by progressive rise in bilirubin, abnormalities of liver enzymes, coagulopathy with raised prothrombin time (PT) and delayed drug metabolism. Ultrasound or CT scan should be performed to exclude localized collections of infected fluid or biliary tract obstruction. The management is essentially supportive. Hepatotoxic drugs should be stopped. Liver function should improve as the patient's general condition improves.

Cholestasis and cholangitis

Cholestasis is common in the critically ill, particularly in the absence of enteral feed, and may result in jaundice. The alkaline phosphatase may be raised. This usually resolves as the patient's condition improves and enteral feeds are established. Abdominal ultrasound and endoscopic retrograde cholangiopancreatography (ERCP) may be necessary to exclude mechanical causes of biliary obstruction. Agents such as ursodeoxycholic acid may be used but there is little evidence for their benefit. Occasionally cholestasis leads to ascending cholangitis, which may require antibiotic treatment.

Acalculous cholecystitis

Rarely, critically ill patients may develop an acute, necrotizing inflammation of the gallbladder, known as acalculous cholecystitis. The aetiology of this is multifactorial, but includes bile stasis and splanchnic hypoperfusion. It should be considered in any patient with right upper quadrant pain, jaundice, raised alkaline phosphatase, abdominal signs and evidence of sepsis. There is no definitive test. Abdominal ultrasound or CT may demonstrate an enlarged, oedematous gallbladder with thickened wall and free fluid around the site. Management options include CT-guided drainage and acute cholecystectomy. Seek surgical opinion.

HEPATIC FAILURE

Liver failure is defined as hyperacute where the onset of encephalopathy occurs within 7 days of the onset of jaundice, acute where the interval is 7–28 days, and subacute where it is between 28 days and 6 months. Longer intervals represent chronic liver failure. The term fulminant liver failure refers to an earlier classification where encephalopathy occurs within 8 weeks of the onset of jaundice. It thus encompasses acute and hyperacute liver failure.

Aetiology

The commonest cause worldwide remains hepatitis B. In the UK, this is second to paracetamol poisoning. Other common causes include hepatitis A, drug idiosyncrasy and non-A non-B viral hepatitis. (Note: this does not equate to hepatitis C, which is not thought to be a cause of fulminant liver failure. Up to 20% of cases may, however, be hepatitis E.)

Pathophysiology

The final common pathway is hepatocellular failure, with a reduction or loss of the synthetic, homeostatic and filter functions of the liver. This results in a failure of carbohydrate metabolism, depletion of glycogen stores and consequent hypoglycaemia. Deranged amino acid metabolism results in accumulation of ammonia and other intermediate compounds, which account in part for the development of encephalopathy.

Protein synthesis is arrested, and this includes the synthesis of albumin and clotting factors. Coagulopathy is invariable. PT is the most sensitive index of hepatocellular failure and recovery. The coagulopathy may be exacerbated by activated fibrinolysis.

The filter (reticuloendothelial) functions of the hepatic Kupffer cells are central to the prevention of translocation of gut-derived endotoxin to the systemic circulation. In acute liver failure, there is systemic endotoxaemia. Further, the massive necrosis of hepatocytes releases high levels of tumour necrosis factor (TNF), platelet-activating factor (PAF) and other proinflammatory cytokines. Systemic inflammatory response syndrome (SIRS) and multisystem organ failure (MOF) follow. Moreover, there is a steep rise in circulating ammonia concentration. This is thought to mediate an increase in excitatory neurotransmitters in the central nervous system. The combination of these effects gives rise to failure of the blood–brain barrier, with cerebral oedema and altered consciousness (encephalopathy).

Clinical features

Hypoglycaemia is common and develops any time in the first few days of the condition. It gradually resolves as the

TABLE 6.1 Grading of hepatic encephalopathy	
Grade 0	Normal
Grade 1	Mild confusion (may not be immediately evident)
Grade 2	Drowsiness
Grade 3	Severe drowsiness, inappropriate words/phrases, grinding teeth
Grade 4	Unrousable

liver failure improves. Acid – base homeostasis is altered and either alkalosis or acidosis may complicate this. A metabolic acidosis is the more sinister. Concurrently with the development of the metabolic derangement, conscious level may become impaired. Encephalopathy is graded as in Table 6.1.

The onset of encephalopathy is followed in some patients by cerebral oedema and raised intracranial pressure (ICP). The risk of raised ICP is greatest in hyperacute liver failure (in excess of 50% of cases), and much lower in acute failure. It is much less common in subacute failure (around 4%). A baseline elevation in ICP up to 20–25 mmHg may be followed by surges, which are transient but severe (up to 80–90 mmHg). This stage may be followed by inexorably rising ICP and brain death.

The haemodynamics of SIRS develop as conscious level reaches grade III–IV. The characteristic hypotension is associated with a high cardiac index and low systemic vascular resistance. Vasodilatation and increased capillary permeability contribute to reduced circulating volume and may predispose to renal failure. Acute tubular necrosis may also occur as a result of SIRS or directly as a result of the precipitating insult, e.g. paracetamol-induced renal damage.

The coagulopathy seldom gives rise to de novo bleeding, even though very high PT values are seen (>100 s). Generalized oozing around cannulation sites is common but is seldom of great significance. Thrombocytopenia may also occur, either due to DIC or hypersplenism. It is occasionally necessary to perform invasive procedures under platelet cover.

True 'infective' sepsis may occur. A rising WCC, falling platelet count, a PT whose recovery becomes arrested or a worsening acidosis should all be regarded as suspicious.

Management

> ⚠ **Acute hepatic failure carries a high mortality and treatment options include transplantation. Early discussion with a specialist centre is therefore mandatory.**

- The development of grade III–IV encephalopathy or the onset of SIRS is an indication for tracheal intubation and mechanical ventilation. This protects the airway, reduces the work of breathing and protects against the risk of secondary hypoxic damage.
- Fluid and haemodynamic management is guided by invasive monitoring. Maintain adequate filling to ensure optimal CO while avoiding the risk of interstitial oedema of the lung, brain and gut.
- Noradrenaline (norepinephrine) is used to keep the mean arterial pressure above 70–80 mmHg and the CPP >50 mmHg (see below).
- Renal failure can make fluid balance difficult. Continuous renal replacement therapy is frequently necessary, but is often associated with transient haemodynamic instability and ICP surges.
- All patients should receive continuous N-acetylcysteine infusion (100 mg/kg per 24 h). This has been shown to improve outcome in fulminant liver failure irrespective of aetiology, even when instituted relatively late in the disease process.
- Stress ulcer prophylaxis with an H_2 antagonist or proton pump inhibitor should be prescribed.
- Prevention of sepsis is a major problem. Prophylactic antibiotics should be discussed with a microbiologist. Selective decontamination of the digestive tract is practised in some centres, but is probably of marginal value.

> ⚠ **The prothrombin time (PT) is one of the key prognostic factors determining whether the optimal treatment of acute liver failure is likely to be medical or surgical. Therefore, do not treat coagulopathy (by, for example, giving fresh frozen plasma) except in cases of life threatening haemorrhage.**

Metabolic issues

- Hypoglycaemia is common. All infusions should be made up in dextrose solutions (5–20%), and dextrose (5–50%) infused to maintain a normal blood sugar.
- Nitrogenous feeds are avoided (no TPN or nasogastric feed should be administered until metabolic resolution of acute liver failure).

- Sodium and potassium are maintained within the normal range; this may involve judicious use of potassium infusions at 10–40 mmol/h.
- The liver is unable to metabolize citrate used as an anticoagulant in blood products. Consequently, persisting citrate chelates calcium, and may drastically reduce ionized calcium levels. Calcium chloride 10 mmol may be given by slow bolus to maintain the ionized calcium to above 0.8 mmol/L.
- Metabolic acidosis is a useful prognostic indicator and is in any case best left untreated on theoretical grounds. The exception to this is where a severe acidosis is associated with haemodynamic instability. It is acceptable to correct the pH slowly to 7.2 if this improves the haemodynamic status. Rapid correction of acidosis with boluses of sodium bicarbonate should be avoided. The use of sodium bicarbonate can result in a transient dramatic elevation in the carbon dioxide tension, with consequent cerebral vasodilatation and a surge in ICP.

Control of ICP
- Nurse patient at a 20° head-up tilt.
- Keep physiotherapy, tracheal suctioning and turning to a minimum until the risk of ICP surges resolves (usually 5 days after the onset of grade IV encephalopathy).
- Ensure adequate sedation and paralysis.
- Primary surges in ICP (often followed by a reflex rise in arterial pressure) are treated acutely by hyperventilation. The response to hyperventilation is not maintained, so it should be discontinued as soon as a fall in ICP is seen. Mannitol 20% 100 ml is used to sustain the reduction in ICP and also where the baseline ICP remains above 25 mmHg. Other hyperosmolar therapies, for example hyperosmolar saline are also of value. The use of these agents should be discussed with your regional centre.
- Cooling the patient and liver support systems have been shown to help control ICP.

Even where the ICP remains very high, a good neurological outcome is possible provided CPP is maintained at or above 40–50 mmHg.

Prognosis
Without transplantation, the prognosis is poorest in the subacute group and best in the hyperacute group. Within this group, the prognosis is poorer in those at the extremes of age, those with non-A, non-B hepatitis and drug dyscrasia. The overall mortality in patients with grade IV encephalopathy is 70%.

With liver transplantation (i.e. in those patients at the highest risk of death with optimal medical management), the 1-year mortality is between 30 and 50%.

ACUTE PANCREATITIS

Inflammation of the pancreas and autodigestion may be precipitated by a number of triggers, some of which are listed in Box 6.3. The commonest causes are alcohol and biliary obstruction. Frequently no cause can be identified.

Clinical features

A spectrum of severity exists from mild pain to severe shock. Epigastric pain radiating to the back and a history of risk factors (including previous episodes) suggest the diagnosis. Examination may reveal flank discoloration (Grey – Turner sign) and peritonism. SIRS, ARDS, coagulopathy and renal failure may develop. The action of digestive enzymes on fat leads to 'soap formation' hypocalcaemia and hypomagnesaemia. Diabetes mellitus arising de novo may be permanent.

Investigations

A raised serum amylase ($>1000\,IU/1$) is diagnostic but is often absent. Values in the range 100–1000 suggest alternative intra-abdominal pathologies, including perforated viscus. CT imaging investigation of first choice. MRI is also useful in more difficult cases. Culture of aspirated fluid can be used to guide surgical drainage, i.e. if heavily infected indication for surgery or drainage.

Localized posterior perforations of duodenum or stomach may be difficult to distinguish. Chest and abdominal plain films should confirm the absence of free gas or pneumonia, and may show calcium deposition. In severe cases the typical radiographic

---

Box 6.3 Common causes of pancreatitis

Alcohol

Biliary obstruction (gallstones)/ERCP

Viral infection (CMV, EBV, etc.)

Surgical injury or trauma

Hypothermia

Cardiopulmonary bypass

Corticosteroids

Oral contraceptives

features of ARDS may be present. Plain film and ultrasound may confirm the presence of gallstones or other underlying biliary lesion. Blood glucose and arterial gases should be closely monitored. As the condition progresses, serial CT scanning is valuable to monitor pancreatic viability and to diagnose pancreatic cysts and pseudocysts.

Management

Severe cases should be referred to specialist centres. In milder cases supportive treatment and analgesia are the main requirements. Pethidine theoretically causes less spasm of the sphincter of Oddi than morphine. Hyperglycaemia is managed by sliding scale insulin infusion. Traditionally, the GI tract is rested by insertion of a nasogastric tube and regular drainage/aspiration. Total parenteral nutrition is frequently introduced early in the condition. These views are currently undergoing reappraisal; some studies suggest that very early enteral feeding reduces mortality.

In some centres, octreotide ($25\mu g$ hourly by infusion) or lanreotide are used to reduce exocrine activity. Patients who develop SIRS/ARDS require intubation, ventilation and haemodynamic optimization. These patients may benefit from antioxidant regimens. Acute renal failure may require renal replacement therapy. Particular attention should be paid to acid–base balance and electrolyte disorders. Repeated calcium, phosphate and magnesium supplementation are often required.

Pancreatic cyst/pseudocyst formation requires expert surgical intervention. Treatment may be conservative, by radiologically guided drainage, or by surgical excision. The latter may require repeated laparotomy for intra-abdominal sepsis.

The role of prophylactic antibiotics in severe pancreatitis has been widely debated and controversial in recent years. The best evidence currently available suggests that prophylactic use of antibiotics is associated with an increased mortality, and that antibiotic use should be guided according to culture results. Because pancreatitis is associated with a brisk SIRS response, it is tempting to introduce antibiotics in the absence of infection. This temptation should be resisted!

Prognosis

This depends on the severity and duration of the disease and the occurrence of complications including SIRS, ARDS and ARF. In general, the prognosis is poorer in the elderly, in those with pre-existing diabetes mellitus and those with alcohol-related disease.

CHAPTER 7

RENAL SYSTEM

Renal dysfunction in
  critical illness   184

Investigation of acute
  renal dysfunction   185

Oliguria   188

Management   188

Acute renal failure   189

Renal replacement
  therapy   190

Peritoneal dialysis   194

Outcome from acute
  renal failure in
  intensive care   195

Management of patients
  with chronic renal
  failure   195

Prescribing in renal
  failure   196

Plasma exchange   199

RENAL DYSFUNCTION IN CRITICAL ILLNESS

Renal dysfunction is common in the ICU and frequently occurs as part of a syndrome of multiple organ failure. The cause of renal dysfunction is often multifactorial. Pre-existing renal impairment may be worsened by the effects of critical illness, including release of cytokines, activation of inflammatory cascades, hypoperfusion, altered tissue oxygen delivery and extraction, and altered cellular function. In addition, many drugs used in intensive care are predictably nephrotoxic, while others have been implicated in idiosyncratic nephrotoxic reactions.

Classically, the causes of acute renal dysfunction are divided into prerenal (inadequate perfusion), renal (intrinsic renal disease) and postrenal (obstruction). These are summarized in Box 7.1.

Clinically, renal dysfunction is usually manifest as oliguria progressing to anuria, and so water retention is a key feature, although high-output renal failure, in which there are large volumes of poorly concentrated urine, may also occur. Renal dysfunction is associated with a reduction in creatinine clearance, and an accumulation of toxic molecules within the patient including potassium, urea, so called middle molecules and drug metabolites.

Three terms are commonly used in relation to different patterns of renal dysfunction/failure

Prerenal failure

This refers to decreased glomerular filtration rate (GFR) due to reduced renal perfusion. There is no tubular damage. May be reversed by adequate fluid resuscitation and reperfusion of the kidney.

Box 7.1 Causes of renal dysfunction*

Pre-renal	Renal	Post renal
Dehydration	Renovascular disease	Kidney outflow obstruction
Hypovolaemia	Autoimmune disease	Ureteric obstruction
Hypotension	SIRS and sepsis	Bladder outlet obstruction (blocked catheter)
	Hepatorenal syndrome	
	Crush injury (myoglobinuria)	
	Nephrotoxic drugs	

*In many patients the cause of renal failure will be multifactorial.

Acute tubular necrosis (ATN)

Decreased GFR is due to reduced perfusion, resulting in ischaemic renal tubular damage. There is no immediate reversal on restoration of perfusion, but it usually improves over time. This is the commonest pattern of ARF (requiring renal replacement therapy, e.g. haemofiltration) seen on ICU.

Acute cortical necrosis (ACN)

Total and irreversible loss of renal function results from severe prolonged ischaemia of kidneys. This is rare. It is seen occasionally in obstetric patients following placental abruption and haemorrhage where combination of a hypotension, hypercoagulable state and endothelial injury leads to thrombosis of renal vessels.

INVESTIGATION OF ACUTE RENAL DYSFUNCTION

In many cases, the causes of acute renal dysfunction in the ICU can be determined from knowledge of the clinical background of the patient, and by simple history and examination. Most cases of ARF will prove to be prerenal or ATN. Up to 10% of cases, however, will have other significant underlying pathologies.

History and examination

- Is there any indication of pre-existing renal disease? Vascular disease, diabetes, multisystem disease/vasculitis, chronic anaemia or previously abnormal U&Es are all suggestive. (Look for small shrunken kidneys on ultrasound or CT.)
- Is there any evidence for prerenal impairment, e.g. dehydration, hypovolaemia or hypotension?
- Is there any evidence for new intrinsic renal impairment, e.g. sepsis, nephrotoxic drugs?
- Is there any history or evidence of trauma or obstruction to the GU tract?

Investigations

Serum urea, electrolytes and creatinine
Serial measurements are used to monitor renal function and predict the need for renal replacement therapy. Avoid placing undue significance on single results. Take serial samples and look at trends.

Creatinine clearance

Creatinine clearance is a surrogate measure for glomerular filtration rate and may be required to guide dose reduction of drugs in renal failure. Creatinine clearance estimates are provided by a number of hospital laboratories based on formulae. These may, however, be misleading in critical illness, particularly where large fluid shifts and renal support are confounders. Formal assessment of creatinine clearance requires a 24-h urine collection, but may be extremely helpful. (See Prescribing in renal failure, p. 196.)

Urinary biochemistry

Urine output should be monitored hourly. A low urine output should alert suspicion, but is not pathognomonic of renal failure. Urine output should be interpreted in the context of urinary biochemistry. Three simple investigations are helpful in distinguishing prerenal from intrinsic renal failure:

● Urinary U&Es.
● Urine and plasma osmolality.
● Urine microscopy: are there casts, red cells, crystals?

Normal urine osmolality depends on the patient's hydration status, and may vary from hypo-osmolar (less than normal plasma osmolality 280 mosmol/L) to highly concentrated hyperosmolar (>1000 mosmol/L).

In prerenal failure, the kidney functions maximally to retain sodium and water in order to re-expand plasma volume. The urine sodium concentration is low and the urine is maximally concentrated, as indicated by high osmolality (600–900 mosmol/L), and a urine to plasma urea ratio greater than 10.

As ATN develops, the renal tubules are no longer able to function normally, and are unable to retain sodium or concentrate the urine. The urinary sodium rises, urinary osmolality falls, and the urine to plasma urea ratio also falls. Eventually the urinary sodium and osmolality approach that of plasma. Renal tubular debris or casts may be seen in the urine. The distinguishing features of prerenal and renal failure are summarized in Table 7.1.

Other investigations may be indicated depending on circumstances:

Creatine kinase (CK)/urinary myoglobin. A raised serum creatine kinase and raised urinary myoglobin (early sign only) are indicative of rhabdomyolysis, for example following trauma, crush injury (see Rhabdomyolysis, p. 320.)

TABLE 7.1 Distinguishing features of prerenal and renal failure

	Prerenal	Renal (ATN)
Urinary sodium*	<10 mmol/L	>30 mmol/L
Urinary osmolality*	High	Low
Urine : plasma urea ratio	>10:1	<8:1
Urine microscopy	Normal	Tubular casts

*If patients have received diuretics, urinary sodium and osmolality are difficult to interpret.

TABLE 7.2 Investigations for autoimmune disease in renal failure

Vasculitis	Antineutrophil cytoplasmic antibodies (ANCA)
Goodpasture's syndrome	Antiglomerular basement membrane antibodies
Systemic lupus erythematosus (SLE)	Antinuclear antibodies (ANA) Anti-double-stranded DNA antibodies
Rheumatoid disease	Rheumatoid factor

Vasculitis screen. Renal disease may be associated with autoimmune conditions and vasculitis. An autoimmune/vasculitis screen may be appropriate, particularly in the presence of coexisting pulmonary disease. Seek advice. Investigations are listed in Table 7.2.

Imaging. Plain abdominal films may show calcification or stones. Intravenous pyelogram (IVP) is not usually performed in ARF. Renal ultrasound may demonstrate small shrunken kidneys in cases with CRF and is useful to show obstruction (e.g. dilated ureters or renal pelvis). Although renal ultrasound is seldom indicated as an emergency investigation in the intensive care patient with renal failure, it should be a routine investigation during daylight hours to rule out renal obstruction or vascular causes.

CT scan with contrast may be useful in trauma/obstruction.

Renal biopsy and radioisotope perfusion scans may be useful in difficult cases.

OLIGURIA

Oliguria is defined as a urine output of less than $0.5\,\text{mL}\,\text{kg}^{-1}\,\text{h}^{-1}$ for at least 2 consecutive hours. Most cases of oliguria do not progress to ARF if adequate steps are taken.

- Review the biochemistry results. Is there evidence of deteriorating renal function over time (i.e. increasing serum urea and creatinine)?
- Review the clinical status of the patient. Is there evidence of dehydration/hypovolaemia suggested by: thirst, poor tissue turgor (pinch skin on back of hand), dry mouth, cool pale limbs, large respiratory swing on arterial line, low CVP or low stroke volume index?
- Are CO and blood pressure adequate?
- Is there any obvious cause for renal failure, e.g. chronic renal insufficiency, nephrotoxic drugs, rhabdomyolysis?
- Is there an occult source of sepsis?

MANAGEMENT

- If there is evidence of hypovolaemia, give a fluid challenge. Even if the patient is apparently normovolaemic it is generally worth giving a fluid challenge (e.g. 500 mL colloid). Any response may not be immediate. If there is no response consider the need for invasive monitoring to further assess volume status.
- Renal filtration is a pressure-dependent process. Elderly patients, in particular, those with hypertensive vascular disease, may require a higher than expected mean blood pressure. Consider the use of inotropes or vasopressors as appropriate to increase blood pressure towards the normal or preadmission blood pressure for the patient.
- If the cause of the oliguria is not clear from clinical evaluation and there is no response to simple measures, consider further investigations as above.
- Review the prescription chart. Decide whether to stop any potentially nephrotoxic drugs (aminoglycosides, non-steroidal anti-inflammatory drugs, immunosuppressant agents).
- Look for any sources of sepsis, necrotic muscle (rhabdomyolysis) and ischaemic gut.
- If the patient remains oliguric, give bumetanide 1–2 mg bolus i.v. or furosemide (frusemide) 20–40 mg bolus i.v. (bumetanide may be preferable to furosemide, as it does not need to be filtered by the glomerulus to achieve its effect). If there is a

response, consider the use of an infusion to maintain urine output: bumetanide 1–2 mg/h or furosemide 20–40 mg/h.

- If there is no response, consider high-dose diuretics, e.g. bumetanide 5 mg or furosemide 250 mg over 1 h, followed, if there is a response, by an infusion.
- If there is still no response, then ARF is established and renal replacement therapy is likely to be needed. Restrict fluid intake to the previous hour's urine output plus 30–50 mL to allow for insensible losses. Seek advice.

(See Renal replacement therapy, p. 190.)

ACUTE RENAL FAILURE

The management of patients in renal failure may benefit from a multidisciplinary approach. Seek senior advice and consider referral to renal physicians or your local renal unit.

Oliguric renal failure

The main problems associated with acute renal failure (ARF) are inability to excrete fluid, impaired acid–base regulation, hyperkalaemia and accumulation of waste products.

- Inability to excrete fluid may result in progressive fluid overload. This may be manifest as hypertension, tissue and pulmonary oedema.
- Impaired acid–base balance results in progressive accumulation of hydrogen ions and metabolic acidosis. This may be exacerbated by the effects of excess chloride load (from use of 0.9% sodium chloride containing fluids) resulting in hyperchloraemic acidosis (see hyperchloraemic acidosis, p. 53).
- Impaired excretion of potassium leads to hyperkalaemia. This can develop rapidly, particularly in critically ill patients, and is a medical emergency. Other problems of electrolyte disturbance include abnormalities of sodium, phosphate and calcium balance.
- Accumulation of creatinine, urea and other molecules may produce clouding of conscious level, metabolic encephalopathy and myocardial depression. GIT side effects include gastric stasis and ileus. Coagulopathy may result from effects on platelet function.

Control of hyperkalaemia

The main concern in the acute phase is the development of ventricular dysrhythmias associated with hyperkalaemia. Potassium levels can rise quickly in the presence of severe sepsis

Box 7.2 Indications for renal replacement therapy (RRT)

Acute	Within 24 h
$K^+ > 6.5$ mmol/L	Urea > 40–50 mmol/L and rising[*]
pH < 7.2	Creatinine $> 400 \mu$mol/L and rising[*]
Fluid overload/pulmonary oedema	Hypercatabolism, severe sepsis

[*]These are nominal values only, which are a guide to the probable need for RRT in acute illness. Patients in chronic renal failure will tolerate higher values. If values plateau and the patient is passing adequate volumes of urine, RRT may be delayed in the hope that renal function may recover.

and hypercatabolism. Patients with chronic renal failure (CRF) may tolerate hyperkalaemia much better than patients with ARF. A serum potassium greater than 6–6.5 mmol/L requires urgent treatment. Calcium, bicarbonate and dextrose/insulin buy time prior to dialysis but do not alter the underlying problem. (See Hyperkalaemia, p. 206.)

Indications for renal replacement therapy (RRT)

Typical indications for instituting renal replacement therapy in acute renal failure are shown in Box 7.2.

High output (non-oliguric) renal failure

This is characterized by rising serum urea and creatinine despite adequate urine volumes. Urine biochemistry demonstrates a failure to concentrate urine. Indications for dialysis are as for oliguric renal failure but there are generally fewer problems with high potassium and fluid overload. Non-oliguric renal failure is said to have a better outcome than oliguric renal failure. It often accompanies the recovery phase of ATN.

RENAL REPLACEMENT THERAPY

Patients with chronic renal failure who require long-term renal replacement therapy usually undergo intermittent haemodialysis 2 or 3 times a week or alternatively receive long-term peritoneal dialysis. These modes are inappropriate for critically ill patients during the acute phase of a critical illness in intensive care.

Intermittent haemodialysis is associated with significant haemodynamic instability in critically ill patients. Continuous renal replacement systems that allow more gradual correction of biochemical abnormalities and removal of fluid are therefore preferred, at least during the acute phase of the illness. These systems also have the advantage that they can be safely used outside specialist renal dialysis centres.

Continuous venovenous haemofiltration (CVVHF)

The simplest form of continuous renal replacement is continuous venovenous haemofiltration (Fig. 7.1).

Blood from the patient is passed through a filter, which allows plasma water, electrolytes and small molecular weight molecules to pass through down a pressure gradient. This filtrate is discarded and replaced by a balanced electrolyte solution. Typically 200–500 mL/h of filtrate are removed and replaced. Overall negative fluid balance can be achieved by replacing less fluid than is removed.

There has been a great deal of interest recently in the role of CVVHF in sepsis. Many of the proinflammatory molecules, toxins and cytokines, which are implicated in the pathogenesis of the systemic inflammatory response syndrome, are removed by haemofiltration. There is anecdotal evidence that some unstable

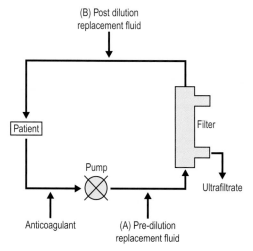

Fig. 7.1 Continuous venovenous haemofiltration. Replacement fluid may be delivered either (A) before the filter (pre-dilution) or (B) after the filter (post dilution). Pre-dilution may reduce clotting within the filter and prolong filter life.

patients have improved following the institution of CVVHF and many units now routinely haemofilter septic patients. There is some limited evidence that high volume haemofiltration, e.g. 2000 mL/h may stabilize the critically ill septic patient. (See Sepsis, p. 331.)

Continuous venovenous haemodialysis (CVVHD)

One problem with CVVHF is that clearance of small molecules and solutes is inefficient, and this can require large volumes of filtrate to be removed and replaced in order to achieve acceptable creatinine clearance.

In continuous haemodialysis (Fig. 7.2), dialysis fluid is passed over the filter membrane in a countercurrent manner. Fluids, electrolytes and small products can move in both directions across the filter, depending on hydrostatic pressure, ionic binding and osmotic gradients. Overall creatinine clearance is greatly improved compared with haemofiltration alone.

In CVVHD, provided the volume of dialysis fluid passing out from the system matches the volume of dialysis fluid passing in, there is no net gain or loss of fluid to the patient. By allowing more dialysate fluid to pass out of the filter than passes in, fluid can be effectively removed from the patient. Rates of fluid removal up to 200 mL/h can be achieved. In most CVVHD machines fluid removal is achieved by increasing the rate of the dialysis pump controlling the exit side of the filter by the amount of fluid to be removed (Fig. 7.2).

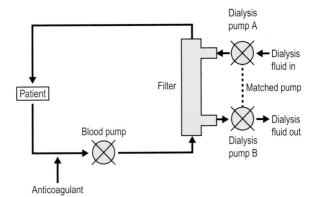

Fig. 7.2 Continuous venovenous haemodialysis (CVVHD). If dialysis machine is not set to remove any fluid, dialysis pumps A and B run at the same rate. If dialysis machine is set to remove fluid, dialysis pump B runs faster than pump A by the amount required to remove the fluid.

Continuous venovenous haemodiafiltration (CVVHDF)

This term is best used for systems that intentionally combine both haemodialysis and haemofiltration. Dialysis fluid is passed across the filter to remove solutes by osmosis but at the same time ultrafiltrate is removed and replaced.

Venous access for renal replacement therapy

Venous access for venovenous renal replacement therapy is generally achieved using a large-bore double-lumen catheter (typically 11.5 Fr). These are sited using a Seldinger technique with the aid of a large, 'stiff' dilator. Care must be taken to avoid damage to the vessels and surrounding structures. Avoid siting in vessels with obvious tight corners, e.g. left internal jugular. Ideally, use right internal jugular or femoral veins. Ensure an appropriate length catheter is inserted to reach IVC or SVC/RA to give adequate flows and extended catheter life. (See Central venous access, p. 387.)

These large-bore catheters are prone to 'clotting off' when not in use. When the catheters are inserted, or when extracorporeal circuits are discontinued, catheters should be flushed with heparin (1000 units/mL) to the priming volume of the catheter, as printed on the hub.

Anticoagulant

In systems where blood passes through an extracorporeal circuit, anticoagulation is needed to prevent clotting, unless the patient has a severe underlying coagulopathy. Typical regimens are heparin 1000 units loading dose then 100–500 units/h or epoprostenol (prostacyclin) $5 \, \text{ng} \, \text{kg}^{-1} \, \text{min}^{-1}$. Infusions are run directly into the dialysis circuit. The effects of anticoagulation should be monitored regularly using activated clotting time (ACT) or activated partial thromboplastin time (APTT) and the anticoagulant regimen adjusted as necessary.

Excessive anticoagulation can result in bleeding problems. One approach to this has been the introduction of citrate as an anticoagulant for renal replacement therapy. As blood leaves the patient and enters the extracorporeal circuit, citrate is added. As the blood leaves the circuit, the calcium is added to reverse the effects of the citrate and prevent the patient becoming systemically anticoagulated.

Problems associated with renal replacement therapy

The problems associated with renal replacement therapy are listed in Box 7.3.

Box 7.3 Complications of renal replacement therapy

Hypotension

Dysrhythmias

Haemorrhage

Platelet consumption

Errors of fluid balance

Infection

Rise in ICP

Air embolism

It is common to see a fall in blood pressure and CO, and deterioration in oxygenation when blood enters any extracorporeal circuit. Factors which may contribute to this include fluid shifts, haemodilution and complement/cytokine activation from blood in the dialysis circuit. Hypotension generally responds to simple fluid loading, but may require vasopressor/inotrope infusion. Consider reducing the rate of fluid removal by the system if hypotension persists.

The so-called dialysis disequilibration syndrome may occur when biochemical abnormalities are corrected too quickly. The rapid removal of plasma solute renders the plasma hypotonic with respect to the brain and acute cerebral oedema develops. It is usually associated with conventional intermittent haemodialysis and is rare with modern practice.

PERITONEAL DIALYSIS

Peritoneal dialysis is commonly used in children and adults for the management of CRF. In children it is frequently also used in the management of ARF because of the difficulties of venous access. The potential advantages of peritoneal dialysis over other forms of renal replacement therapy are shown in Box 7.4.

Box 7.4 Potential advantages of peritoneal dialysis

No requirement for vascular access

No extracorporeal circuit

No need for anticoagulation

Little cardiovascular instability

Minimal direct effects on gas exchange in the lung

Patients can remain ambulatory

In adult intensive care, peritoneal dialysis is rarely used for the management of ARF except in patients already established on this mode of dialysis. It is generally ineffective at controlling fluid and electrolyte balance in the septic, catabolic patient. Intra-abdominal pathology, particularly sepsis, is common, making peritoneal dialysis impractical. Fluid in the peritoneum can result in diaphragmatic splinting, which may impair ventilation.

OUTCOME FROM ACUTE RENAL FAILURE IN INTENSIVE CARE

Most cases of acute renal failure occurring on the intensive care unit result from ATN and recover relatively quickly, as the overall condition of the patient improves. Re-establishment of a spontaneous urine output is generally followed by a polyuric phase. Large volumes of dilute urine may be produced, which require replacement. Measure electrolyte losses in the urine to guide this fluid and electrolyte replacement. During this polyuric phase the creatinine clearance is initially low, but progressively improves. It often reaches values sufficient that the patient needs no further ongoing organ renal support, even though it may not return to normal 'healthy' values.

A proportion of patients, however, fail to regain adequate renal function. In some recovery is delayed, while in others, severe renal impairment may be permanent. Patients with persisting renal dysfunction should be referred to a renal physician while still in the intensive care unit, who can advise on further investigation and on-going management, including the role of intermittent haemodialysis on the ICU/HDU. In this period, following the acute phase of critical care, intermittent haemodialysis rather than continuous renal replacement may have the advantages of intermittent anticoagulation, less platelet consumption, improved patient mobility, reduced staff workload and lower overall costs. Some patients will require a period in the renal unit during a prolonged phase of renal recovery, and a few will go on to require long-term renal supervision and dialysis.

MANAGEMENT OF PATIENTS WITH CHRONIC RENAL FAILURE

Patients with chronic dialysis dependent renal failure (CRF) may present to the ICU with intercurrent disease. The principles for managing these patients are very similar to those for managing

---

Box 7.5 Problems associated with chronic renal failure

Anaemia
Bone disease
Limited fluid tolerance
Hypertension
Accelerated CVS disease
Difficult vascular access

---

patients with ARF. These patients, however, have a number of specific problems (Box 7.5).

Patients with CRF are invariably anaemic, but are generally well compensated (may be on erythropoietin, EPO). In the intensive care setting, the need for transfusion will depend on the overall clinical picture and the need for increased oxygen delivery. An Hb of less than 8 g/dL is a reasonable threshold for transfusion.

Patients with CRF who survive intensive care will need to return to long-term dialysis. This will require long-term AV access. Take great care to protect existing AV fistulae and avoid damage to potential future fistula sites. Minimize the number of arterial and venous punctures made. If central venous access is required, avoid the subclavian vein on the side of the fistula, due to risk of bleeding from the venepuncture site (arterialized high-pressure vessel) and because of the risk of late vein stenosis leading to blockage of the fistula. Radial artery lines may be best avoided.

PRESCRIBING IN RENAL FAILURE

Renal failure results in changes to both the pharmacodynamics (what the drug does to the body) and pharmacokinetics (what the body does to the drug) of many agents. Problems include:

- Altered clearance of drugs and their metabolites.
- Altered sensitivity to some drugs even if clearance is unaltered.
- Reduced effectiveness of some drugs in the presence of renal failure.
- Poor tolerance of side-effects.

Prescribing drugs to patients in renal failure is therefore a complex issue, and you should seek advice from your pharmacist and/or renal physicians. Where possible, nephrotoxic drugs should be avoided and alternative agents prescribed. Where either no alternative exists or none is suitable, close monitoring

---

Box 7.6 Commonly used drugs which impair renal function

ACE inhibitors

Aminoglycosides

NSAIDs

Ciclosporin

X-ray contrast media

Amphotericin

Cancer chemotherapy drugs

Gancyclovir

Box 7.7 Cockcroft–Gault formula for estimating creatinine clearance

Creatinine clearance (mL/min) [adult male] = (140−age in years)− lean body mass (kg) ÷ serum creatinine (μmol/L) × 0.815

For females multiply by 0.85.

Normal creatinine clearance   >100 mL/min

Significant impairment   <50 mL/min

(e.g. of plasma levels) may be required and the risks and benefits of continuing treatment considered daily. A list of commonly prescribed nephrotoxic drugs is given in Box 7.6.

The dose and/or frequency of many drugs vary according to the renal function, based on estimates of creatine clearance. The most commonly used formula for calculating creatinine clearance is the Cockcroft–Gault formula, shown in Box 7.7.

These calculations provide an accurate estimate of creatinine clearance in most patients but are unreliable in the presence of malnutrition, obesity, and critical illness (rapidly changing renal function). Seek senior advice.

Drug clearance during RRT

For the purpose of prescribing, creatinine clearance during renal replacement therapy can be considered as being greatly reduced. (<10 mL/min). Drug clearance is dependent on molecular size, charge, volume of distribution and water solubility. In general, non-ionized drugs with high fat solubility and large volume of distribution will not be cleared efficiently by dialysis (e.g. CNS-acting sedative and analgesic drugs).

Opioids

The morphine metabolites (morphine-3-glucuronide and morphine-6-glucuronide) are both active and accumulate in renal failure. It is reasonable to give morphine derivatives as small intermittent intravenous injections but avoid infusing them over long periods of time. Pethidine is metabolized to norpethidine, which accumulates and may produce cerebral excitation and fits. Fentanyl, alfentanil and remifentanil accumulate less and may be used for continuous infusions.

Benzodiazepines

The two most commonly used benzodiazepines in intensive care are midazolam and diazepam. Both are metabolized by the liver, but diazepam has an active metabolite that is excreted by the kidneys and may accumulate in renal failure.

Muscle relaxants

Suxamethonium causes a transient elevation in serum potassium that is likely to be clinically relevant and potentially dangerous in patients with renal failure, particularly when this is associated with muscle damage. The use of suxamethonium should be carefully considered on balance of risks, as the risk of aspiration of gastric contents into the airway may be less than the risk of cardiac arrest due to hyperkalaemia (see Suxamethonium, p. 34).

Some non-depolarizing muscle relaxants may accumulate in renal failure. Atracurium and its isomer cis-atracurium undergo spontaneous (non-metabolic) degradation at body pH and temperature and are generally the most suitable for use in the critically ill (see Sedation and analgesia, p. 43).

Antibiotics

The clearance of aminoglycosides is reduced in renal failure, and high levels are both nephrotoxic and cause deafness if maintained over time. Reduce the dosage/frequency and monitor levels (see Appendix 1, p. 449). Penicillins may accumulate and produce seizures at high concentrations. Dose and frequency should be reduced after loading doses have been given. Carbipenems, cephalosporins and other antibiotics may also need dose reduction. Seek advice.

Digoxin

Digoxin is unpredictable in renal failure. Levels may be substantially elevated compared with healthy patients. It is cleared to a variable extent by dialysis. Consider alternative agents, e.g. amiodarone.

PLASMA EXCHANGE

Plasma exchange is a therapy used in some acute, immune mediated conditions to reduce the load of circulating immunologically active proteins. Simplistically, plasma containing such active proteins is removed and its volume replaced with 4.5% albumin solution or FFP. There are a number of established indications and it is occasionally used in ICU patients (Box 7.8).

Box 7.8 Indications for plasma exchange	
Established indications include:	*Speculative uses include:*
Guillain–Barré syndrome	Severe sepsis
Myasthenia gravis	Pancreatitis
Systemic lupus erythematosus	
Other vasculitis (e.g. Goodpasture's syndrome)	
Thrombotic thrombocytopenic purpura (TTP–HUS)	

Plasma exchange is usually performed by the blood transfusion service or by renal medicine. Typically in an adult a 40–50 mL/kg plasma exchange is performed daily (or alternate days) over 5–7 days using an extracorporeal circuit as in dialysis/haemofiltration. The problems associated with plasma exchange are similar to haemodialysis, i.e. need for large-bore venous access, hypotension, anticoagulation, fluid shifts and deterioration in oxygenation. Seek expert help and advice. In general, most benefit is obtained if performed in the first few days after presentation.

In some inflammatory conditions (e.g. Guillain–Barré syndrome) immunoglobulin solutions may be given as a simpler alternative to plasma exchange (see Guillain–Barré syndrome, p. 303).

CHAPTER 8

METABOLIC AND ENDOCRINE PROBLEMS

Introduction 202
Sodium 202
Potassium 204
Calcium 207
Phosphate 209
Magnesium 210
Albumin 210
Metabolic acidosis 212
Metabolic alkalosis 215
**Disturbances of blood
    glucose** 215
Diabetic emergencies 217
Adrenal insufficiency 221
Phaeochromocytoma 222
Thyroid dysfunction 223
Temperature control 224

INTRODUCTION

Metabolic and endocrine disturbances are common in the ICU. They may be the patient's primary presenting condition, or a consequence of the response to the primary disease process, the physiological stress response, fluid management and/or the effects of prescribed or illicit drugs.

Some typical electrolyte disturbances seen on the intensive care unit are discussed below. Long lists of possible causes have been deliberately omitted. In general, aim for slow correction of most abnormalities over a 24- to 48-h period to avoid major fluid shifts.

SODIUM

(Normal range serum sodium 135–145 mmol/L.)

Sodium is primarily an extracellular ion. Plasma or serum sodium concentrations are a result of the balance between the sodium and water content of the extracellular compartments. Most acute disturbances of sodium concentration represent changes in water balance rather than total body sodium.

Hyponatraemia

The causes of hyponatraemia are shown in Table 8.1.

Hyponatraemia is most commonly due to an excess of extracellular fluid (rather than sodium loss). This is often the result of excessive use of hypotonic intravenous fluids. Hyponatraemia may also result from the chronic use of some diuretic drugs; this is

TABLE 8.1 Causes of hyponatraemia	
Excess water intake	Hypotonic fluids
	TURP syndrome
	Water intoxication
Reduced free water clearance	Stress response with raised ADH
	Syndrome of inappropriate ADH secretion
	Renal impairment
	Cardiac failure
Loss of body sodium	GI tract losses
	Renal losses including diuretic therapy
	Adrenal insufficiency
	Hyperpyrexia and sweating (inadequate salt replacement)

more commonly seen in the elderly. More rarely, hyponatraemia is associated with other forms of organ dysfunction, including renal dysfunction and hepatic cirrhosis (where it is seen in association with secondary hyperaldosteronism). Treatment is not usually necessary unless the serum sodium falls below 130 mmol/L. Serum sodium below 120 mmol/L may be associated with altered conscious level and fits. Symptoms are related as much to the speed of change in concentration as to the actual measured level.

- Consider the underlying cause.
- Change maintenance fluids to 0.9% saline.
- Restrict total fluid intake. Allow the kidneys to clear excess fluid.
- If oliguric, consider the need for renal replacement therapy to remove excess fluid.

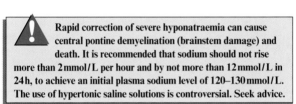

Rapid correction of severe hyponatraemia can cause central pontine demyelination (brainstem damage) and death. It is recommended that sodium should not rise more than 2 mmol/L per hour and by not more than 12 mmol/L in 24 h, to achieve an initial plasma sodium level of 120–130 mmol/L. The use of hypertonic saline solutions is controversial. Seek advice.

Excessive antidiuretic hormone (ADH) secretion

This is a cause of dilutional hyponatraemia due to reduced free water clearance. It is most commonly seen as part of the syndrome of inappropriate ADH secretion (SIADH), which may accompany the neuroendocrine stress response to trauma, surgery and critical illness. Rarely, ectopic ADH secretion by tumours may produce a similar picture. Oliguria is accompanied by increased urine osmolality (>500 mosmol/L) and reduced plasma osmolality (<280 mosmol/L).

- Restrict fluids.
- Consider a trial of diuretic therapy.

Hyponatraemia due to sodium loss

Significant sodium depletion is associated with a reduction in extracellular fluid volume. This stimulates the release of aldosterone and causes the kidneys to retain salt and water and lose potassium. Urinary osmolality is raised and urinary sodium is low, less than 10 mmol/L (unless there is an intrinsic renal problem or use of diuretics).

- Replace sodium and ECF with isotonic (0.9%) saline.

Pseudohyponatraemia

Electrolytes are present and measured only in the aqueous phase of plasma, but the concentration is expressed according to the total plasma volume. If there is a raised lipid or protein content in the plasma this can produce a spurious result.

Hypernatraemia

High serum sodium usually represents free water depletion. This is associated with a raised serum urea (without a significant corresponding rise in serum creatinine) and an increased serum osmolality (>290 mosmol/L). In critically ill patients, this situation can arise despite the apparent appearance of widespread oedema and 'fluid overload' as a result of fluid shifting between 'compartments'.

- Assess patient's clinical volume status (tissue turgor, sunken eyes, CVP, etc.).
- Review fluid balance regimen.
- Give additional free water as 5% dextrose (e.g. 1 L over 6–12 h) or water via NG tube. Consider diluting enteral feeds with sterile water.
- If additional fluid is contraindicated or undesirable, consider renal replacement therapy. This should be discussed with the nephrologists, on a case-by-case basis.

Hypernatraemia due to genuine sodium overload is uncommon. It is usually due to excess sodium chloride ingestion or administration, and is therefore accompanied by a high serum chloride and a hyperchloraemic acidosis. Management is essentially the same. Increase free water intake to allow the kidneys to excrete the additional solute load.

 Rapid correction of hypernatraemia, particularly if serum sodium is >160 mmol/L, can result in cerebral oedema as water enters the brain. As with hyponatraemia, correct slowly over 24–48 h.

POTASSIUM

(Normal range serum potassium 3.5–5 mmol/L.)

Potassium is primarily an intracellular ion. Small changes in serum concentration have significant effects on nerve conduction and muscle contraction.

Hypokalaemia

Causes of hypokalaemia are shown in Box 8.1.

Hypokalaemia is relatively common in the ICU. ECG changes include ST depression, flattening of the T wave and prominent U wave. If severe (<2 mmol/L), cardiac arrhythmias, including supraventricular and ventricular extrasystoles, tachycardias, atrial fibrillation, and ventricular fibrillation, may occur (Fig. 8.1).

Ensure adequate potassium concentration in maintenance fluids. The maximum safe concentration of potassium in peripheral fluid infusions is usually taken to be 60 mmol/L. In the intensive care unit where continuous monitoring is in place, a stronger potassium solution may be infused through a central line using a volumetric infusion pump or syringe driver

If additional potassium is required:

● Do not give a rapid bolus injections of potassium, as there is a risk of sudden death.

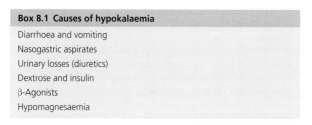

Box 8.1 Causes of hypokalaemia

Diarrhoea and vomiting
Nasogastric aspirates
Urinary losses (diuretics)
Dextrose and insulin
β-Agonists
Hypomagnesaemia

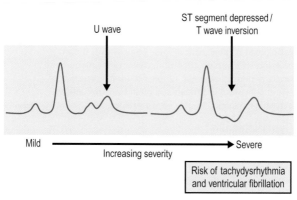

U wave

ST segment depressed / T wave inversion

Mild ———————————————→ Severe
Increasing severity

Risk of tachydysrhythmia and ventricular fibrillation

Fig. 8.1 ECG changes associated with hypokalaemia.

Box 8.2 Causes of hyperkalaemia

Spurious (e.g. haemolysed blood sample, check result)

Iatrogenic (excess administration)

Renal failure

Acidosis

Muscle injury (including suxamethonium, crush injury, compartment syndrome)

Tumour lysis syndrome (following chemotherapy)

Addison's disease

Ischaemia reperfusion

- Give 20 mmol of K^+ in 20–40 mL of saline over 1 h via a central venous catheter using an infusion pump. Repeat as necessary.
- Monitor the ECG during infusion.

 Inadvertent and inappropriate injection of strong potassium solutions has been associated with death. These solutions should be treated as a controlled drug, and use should be governed by local protocols. Ideally, strong potassium infusions should be prepared by a pharmacy aseptic service. If you are required to prepare potassium infusions, ensure that fluids are thoroughly mixed before administration. Strong potassium chloride solution has a higher specific gravity than standard i.v. solutions and can 'layer' at the bottom of a bag/syringe. Administration should be via a central venous cannula to avoid the risk of extravasation injury. During infusion continuous ECG monitoring and regular blood sampling are mandatory.

In many patients, hypokalaemia is a reflection of a more widespread derangement of ionic homeostasis. It may be associated with an attempt to conserve magnesium in severe hypomagnesaemia. In this situation, correction of serum potassium is difficult and often transient until the hypomagnesaemia has also been corrected.

Hyperkalaemia

Causes of hyperkalaemia are shown in Box 8.2.

ECG changes include peaked T waves, broad QRS complexes and conduction defects (Fig. 8.2). Asystole may occur. Urgent treatment is usually required, although patients with long-term end-stage renal failure may be more tolerant of hyperkalaemia than the general intensive care patient population.

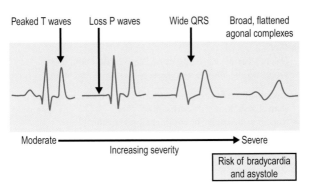

Fig. 8.2 ECG changes in hyperkalaemia.

Treatment to reduce risk of immediate arrhythmia
- 10 mL of 10% calcium chloride as a slow i.v. bolus will help to stabilize cardiac muscle.
- In the presence of metabolic acidosis, give 50 mL 8.4% bicarbonate.

Treatment to lower serum potassium:
- Nebulized salbutamol 2.5 mg, repeated as necessary.
- 50 mL of 8.4% bicarbonate, particularly in the presence of metabolic acidosis.
- 20% dextrose infusion plus 10 units of short-acting insulin i.v. (e.g. Actrapid).
- Oral/rectal calcium resonium (chelating agent).
- Consider the need for urgent renal replacement therapy.

CALCIUM

(Normal range standard serum calcium 2.12–2.62 mmol/L.)
(Normal range ionized serum calcium 0.84–1 mmol/L.)

Most laboratories measure total calcium, which includes bound and unbound fractions. The unbound fraction (ionized Ca^{2+}), which is the physiologically active component, varies with the albumin concentration. Therefore, look at the corrected figure, which takes account of protein binding. Alternatively, many blood gas analysers now measure ionized Ca^{2+} directly.

Hypocalcaemia

Hypocalcaemia is common on the ICU. Typical causes are shown in Box 8.3.

Hypocalcaemia causes depressed cardiac function, loss of vasomotor tone, muscle weakness, paraesthesia and tetany.

- Give 10 mL of 10% calcium chloride as slow i.v. bolus (into central vein, as it is a sclerosant).
- Repeat as necessary or consider slow infusion.

In hypocalcaemia secondary to phosphate accumulation, there are risks of calcium phosphate deposition in tissues with overzealous calcium administration. Seek specialist advice.

Hypercalcaemia

This occurs less commonly, and is generally due to an underlying disease process. Typical causes are listed in Box 8.4.

Symptoms include GI disturbance, confusion and polyuria. Treatment is by rehydration and the use of calcium-binding agents.

- Give 0.9% saline to rehydrate the patient. Check plasma osmolality is within the normal range (280–290 mosmol/L).
- A forced diuresis may be used to aid excretion. Furosemide (frusemide) is administered and the urine output replaced with alternating 0.9% saline and 5% dextrose.

Box 8.3 Causes of hypocalcaemia

Citrate accumulation (massive transfusion/liver failure)
Generalized failure of Ca^{2+} homeostasis in severe sepsis
Pancreatitis
Secondary to phosphate accumulation in renal failure
Parathyroid damage after head and neck surgery

Box 8.4 Causes of hypercalcaemia

Hyperparathyroidism
Excessive intake vitamin D or calcium
Malignancy
Sarcoidosis
Bone disease
Drug-induced (thiazide diuretics)

- Calcitonin reduces the rate of calcium and phosphate release from the bones. It is useful in patients with hypercalcaemia associated with malignancy, and generally reduces the calcium level within 2 h.
- Bisphosphonates (e.g. disodium etidronate) also reduce release of calcium from bones but generally take a few days to achieve maximum effect.
- Corticosteroids may be helpful in hypercalcaemia associated with sarcoidosis and malignancy.

PHOSPHATE

(Normal range serum phosphate 0.7–1.25 mmol/L.)

Hypophosphataemia

This is common in the ICU. It is usually multifactorial, resulting from reduced intake (particularly in patients receiving TPN), redistribution and increased losses (especially patients on renal replacement therapy). Hypophosphataemia causes muscle weakness, which may lead to heart failure or difficulty in weaning from artificial ventilation. It also contributes to failure of many metabolic processes and, if severe, results in depressed conscious level and seizures. It has also been associated with insulin resistance.

It is debatable at what level replacement is required. In most cases, as the patient's overall condition improves, phosphate balance returns. Patients whose levels are below 0.8 mmol/L, particularly if symptomatic, may benefit from additional phosphate either in feeds or intravenously.

- Use sodium phosphate or potassium phosphate depending upon requirements.
- Give 30–60 mmol phosphate diluted in 100–500 mL 5% dextrose over 24 h.

Hyperphosphataemia

Hyperphosphataemia is caused by excessive intake or decreased excretion (e.g. renal failure). Maintain adequate hydration with 5% dextrose. If severe, consider the need for renal replacement therapy. Phosphate is effectively removed by continuous RRT techniques, with haemodialysis and haemodiafiltration performing better than simple filtration techniques.

Box 8.5 Causes of hypomagnesaemia

Diuretics

Insulin

Gastrointestinal tract losses

Parenteral nutrition

MAGNESIUM

(Normal range serum magnesium 0.7–1 mmol/L.)

Hypomagnesaemia

Magnesium is the second most common intracellular cation and as such, serum levels are a poor guide to the need for replacement. Serum magnesium is frequently depleted in critical illness. Common causes of hypomagnesaemia are shown in Box 8.5.

Hypomagnesaemia is usually asymptomatic, but can give rise to muscle weakness and cardiac arrhythmias (hypomagnesaemia exacerbates the effects of hypokalaemia, see above.). The treatment is by magnesium supplementation.

- Give 10 mmol magnesium sulphate i.v. over 30 min.
- If severe can be followed by 50–100 mmol over 24 h.

Hypermagnesaemia

This is less common and generally results from excessive administration, particularly in the presence of renal failure. Consciousness level may be reduced. Cardiac conduction may be impaired with prolongation of the PR interval and broadening of the QRS complexes. At extreme levels, this may result in cardiac arrest.

- 10 mL calcium chloride i.v. will temporarily improve cardiac conduction.
- Consider the need for urgent haemofiltration or haemodialysis.

ALBUMIN

Albumin is a plasma protein which is important in contributing to colloid oncotic pressure and as a binding protein for drugs and other substances.

Hypoalbuminaemia

Low serum albumin is common in critically ill patients. Common causes of hypoalbuminaemia are shown in Box 8.6.

> **Box 8.6 Causes of hypoalbuminaemia**
>
> Malnutrition
>
> Impaired protein synthesis (liver disease)
>
> Redistribution from generalised capillary leakage
>
> Increased losses; renal disease (nephrotic syndrome)

Low albumin concentration is generally a marker of disease severity rather than a problem in its own right. There is no benefit in giving albumin solely to raise the albumin concentration. Concentrations will recover as the patient's condition improves, and synthesis of albumin by the liver increases while capillary leak is reduced. Ensure adequate nutrition in order to encourage protein synthesis and treat the underlying condition.

Use of albumin solutions

There are two albumin preparations that are readily available: 4.5% albumin (contains Na^+ 140 mmol/L) and 20% albumin (contains Na^+ 60 mmol/L).

There has been considerable debate over recent years regarding the use of these solutions in critically ill patients. A meta-analysis suggested that the use of albumin-containing solutions may increase mortality The subsequent SAFE study showed no difference in 28-day outcome of patients admitted to ICU and receiving either 4% albumin or normal saline for fluid resuscitation. Nonetheless, the use of 4.5% albumin solution purely for volume expansion purposes has declined. Synthetic colloids are as effective and cheaper.

Use of 20% albumin

Given as a bolus, 20% albumin effectively raises the plasma oncotic pressure and expands the intravascular space by factor of up to 5 times the volume given, by drawing fluid in from extravascular spaces. Depending on vascular permeability and metabolism of albumin, this effect is likely to be transient (lasting less than 4 h). This effect has, however, been used in conjunction with diuretics in an attempt to correct oedema secondary to severe hypoalbuminaemia. Similar strategies have been used in treatment of hepatorenal failure (together with terlipressin) and to try to avert impending renal failure. Although relatively widely practised, the evidence for such strategies is limited. Twenty percent albumin is used to replace protein losses in the nephrotic syndrome.

METABOLIC ACIDOSIS

(See Interpretation of blood gases, p. 114, and Sepsis, p. 331.)

Metabolic acidosis is common in patients requiring intensive care. The causes can be simply understood in terms of either excess accumulation of non-carbonic acid or loss of bicarbonate buffering capacity. These processes may be present separately or together. Calculation of the anion gap provides a simple guide to the underlying process. The anion gap can be calculated as follows:

$$\text{Anion gap} = [Na^+ + K^+] - [HCO_3^- + Cl^-]$$

Normal anion gap is $< 18\,mmol/L$. In the presence of a metabolic acidosis, an anion gap $>18\,mmol/L$ implies the presence of an excess of non-carbonic acid, while an anion gap $<18\,mmol/L$ implies the loss of bicarbonate buffering capacity.

Common causes of metabolic acidosis classified according to anion gap are shown in Box 8.7.

In critical illness, the cause of metabolic acidosis is often multifactorial. Poor tissue perfusion combined with multiorgan dysfunction may lead to accumulation of acid moieties whilst at the same time there may be reduced buffering capacity. The use of β-agonist inotropes is associated with increased metabolic acidosis. Hyperchloraemic acidosis from the administration of excess chloride containing intravenous fluids is common (see below).

The effects of acidosis are increased respiratory drive (unless the patient is sedated/paralysed), and at low pH < 7.1 reduced CO, and reduced response to inotropes. Hydrogen ions move into cells and K^+ moves out in an attempt to buffer the acidosis, so hyperkalaemia may occur. Treatment depends on the severity, underlying cause and speed of response to interventions.

Box 8.7 Causes of metabolic acidosis

Accumulation of H+ (anion gap >18 mmol/L)	Loss of bicarbonate (anion gap < 18 mmol/L)
Lactic acidosis (shock and tissue ischaemia)	Vomiting or diarrhoea
Ketoacidosis	Small bowel fistula
Liver failure	Renal tubular acidosis
Acute renal failure	Hyperchloraemic acidosis
Salicylate poisoning	

In most cases, the metabolic acidosis will correct as the underlying condition improves.

- Treat the underlying cause. (See Lactic acidosis below, Diabetic ketoacidosis, p. 218, and Poisoning p. 230.)
- If pH < 7.1 or the patient's clinical condition is deteriorating, either give 50 mL 8.4% (50 mmol) sodium bicarbonate i.v., or for lower body weight individuals, calculate the dose of bicarbonate as follows:

Sodium bicarbonate = [1/2 × base deficit (mmol/L × weight kg)]/3

- Check blood gases and repeat as necessary.

 The evidence of benefit from bicarbonate solutions to treat acidosis is limited with some evidence that it actually worsens intracellular pH. Other disadvantages include large sodium load (particularly if used repeatedly). Therefore only consider if the pH < 7.2 in an inotrope resistant, hypotensive patient.

There are a number of other alkalizing solutions commercially available, including Tris buffered bicarbonate solution (THAM). Despite theoretical advantages, they are not widely used. Ask for advice and seek local guidelines in your unit.

Lactic acidosis

Lactate measurements are increasingly available from blood gas analysers. There is considerable argument as to their value. Lactate levels >2 mmol/L are abnormal. There are two situations in which lactic acidosis may occur.

Type A

This is the commonest type of metabolic acidosis seen in the ICU and is due to inadequate delivery of oxygen to the tissue. This may occur, for example, as a result of cardiorespiratory arrest or from inadequate tissue perfusion, as seen in shock states. Inadequate oxygen delivery leads to anaerobic metabolism and the accumulation of lactate. It is not uncommon, however, for patients with severe shock and acidosis to have a normal lactate.

- Restore adequate oxygen delivery and tissue perfusion.
- Give bicarbonate as above if necessary.

- Consider the need for renal replacement therapy. If already on RRT using lactate buffered replacement/dialysis fluid, consider changing to bicarbonate buffered solutions. Seek senior advice.
- Lactate levels usually return to normal with adequate resuscitation. Failure to do so implies either a failure of resuscitation or critically ischaemic or dead tissue. Look for hidden areas of ischaemic tissues, e.g. ischaemic bowel.
- Where lactic acidosis is sustained and refractory to treatment, the prognosis is poor.

Type B

This is uncommon, and is due to the accumulation of lactate without evidence of tissue hypoxia. It may be precipitated by drugs, ingestion of ethylene glycol or methanol, liver failure and some rare hereditary disorders, including disorders of mitochondrial function.

- Treat the underlying condition if possible. The acidosis should be corrected. This may be possible simply by removing the underlying precipitating cause, but may require vigorous resuscitation.
- Infusion of bicarbonate solution (potentially in large volumes) may be necessary as part of the initial resuscitation.
- Renal replacement therapy may be necessary, and should be considered early. (See Methanol/ethylene glycol poisoning, p. 240.)

Hyperchloraemic acidosis

Elevated serum chloride levels, for example following resuscitation with large volumes of normal saline, produce a corresponding decrease in bicarbonate levels (in order to maintain anion balance) and hyperchloraemic acidosis. This usually resolves without the need for treatment as the chloride levels correct (see choice of fluids, p. 49).

Renal tubular acidosis (RTA)

This is a metabolic acidosis arising from renal tubular dysfunction, in which there is excess loss of bicarbonate through the kidneys, with a corresponding increased serum chloride (normal anion gap). This may present as a feature of renal disease, or may result as a side-effect from drugs (e.g. amphotericin). If you suspect renal tubular acidosis, test the urine pH. A systemic acidosis accompanied by a non acid urine (pH > 6) is highly suggestive. Type 1 (distal convoluted tubule) and type 2 (proximal convoluted tubule) are associated with hypokalaemia. Type 4 results from hypoaldosteronism or aldosterone resistance, and is associated with hyperkalaemia and metabolic acidosis. (Type 3 is no longer recognized.)

METABOLIC ALKALOSIS

This is relatively uncommon and is due either to the loss of acid (e.g. from vomiting of gastric acid), or from the excessive administration of alkali (e.g. sodium bicarbonate). The metabolism of citrate (an anticoagulant in transfused blood) may also produce metabolic alkalosis. (See Hepatic failure, p. 176.) Significant potassium loss alone (e.g. diuretic therapy) may also induce a metabolic alkalosis.

Metabolic alkalosis typically occurs in young children following protracted vomiting (e.g. secondary to pyloric stenosis), but is also occasionally seen in adults. Massive losses of fluid, H^+, Cl^- and K^+ lead to a marked alkalosis and shock state. Profound hypoventilation occurs as the body retains CO_2 as a compensatory mechanism. The treatment is by volume resuscitation with 0.9% saline and added potassium. The use of acidifying agents such as HCl or arginine hydrochloride is controversial and usually unnecessary. Seek advice.

 If assisted ventilation is considered, beware of cardiovascular collapse when using sedative agents in profoundly dehydrated patients. Avoid hyperventilation, which will exacerbate the alkalosis.

DISTURBANCES OF BLOOD GLUCOSE

Disturbances of blood glucose are common in the critically ill, even in those patients who are not normally known to be diabetic, and both hypoglycaemia and hyperglycaemia may occur. It is therefore vital to monitor blood glucose regularly even if the patient is not diabetic.

Tight glycaemic control regimens have become standard practice in critical care units in recent years because of the apparent reduction in overall intensive care mortality, particularly in post-surgical patients. They are associated, however with a greatly increased risk of hypoglycaemia (due to the use of insulin to control hyperglycaemia), and more recent studies have challenged their efficacy.

Box 8.8 Causes of hypoglycaemia

Insulin administration

Oral hypoglycaemics

Hepatic failure

Adrenal cortical failure

Hypopituitarism

Excess insulin secretion (insulinoma)

Hypothermia

Hypoglycaemia

Hypoglycaemia can be defined as a blood glucose <3 mmol/L. It occurs most commonly as a consequence of insulin or oral hypoglycaemic therapy in diabetic patients, but may also be associated with some disease states. Typical causes are shown in Box 8.8.

> ⚠ **When measuring blood glucose, be careful that the sampling line used is not contaminated with glucose solutions. There have been cases of samples drawn from lines that have been contaminated with glucose inadvertently used to flush the line, leading to spuriously high serum glucose levels, followed by excessive insulin administration and profound hypoglycaemia.**

Clinical signs of hypoglycaemia include confusion, sweating, tachycardia and seizures, leading if untreated to coma and brain damage. Such signs may be masked or absent in the critically ill or sedated patient, so great care and regular glucose monitoring are required in patients receiving insulin infusions. It should be appreciated that at present there is no clinically available real time technique for monitoring blood glucose, and plasma glucose concentrations can fall to dangerously low levels very quickly after the administration of insulin. This means that there is a real chance of missing hypoglycaemia between intermittent (e.g. hourly) glucose measurements.

- Consider the cause. Reduce or discontinue hypoglycaemic agents as appropriate.
- Give 50 mL of IV 20% dextrose and repeat as necessary. Boluses of 50% dextrose have been associated with significant disturbances of osmolality, and are best avoided.

- Commence infusion of 10–20% dextrose (with potassium) as necessary to maintain blood sugar.

(See Hepatic failure, p. 176.)

Hyperglycaemia

This is common in the critically ill, and may result from pre-existing diabetes or glucose intolerance. The effects of critical illness, the associated stress response and the effects of drugs such as exogenous catecholamines and steroids can all lead to glucose intolerance. This may be further compounded by the use of high glucose loads in TPN. Consequently, hyperglycaemia is common and frequently requires the use of insulin infusions to control the blood sugar, even in the non-diabetic patient.

- Start a sliding scale insulin infusion.
- Monitor potassium – insulin drives K^+ into cells.

It may be impossible to achieve normal blood glucose levels in very sick patients. In this case, avoid peaks and troughs in glucose levels caused by repeated changes in insulin dosage. It was previously considered that perfect glucose control was not necessary in the critically ill, but recent evidence suggested that the outcome of critically ill patients, particularly those with sepsis, may be improved by tightly controlling blood glucose within the normal range (see Sepsis, p. 329). More recent analysis has suggested that such benefit is more questionable, and there is a very real risk of dangerous hypoglycaemia with more aggressive glucose control. Therefore, seek reasonable control aiming to get within the upper range of the normal limit within a few hours rather than minutes Brain injury is worsened in the presence of hyperglycaemia.

DIABETIC EMERGENCIES

Both insulin and non-insulin dependent diabetes are common in hospitalized patients. In most cases, oral hypoglycaemic agents should be discontinued while patients are on the ICU. There are no directly comparable parenteral alternatives to such drugs. Blood sugar should be monitored closely, and if necessary an insulin infusion commenced.

Most diabetic emergencies are managed on general wards or HDU rather than ICU. Occasionally patients are moribund or have associated features, such as sepsis, which require intensive care. The source of sepsis may be occult (e.g. renal abscess). Abdominal ultrasound or a CT scan may be required.

Patients with hyperglycaemia or hyperosmolar coma have large deficits of water, sodium, potassium and other electrolytes. Manage these according to basic principles with rehydration, and control of blood sugar and other metabolic derangements with insulin. Aim for a gradual correction of deficits over 24–48 h. There is a small but definite risk of cerebral oedema, which may in part be caused by over-rapid correction of electrolyte/fluid abnormalities.

DIABETIC KETOACIDOSIS

Diabetic ketoacidosis (DKA) is the most common diabetic emergency. It may be the presenting episode in a newly diagnosed diabetic, or may be precipitated in existing diabetic patients by intercurrent illness (increased insulin requirements) or by reduced insulin dosage.

Pathophysiology
Absolute or relative deficiency of insulin leads to an imbalance between the hyperglycaemic effects of stress hormones and the hypoglycaemic effects of insulin. Increased hepatic glycogen breakdown and gluconeogenesis coupled with reduced cellular uptake of glucose results in hyperglycaemia. This in turn leads to polyuria, with loss of water, sodium and potassium. The hormonal changes also result in lipolysis with release of triglycerides and fatty acids, which are metabolized by the liver to ketones, which exacerbate the metabolic acidosis.

Clinical features
- Polyuria.
- Polydipsia initially followed by anorexia, nausea and vomiting.
- Ketones on breath. (Note that not everyone can smell ketones.)
- Kussmaul respiration (hyperventilation in response to metabolic acidosis).
- Abdominal pain and tenderness – an important differential diagnosis of the acute abdomen!
- Severe dehydration and shock.

Management
- Give oxygen. Despite profound acidosis, most patients manage to compensate well by hyperventilation and do not require artificial ventilation. If there is evidence of hypoxia,

hypoventilation or compromised airway, intubate and establish ventilation, but beware of cardiovascular collapse!

- The need for invasive cardiovascular monitoring will depend on the severity of the condition but in general arterial access and CVP lines are appropriate.
- If the patient is severely shocked, colloid boluses and inotropic support may be required.
- Pass a urinary catheter and consider the need for an NG tube.
- Take base line investigations. FBC, urea and electrolytes (sodium and potassium), glucose, and blood gases. Monitor glucose, potassium and arterial blood gases hourly.
- Look for a precipitating cause. Send blood, urine and sputum for culture. ECG, CXR and troponin if indicated. Abdominal pain is a common feature of DKA; consider abdominal ultrasound/CT and send blood for amylase.
- Start i.v. infusion of 0.9% normal saline and aim to correct dehydration over 24 h. The volume required can be estimated from the percent dehydration (Table 8.2). These are estimates only and should be viewed in the context of the overall clinical picture.
- Typically give 1 L in the first 30 min and then 1 L/h over the next 2 h, and assess response. Give the rest over the remaining 22 h. If serum sodium is >150 mmol/L consider 0.45% saline as an alternative.

TABLE 8.2 Estimation of percent dehydration

	Mild (<5%)	Moderate (5–10%)	Severe (>10%)
Dry mucous membranes	+	++	+++
Reduced tissue turgor	+	++	+++
Reduced urine output	+	++	+++
Pulse	Normal	Tachycardia	Tachycardia
Blood pressure	Normal	Normal/mild hypotension	Significant hypotension
Conscious level	Normal	Normal	Reduced

Fluid requirement (mL) is calculated as:
percent dehydration × weight in kg × 10.
Example: 70 kg patient 10% dehydrated deficit = 7000 mL.

- In addition to resuscitation fluid volume above, give maintenance fluids to provide the patient's normal daily requirements. Give this as a separate infusion. Initially give as 0.9% normal saline. This can be changed to a dextrose solution when the blood glucose is under control (see below).
- Give 10 units of short-acting insulin i.v. Follow this with an insulin infusion of 6–10 units/h as necessary. The aim should be to reduce the blood sugar slowly over a number of hours.
- The acidosis will usually correct as the patient's overall condition improves. If there is a severe metabolic acidosis pH < 7.1, and the patient's condition is not improving, consider bicarbonate (see above).
- Monitor the potassium carefully. As the acidosis corrects, the potassium will fall. Start a potassium infusion at 20 mmol/h as required.
- When plasma glucose falls to 12–14 mmol/L change maintenance fluids to dextrose 4%/saline 0.18% to prevent hypoglycaemia. Continue insulin as a sliding scale infusion and potassium replacement as necessary.

HYPEROSMOLAR NON-KETOTIC STATES

Some diabetic patients may have sufficient residual insulin activity to prevent ketogenesis but not to prevent hyperglycaemia. Polyuria develops, which leads to dehydration and hyperosmolar states. Hyperglycaemia, hyperosmolality and hypernatraemia are typical and these eventually lead to reduced conscious level and seizure activity. Severe dehydration may lead to raised haematocrit and increased risk of thromboembolic disease. Hyperosmolar non-ketotic states are more common in the elderly. They may be precipitated by the stress response to surgery or infection, and the effects of some drugs, including diuretics, phenytoin and glucocorticoids.

Management
- Similar to DKA above.
- Give oxygen. Secure the airway and institute ventilation if necessary.
- Invasive cardiovascular monitoring. NG tube. Urinary catheter.
- If severely shocked, colloid bolus and inotropic support may be required.
- Use 0.9% saline as rehydration fluid (0.45% saline in severe cases). Correct dehydration more slowly than in DKA, typically

over 24–48 h. Rapid correction may be associated with cerebral oedema.

- Insulin as in DKA but typically give lower doses, e.g. 3 units/h.
- Monitor potassium and replace as necessary. Potassium requirements are usually less than for DKA because of the absence of significant acidosis.

Patients with diabetic hyperosmolar states are at high risk of deep vein thrombosis. You should play close attention to the prophylaxis of deep vein thrombosis. This should include all the usual measures, such as support stockings and the use of a low molecular weight heparin; early mobilization and physiotherapy.

ADRENAL INSUFFICIENCY

Addison's disease

Addison's disease (primary adrenal cortical failure) is rare, but should be considered as a differential diagnosis in critically ill patients. It is easily missed due to the non-specific nature of signs and symptoms

The typical clinical features are increased pigmentation, weakness, abdominal pain (may be mistaken as a surgical acute abdomen), vomiting, diarrhoea and hypotension. Biochemical findings include hyponatraemia, hyperkalaemia, hypoglycaemia and hypercalcaemia. Aside from general support measures:

- If possible perform a short Synacthen test (Synacthen is an ACTH analogue). Give Synacthen 0.25 mg i.m. Measure plasma cortisol before and 30 min after. Cortisol level should rise by 2–3 times the basal level.
- Give steroid replacement therapy. Basal replacement doses hydrocortisone 20 mg a.m., 10 mg p.m. In stress states give larger doses, e.g. 100 mg 3 times daily.
- Consider mineralocorticoid replacement, e.g. fludrocortisone 50–300 μg daily (only available as an enteral preparation).

Patients on long-term steroid therapy

Many patients will already be on long-term corticosteroids for management of various disease processes. The true significance of pituitary adrenal suppression by longer term steroid therapy is still debatable but most authorities recommend increasing doses of steroids during critical illness and major surgical interventions.

Box 8.9 Conditions in which steroids may be indicated

Asthma, COPD

Cerebral tumours

Autoimmune conditions

Airway swelling

Spinal cord injury

Meningitis

Pneumocystis pneumonia

Fibroproliferative ARDS

Equivalent anti-inflammatory doses for a change from oral steroids to i.v. hydrocortisone are:

$$\text{hydrocortisone } 20\,\text{mg} = \text{prednisolone } 5\,\text{mg}$$

Functional adrenal insufficiency

Whist primary adrenal failure is rare, it is increasingly recognized that critically ill patients may have inadequate levels of cortisol production for their needs. This can contribute to refractory shock. Low-dose steroid replacement may improve outcomes in these patients and there are a number of conflicting large clinical trials. At the time of writing there is little evidence for the routine use of steroids in this situation, but if the patient is deteriorating despite all other measures it is probably reasonable to assess the effects of low dose steroids.

● Measure random cortisol or perform short Synacthen test (above).
● Give low (physiological) replacement doses of hydrocortisone, e.g. 50 mg b.d.

High-dose steroid therapy in shock states

High-dose steroid therapy has been trialled in shock states but studies tend to show it worsens outcomes. Likewise there is no benefit in traumatic acute brain injury. Steroids have been reported to improve outcomes in some other conditions (Box 8.9).

PHAEOCHROMOCYTOMA

This adrenal secretory tumour is a rare cause of hypertension/heart failure in young adults and may occasionally be a presenting diagnosis in critical care. Patients are most likely to been seen in ICU situation in the postoperative period. Patients are typically volume depleted due to the long-term effects of endogenous catecholamine secretion. The diagnosis is made by measurement of serum or urinary catecholamines or metabolites, and CT imaging to find the tumour.

Management

- Patients are commenced on α-blocking agents preoperatively. These block the hypertensive effects of catecholamines. Relative hypovolaemia is unmasked and fluid loading is required until postural changes in blood pressure are abolished.
- High dose magnesium may be administered prophylactically to stabilize catecholamine secreting cells.
- If tachycardia develops, β-blockers may be added only after full α-blockade.
- Perioperative dysrhythmias are common and may require magnesium, β-blockers or lidocaine (lignocaine).
- Once the tumour is removed, patients may require replacement of catecholamines [e.g. adrenaline (epinephrine) or noradrenaline (norepinephrine) infusion] to maintain blood pressure. These can then be gradually reduced over 2–3 days.

THYROID DYSFUNCTION

The accurate clinical and laboratory assessment of thyroid function is difficult in a normal outpatient/inpatient setting. Laboratory results are tempered by clinical signs and symptoms. In the ICU, symptoms of thyroid under/over activity are mimicked by many other conditions, making diagnosis difficult.

Most patients with pre-existing thyroid disease will be reasonably controlled. Occasionally previously undiagnosed patients will have their condition unmasked by critical illness. For patients on oral thyroid replacement therapy, the effects of oral thyroxine last 7–10 days, so that it is reasonable in the short term to wait for gut function to return rather than moving to parenteral preparations, which are usually only available as T3. If the oral route cannot be used, change to T3 (20 μg T3 is approximately equivalent to 100 μg T4).

Sick euthyroid syndrome

Thyroid function tests are often abnormal in the critically ill patient. Most sick patients will have results consistent with the so-called sick euthyroid syndrome. The pattern is low T3, low T4, and inappropriately low/normal TSH. This pattern persists until recovery occurs. The current consensus is that it does not reflect true clinical hypothyroidism so thyroid replacement therapy is not usually warranted. Seek expert advice if unclear.

Hypothyroidism

Hypothyroidism should be considered in the elderly patient presenting with hypothermia, coma or other non-specific illness. Treat with replacement therapy in the form of oral/parenteral T3 or thyroxine.

Hyperthyroidism

Uncontrolled hyperthyroidism is rarely seen. It should be considered in cases of AF, other dysrhythmias and metabolic disturbances. Hyperthyroidism may present in patients on ICU with other pathologies. Management includes antithyroid drugs, e.g. carbimazole, β-blockers and general supportive measures.

TEMPERATURE CONTROL

Disturbances in temperature regulation are common in ICU. Often the cause will be multifactorial, combining abnormalities of central temperature control and environmental causes.

Measurement of temperature

Core temperature measurements may be obtained from the tympanic membrane, nasopharynx, oesophagus, bladder and rectum, or from an indwelling vascular catheter. These reflect the patient's true temperature more reliably than axillary, oral or peripheral temperature measurements. The core–peripheral temperature gradient gives an indication of the cardiovascular condition of the patient and the degree of peripheral vasoconstriction. A well-filled, well perfused patient has a core to peripheral temperature gradient of <2°C.

Hyperthermia

Hyperthermia is important as a marker for infection or other disease processes. Causes of hyperthermia are shown in Box 8.10.

The exact mechanisms that produce hyperthermia are not known but in many cases it can be viewed as a physiological response to critical illness rather than a significant part of the disease process. There is debate, therefore, about the need to treat a mildly raised temperature <39°C except in brain-injured patients, where increased temperature is associated with a worse

---

Box 8.10 Causes of hyperthermia

Infection

Systemic inflammatory response syndrome

Adverse reactions to drugs or blood products

Sympathomimetics

Brain injury

Seizures

Malignant hyperthermia*

Heatstroke*

Neuroleptic malignant syndrome*

*Rare

---

outcome. (See Brain injury, p. 272 and Management of cardiac arrest, p. 109.)

In general, however, measures such as regular paracetamol and tepid sponging for low-grade pyrexia may improve patient comfort.

Urgent treatment is required if core temperature exceeds 39°C. Prolonged core temperatures of >42°C are associated with cardiovascular collapse, rigors, seizures, brain injury, coagulopathy, multiple organ failure and death.

- Ensure adequate hydration (increased insensible losses).
- Give regular rectal paracetamol (ibuprofen is also effective if there are no contraindications to NSAIDs).
- Institute passive cooling: wet drapes, ice packs, fans, and gastric, peritoneal or bladder lavage with cold fluids.
- Consider sedation, intubation, ventilation and muscle relaxation to reduce metabolic rate.
- If severe hyperpyrexia, consider an extracorporeal circuit to actively cool the patient. Seek senior advice.

Dantrolene is a muscle relaxant that works distal to the neuromuscular junction. It has an established role in malignant hyperpyrexia, and appears to work after Ecstasy ingestion. It has not been shown to be effective in other conditions; however, it has limited side-effects in ventilated patients so can be tried when other measures fail.

- Dantrolene 1 mg/kg bolus repeated every 10 min up to 10 mg/kg. (See Malignant hyperpyrexia, p. 363.)

Hypothermia

Hypothermia is defined as a core temperature below 35°C. To avoid missing hypothermia, you should always have a high index of suspicion and measure core temperature in at-risk patients. Common causes are given in Box 8.11.

Box 8.11 Common causes of hypothermia

Environmental (particularly elderly)

Exposure (e.g. trauma victims)

Cold water immersion

Drug overdosage

Prolonged surgery with massive fluid/blood losses

Deliberate cooling during cardiac bypass

Brain protection (post-cardiac arrest)

Hypothermia is associated with a number of adverse effects. These include: arrhythmias, myocardial depression, vasoconstriction, coagulopathy, increased risk of wound infections and wound dehiscence, prolonged drug clearance, altered acid–base balance and prolonged ICU stay. In the surgical context, prevention is better than cure. The use of fluid warming devices, warming blankets and heated humidifiers perioperatively all help to reduce the risk.

In severely hypothermic patients from other causes:

● Exclude other injuries, drug ingestions, head injury, myxoedema, pressure necrosis of limbs, compartment syndromes, rhabdomyolysis and renal failure (measure CK). Treat appropriately (see Trauma, p. 306).

● Most patients respond to passive slow rewarming with a slow rise in core temperature of about 1°C per hour. Utilize a warm environment, hot-air warming blankets, and warm i.v. fluids for volume replacement.

● For severely hypothermic patients, with a core temperature below 32°C, consider more active warming measures such as peritoneal lavage with warm fluids, instillation of warm fluids into the bladder, or partial (femoral–femoral) bypass with a heat exchanger.

● Patients may develop dysrhythmias on rewarming, usually at around 31°C, and may need repeated cardioversion. It may, however, be difficult to restore sinus rhythm while the patient remains hypothermic. Occasionally under these circumstances profoundly hypothermic patients can be successfully warmed utilizing cardiopulmonary bypass.

In profoundly hypothermic patients it may be difficult to determine whether the patient has actually died. This follows cases of patients making a full recovery from prolonged circulatory arrest and deep hypothermia after cold water immersion. Therefore, resuscitation efforts should be continued until the patient approaches normothermia. Remember the maxim, 'you can't be dead until you're warm and dead'. Seek senior advice.

CHAPTER 9

OVERDOSE, POISONING AND DRUG ABUSE

Overdose and poisoning 230

Investigations 231

Measures to reduce absorption / increase elimination of drugs 231

Antidotes 233

Intensive care management 234

Paracetamol 235

Salicylates (aspirin) 236

Benzodiazepines and opiods 237

Antidepressants 237

Insulin overdose 238

Carbon monoxide and cyanide poisoning 239

Methanol and ethylene glycol 240

Alcohol 241

Recreational drug abuse 242

Problems associated with intravenous drug abuse 243

OVERDOSE AND POISONING

The problems associated with overdose and poisoning (deliberate or accidental) are responsible for a significant portion of the acute medical workload in hospitals. While most overdoses and poisonings are not serious and can be managed on medical wards, some patients will require admission to intensive care. This may be the result of the specific nature and effects of the substance involved, respiratory or cardiovascular complications or occasionally due to the onset of multiorgan failure. Common complications associated with overdose and poisonings are shown in Table 9.1.

This chapter provides general advice only. The UK National Poisons Information service (http://www.npis.org) operates TOXBASE®, which is an on-line poisons information service available at http://www.toxbase.org. This requires registration but should be available in most centres and should be consulted

TABLE 9.1 Potential complications of overdose	
General	Hypothermia/hyperthermia Pressure sores Crush syndrome/rhabdomyolysis Dehydration
Cardiovascular	Hypotension/hypertension Dysrhythmias Cardiac arrest
Respiratory	Respiratory depression Aspiration Pneumonia
CNS	Coma Hypoxic brain damage Seizures Confusional states/aggression
Renal	ATN secondary to hypotension/dehydration Effects of rhabdomyolysis Direct toxic effects
Gastrointestinal/liver	Diarrhoea/vomiting Acute gastric erosions/ gastrointestinal haemorrhage Acute liver failure

in the first instance. If additional advice is needed, this can be obtained from one of the regional poisons information services by telephone. Telephone numbers will be available through local hospital switch boards, via Toxbase® and from the British National Formulary (BNF: available on line at www.bnf.org).

INVESTIGATIONS

In the unconscious patient it is essential to exclude other treatable causes of loss of consciousness (e.g. head injury, subarachnoid haemorrhage, hypoglycaemia, meningitis), even if the patient has left a suicide note or is known to have taken an overdose previously. If in doubt, organize a CT scan of the brain and consider lumbar puncture and other investigations as appropriate.

The response to a (cautious) challenge of naloxone or flumazenil may occasionally be helpful in identifying opioid and benzodiazepine overdose, respectively (see below).

Aspirin (salicylate) and paracetamol assays should be performed in all cases. Alcohol levels can be measured in most centres and may be useful to distinguish intoxication from brain injury. The majority of other assays are unavailable at short notice, and the samples should be sent to regional centres. Aside from paracetamol, it is rare for assays to alter clinical management. Ask the laboratory to save serum in uncertain cases for later analysis and send urine for a toxicology screen. These samples may be invaluable if the patient subsequently dies and there is a Coroner's inquest or other inquiry.

MEASURES TO REDUCE ABSORPTION/INCREASE ELIMINATION OF DRUGS

Gastric lavage
Historically, gastric lavage was frequently performed in an attempt to remove tablet debris from the stomach. This is no longer a routine procedure, as evidence suggests it is largely ineffective, does not improve survival and is associated with potentially serious adverse events including aspiration, airway compromise, hypoxia and death.

Gastric lavage should therefore only be performed when recommended by a poisons information centre. It is usually only indicated when patients present within one hour of ingestion of life threatening quantities of drugs. Contraindications include ingestion of corrosives or substances liable to cause lipoid pneumonias and refusal of consent. It is not usually performed in children.

In the rare cases where gastric lavage is indicated, the airway should be protected by endotracheal intubation. If necessary, seek help from an experienced anaesthetist.

- If the patient is very obtunded, it may be possible to intubate the trachea without any anaesthetic drugs.
- If not, perform a rapid sequence induction with preoxygenation, cricoid pressure, an intravenous induction agent and suxamethonium.
- Pass the gastric tube under direct vision and then perform lavage.
- Consider extubation in head-down, left lateral position.
- If the patient is not fit to extubate and/or send to the ward, keep the patient intubated and transfer to ICU.
- If respiratory effort is feeble, it is better to support ventilation for a few hours than leave the patient to breathe spontaneously with poor tidal volumes. This helps to maintain lung expansion, minimizes the tendency to atelectasis and provides ongoing airway protection.

Activated charcoal

Activated charcoal (oral or via a nasogastric tube) has two effects. It binds free drug within the lumen of the bowel and also actively absorbs drug from the circulation. It is absorption of ingested drug from the bloodstream that is the rationale for repeated use of activated charcoal in some cases. Indications for multiple-dose activated charcoal are shown in Box 9.1.

Box 9.1 Overdoses for which multiple-dose activated charcoal may be useful

Barbiturates
Carbamazepine
Chlormethiazole
Digoxin
Phenobarbital
Phenytoin
Quinine
Salicylates
Theophylline

TABLE 9.2 Role of haemodialysis and haemoperfusion in overdose	
Haemodialysis	**Haemoperfusion**
Ethylene glycol	Barbiturates
Methanol	Theophylline
Lithium	
Salicylates	

A typical dose regimen is as shown:

- 50 g 4-hourly oral/NG.
- If nausea/vomiting are a problem, it can be given as 12.5 g hourly.

Forced alkaline diuresis

Traditionally, this has been used to increase the renal clearance of soluble, acidic drugs, particularly salicylates and barbiturates. It is now controversial due to problems with fluid overload and acid–base disturbance. Seek senior advice. A typical regimen is as follows:

- Use CVP to guide volume loading with normal saline/colloid.
- Give 0.25–0.5 g/kg mannitol 20% to promote diuresis >200 mL/h.
- Give sodium bicarbonate (8.4%) 1 mmol/kg/h to achieve urinary pH > 7.5.

The role of loop diuretics to increase urine flow in this setting is controversial. Some authors recommend them if the response to mannitol is inadequate. They can, however, produce acidification in the renal tubule and promote precipitation of acid-soluble drugs and compounds such as myoglobin. (See Rhabdomyolysis, p. 320.)

Haemodialysis and haemoperfusion

Haemodialysis and haemoperfusion over activated charcoal are useful for some life-threatening overdoses. These are listed in Table 9.2. Seek specialist advice. There are also some reports of albumin dialysis (e.g. MARS®) being used in the treatment of heavy metal poisoning.

ANTIDOTES

Some overdoses/poisonings have specific antagonists or antidotes which reduce the toxic effects and mortality. These should generally only be used for potentially life-threatening situations when the nature of the overdose or poison is known. Available antagonists/antidotes are shown in Table 9.3.

TABLE 9.3 Commonly available antagonists and antidotes

Drug	Antagonist/antidote
Benzodiazepines	Flumazenil
Copper	Penicillamine
Digoxin	Digoxin-specific antibodies
Ethylene glycol	Ethanol, fomepizole
Heparin (unfractionated)	Protamine
Iron	Desferrioxamine
Lead	Sodium calcium edetate
Methanol	Ethanol, fomepizole
Opioids	Naloxone
Organophosphates	Atropine, pralidoxime
Paracetamol	N-acetylcysteine
Warfarin	Vitamin K, fresh frozen plasma, prothrombin complex concentrate (Beriplex)

INTENSIVE CARE MANAGEMENT

In the majority of overdoses/poisonings there is no specific antidote and care is supportive with the aim of preventing or reversing the onset of complications. Indications for admission to intensive care are shown in Box 9.2.

● Secure the airway and support respiration with IPPV if necessary. Sedative drugs can usually be avoided if the patient is deeply comatose. Muscle relaxants may aid intubation. Extubate once the consciousness level improves.

Box 9.2 Indications for admission to intensive care following overdose/poisoning

Need for tracheal intubation/assisted ventilation

Reduced conscious level (GCS < 8) or seizures

Need for invasive monitoring/cardiovascular support

Dysrhythmias*

2nd or 3rd degree heart block*

QRS > 0.12 s or QTc > 420 ms*

Need for renal replacement therapy or other organ support

*Need for continuous cardiac monitoring. Depending on local policies may be admitted to coronary care unit or HDU.

- Monitor ECG and blood pressure.
- A number of common overdoses are associated with cardiac rhythm disturbances. Where possible avoid procedures or treatments that may precipitate dysrhythmias. Most patients admitted to intensive care following self-poisoning are admitted for a relatively short period, and remain stable (generally suffering only a depressed level of consciousness). It is usually neither necessary nor desirable to insert a central venous catheter. If central venous access is required, avoid precipitating cardiac rhythm disturbances by inserting the guide wire too far.
- Use fluid in the first instance to manage hypotension. Some patients may be severely dehydrated and require significant fluid therapy.
- Monitor body temperature. Hypothermia is common following prolonged unconsciousness and after overdose with some centrally acting drugs while hyperthermia may follow some specific overdoses.
- Single short convulsions do not require treatment. Prolonged seizure activity should be treated; seek specialist advice. (See Seizures, p. 296.)
- Beware of pressure-related injuries from prolonged immobilization. Pressure sores, tissue necrosis and compartment syndromes are common following prolonged unconsciousness. Rhabdomyolysis and myoglobinuria can precipitate renal failure. (See Peripheral compartment syndromes, p. 319 and Rhabdomyolysis, p. 320.)

Typically, a patient who has taken an overdose of sedative or analgesic agents needs between 12 and 24 h of supportive care (possibly including ventilation) before discharge to the ward.

All patients who are admitted following deliberate overdose should be referred to a liaison psychiatrist. The psychiatric consultation will not normally take place until the patient is sufficiently well for this to be meaningful, and this may therefore not occur until after the patient has returned to the ward. Nevertheless, it is important to make the referral at an early stage so that it is not overlooked. This is particularly important as many patients who have taken an overdose may discharge themselves from hospital against medical advice.

PARACETAMOL

Paracetamol poisoning is important, as it is the commonest overdose referred to the UK National Poisons Information Service, accounting for over 1000 calls per year. Despite legislation to reduce the amount of paracetamol which can be bought at any one time,

TABLE 9.4 Indications for liver transplant following paracetamol overdose

Either (any one of the following)	Or (all of the following)
pH < 7.3 after fluid resuscitation	Creatinine > 300 μmol/l
Lactate > 3.5 (pre-resuscitation)	PT > 100 s
Lactate > 3.0 (post-resuscitation)	Grade III or IV encephalopathy

in the UK, 48% of all hospital admissions for poisoning are due to paracetamol. It remains a leading cause of hyperacute liver failure in intensive care units, and results in 300 deaths in the UK annually.

Relatively low doses of drug may produce fatal liver failure in susceptible patients, such as those with pre-existing liver disease. In addition, the ingestion of other drugs (e.g. anticonvulsants) may increase the toxicity of paracetamol.

The need for treatment is determined by plasma paracetamol concentrations. For those who fall above treatment thresholds, intravenous N-acetylcysteine is an effective antidote if started within 10–12 h of ingestion. For treatment thresholds and dosage schedules, see BNF or contact poisons advice centre.

For those patients who present more than 12 h after significant ingestion of paracetamol, N-acetylcysteine may still be of some benefit. Advice should be obtained from the poisons centre and/or the local liver unit.

Patients who develop liver failure often have few visible signs of problems for about 48 hours, and then deteriorate rapidly. Fulminant liver failure follows, with hepatic encephalopathy, increasing prothrombin time and INR, falling platelet count, jaundice, acidosis and renal dysfunction. These patients must be urgently transferred to a regional liver unit for further management, including possible acute transplantation. As patients with fulminant paracetamol-induced liver failure deteriorate extremely quickly, it is important to discuss such cases with your local liver unit as soon as possible, and carry out the transfer before the patient succumbs to multiple organ failure. (See Hepatic failure, p. 176.) Indications for urgent transplantation (within 24 h) are shown in Table 9.4.

SALICYLATES (ASPIRIN)

The features of salicylate poisoning are hyperventilation, tinnitus, deafness, vasodilatation and sweating. Hyperventilation and sweating result in dehydration. Coma is uncommon but indicates severe overdose. Gastric emptying is delayed and gastric lavage is useful to retrieve tablet debris up to 4 h after ingestion. For the same reason, plasma levels may be misleading if taken within 6 h.

Blood gases and electrolytes should be monitored. Treatment is by rehydration. If plasma levels are above 500 mg/L (3.6 mmol/L) in adults or 350 mg/L (2.5 mmol/L) in children then forced alkaline diuresis with 1.26% sodium bicarbonate should be used to improve urinary excretion. In very severe cases, levels above 700 mg/L (5.1 mmol/L), haemodialysis is the treatment of choice.

BENZODIAZEPINES AND OPIODS

Benzodiazepines or opioid overdose generally requires no specific therapy other than supportive care and airway protection, with or without assisted ventilation until conscious level and respiratory drive improve. Flumazenil and naloxone may be used to confirm the diagnosis in benzodiazepine and opioid overdose, but may precipitate seizures, arrhythmias and hypertension. Do not use these antidotes in an attempt to avoid the need for tracheal intubation, assisted ventilation and ICU admission. They are short acting. If the infusion stops or the cannula is pulled out, then the patient's conscious level may rapidly deteriorate, potentially with fatal consequences. Cases have also been reported where, following administration of these antagonist agents, the patient has rapidly woken up, become aggressive and taken hospital discharge, only to collapse again once outside the hospital. (See Intravenous drug abusers, p. 243.)

ANTIDEPRESSANTS

Tricyclic antidepressants
The tricyclic and related antidepressant drugs, in addition to sedative properties, have anticholinergic/sympathomimetic effects, which cause significant problems following overdose. Potential effects are shown in Box 9.3.

Box 9.3 Effects of tricyclic overdose

Confusion

Seizures

Coma

Dehydration

Tachycardia/dysrhythmias

Widely dilated pupils

Hyperthermia

Treatment is supportive, with resuscitation, control of seizures and rehydration. Tachydysrhythmias are common and may require repeated cardioversion. Antidysrhythmic drugs are best avoided. Once hypoxia, acidosis and dehydration are corrected, cardiac rhythm usually settles to a sinus tachycardia. Correction of acidosis with bicarbonate is thought to help by reducing unbound free drug (pKa effect). Typically, even after severe problems (e.g. dysrhythmias requiring repeated cardioversion), patients are stable enough to be extubated after 12–24h. Often the patient will require no sedation for the first few hours. Short-acting sedatives/anticonvulsants (e.g. propofol infusion) may be required for a few hours until the patient is stable.

Selective serotonin reuptake inhibitors (SSI)

Selective serotonin reuptake inhibitors have been increasingly implicated in overdosage in recent years. Overdose with this class of drugs carries a much lower mortality than overdosage with tricyclic antidepressant agents. While all members of the class have presented as overdoses, the commonest is citalopram. Overdose with this class of drugs generally presents with drowsiness, though in severe cases there may be depression of consciousness, fitting, and prolonged QT_C. Very rarely, this leads to significant cardiac dysrhythmias. The literature includes sporadic cases of cardiac arrest. Admission to intensive care for management of the sedative side-effects is recommended. The effects of selective serotonin reuptake inhibitors in overdose may be prolonged, as drug elimination is reduced and normal pharmacokinetics appear not to apply.

INSULIN OVERDOSE

Relative overdose from unintentional mismatch between insulin dosage and insulin requirement is common. If managed in a timely fashion, the resulting mild hypoglycaemia is usually short lived and results in no harm to the patient (see Hypoglycaemia).

Deliberate overdose of insulin either by the patient or by a third party acting with criminal intent, although uncommon has been seen both inside and outside the hospital setting. Protracted severe hypoglycaemia leads to irreversible brain damage and frequently death. Insulin overdose (deliberate or otherwise) should always be considered as a cause of severe hypoglycaemia. Consider taking blood for later insulin assay. Treatment is by dextrose infusion. Survivors with brain damage have similar problems to those with hypoxic brain injury.

Box 9.4 Clinical features of carbon monoxide poisoning

Cherry red colour (unreliable)

Headaches

Nausea and vomiting

Arrhythmias

Seizures

Coma, confusional states

CARBON MONOXIDE AND CYANIDE POISONING

Carbon monoxide

Carbon monoxide is a product of incomplete combustion. Carbon monoxide poisoning may be seen in combination with burns, from smoke inhalation, from inadequately ventilated heating appliances (unexplained collapse) and following suicide attempts (car exhaust). Apparently unburned victims from house fires may present with carbon monoxide poisoning. Carbon monoxide bonds avidly to haemoglobin, resulting in carboxyhaemoglobin, which does not carry oxygen. Severe cases may suffer anoxic brain damage. The clinical features are shown in Box 9.4.

Diagnosis is made by measurement of carboxyhaemoglobin levels. Many blood gas analysers now include a co-oximeter that can measure carboxyhaemoglobin (normal levels <5%). Some pulse oximeters also have this facility.

Treatment is supportive. If the inspired oxygen concentration is increased to 100% the half-life of carboxyhaemoglobin is 1 h; therefore, blood levels will quickly return to normal although tissue levels may remain elevated for longer. There is some evidence that, in patients who have had recorded carboxyhaemoglobin levels >20% and/or neurological symptoms at any time, the incidence of late neurological sequelae may be reduced by hyperbaric oxygen therapy. The benefits of hyperbaric oxygen need to be weighed against the risks of transfer to a specialist centre. Seek senior advice.

 Not all hyperbaric facilities are based on hospital sites: check before agreeing to go, as you may find yourself in an isolated site with limited facilities and no backup.

Cyanide poisoning

Cyanide is a product of combustion of some foam materials. Cyanide poisoning may therefore occur in patients with smoke inhalation/carbon monoxide poisoning. The clinical features, which may be rapid in onset, include anxiety, vomiting, headache and reduced consciousness. Metabolic acidosis is common.

In mild cases, only supportive treatment is required. Give 100% oxygen. In severe cases with loss of consciousness, sodium thiosulphate is used to convert cyanide to thiocyanate. Seek advice. Typically:

● Sodium thiosulphate 150 mg/kg i.v. followed by 30–60 mg/kg/h infusion.

METHANOL AND ETHYLENE GLYCOL

These agents may be ingested accidentally or deliberately.

Methanol

Methanol is available as a solvent, in methylated spirits and is present in de-icers and antifreeze solutions. Methanol may be taken as an alcohol substitute by patients who are unaware of the risks.

Clinical features are progressive confusion, ataxia and visual disturbances. Metabolism to formaldehyde and then formic acid leads to severe metabolic acidosis 12–18 h after ingestion. The direct toxic effects of formate on the optic nerve can result in blindness. Plasma osmolality and anion gap are increased (see Treatment below).

Ethylene glycol

Ethylene glycol is a sweet-tasting liquid used alone or in combination with other alcohols in antifreeze. Clinical features are similar to alcohol intoxication, followed by nausea, vomiting and haematemesis. Focal neurological signs, seizures and a gradual deterioration in conscious level then occur. While most of the ethylene glycol is excreted unchanged in the urine, metabolites include oxalic acid. This accumulates, resulting in severe metabolic acidosis, increased anion gap and hypocalcaemia. Oxalate excretion in the urine leads to the formation of oxalate crystals and renal failure.

Treatment of both methanol and ethylene glycol poisoning is based on supportive care, correction of the underlying acidosis and inhibition of the metabolism with ethanol or fomepizole. Ethanol competes with methanol/ethylene glycol as a substrate in the metabolic pathway. High percentage proof ethanol ampoules are available from most hospital pharmacy departments. Fomepizole is an expensive, newly introduced alcohol dehydrogenase inhibitor. In both cases, the metabolism of methanol/ethylene glycol and the production of toxic metabolites are reduced. Haemodialysis to remove methanol/ethylene glycol should be considered in severe cases. Seek specialist advice.

ALCOHOL

Alcohol (ethanol) is the most commonly used and abused non-prescription drug. Acute alcohol intoxication is a factor in many patients admitted to intensive care, particularly following trauma.

Acute alcohol intoxication

Acute alcohol intoxication produces coma, hypothermia, hypoglycaemia and in severe cases metabolic acidosis. Other causes of coma (e.g. extradural haemorrhage) must be excluded. Other injuries should also be excluded. Treatment is supportive. Consider:

- intubation to protect the airway and ventilation as necessary
- gastric lavage to reduce alcohol absorption (alcohol delays gastric emptying)
- dextrose infusion to correct hypoglycaemia.

In severe life threatening cases of alcohol intoxication, an alcohol dehydrogenase inhibitor such as fomepizole may be of value. Seek specialist advice. Haemodialysis has also been used to remove alcohol, although only sporadic cases have been reported.

Management of alcohol withdrawal on ICU

Acute withdrawal from alcohol may result in insomnia, tremor, agitation and seizures. Delirium tremens, in which patients develop visual hallucinations, is the most serious withdrawal phenomenon. Symptoms develop 1–5 days after withdrawal and may be life-threatening. Treatment comprises adequate sedation, together with supportive care:

- Standard ICU sedative regimens (particularly benzodiazepine based) are usually adequate. Chlormethiazole given by infusion is difficult to titrate, provides a substantial fluid load, and is probably best avoided. (See Sedation and analgesia, p. 34.)

Box 9.5 Problems associated with chronic alcohol abuse

Decreased resistance to infection

Severe chest infections are common (TB should be excluded)

Self-neglect/poor nutrition (give B group vitamins)

Alcoholic cardiomyopathy (atrial fibrillation common)

Cirrhosis/liver failure

Gastrointestinal bleeding

Pancreatitis

Acute confusional states

Autonomic and peripheral neuropathy

Acute withdrawal states/delirium tremens/seizures

Cerebral atrophy

Central pontine myelinosis

Wernicke's encephalopathy

Chronic alcohol abuse

It may not be evident on admission that patients are alcohol abusers, and neither the patient nor friends or relatives may know or disclose this. Chronic alcohol abuse is associated with a number of medical problems (Box 9.5).

● All chronic alcoholics should receive vitamin B supplements parenterally.

RECREATIONAL DRUG ABUSE

The abuse of drugs by all routes is widespread. Some of the commonly abused 'recreational' drugs and their effects are shown in Table 9.5.

Ecstasy

This and other amphetamine derivatives are increasingly seen as a cause of severe toxic reactions. Patients present with signs of sympathetic overactivity similar to tricyclic overdose. These reactions appear more idiosyncratic rather than dose related. It is not clear what triggers the response in a particular individual who may have been exposed to the drug before without problems. Hyperpyrexia, rhabdomyolysis, acute renal failure and multiple organ failure are seen in severe cases. Treatment is supportive with cooling measures, and dantrolene may be helpful. Seek advice from poisons centre. (See Hyperthermia, p. 224.)

TABLE 9.5 Common drugs of abuse and their effects	
Substance	*Effects*
Amphetamines	Stimulant effects, increased metabolic rate, weight loss, tachycardia, hypertension, dysrhythmias, hallucinations, paranoia, aggression
Anabolic steroids	No intoxication effects. Occasional acute psychosis; long-term risks associated with steroids, cardiomyopathy and sudden death
Cannabinoids	Euphoria, slowed reaction time, impaired balance/co-ordination/anxiety and panic attacks
Cocaine	Stimulant effects similar to amphetamines. Tachycardia, hypertension, seizures, CVA, coma
Gamma-hydroxybutyrate (GHB)	Reduced pain and anxiety, feeling of well-being, drowsiness, nausea/vomiting, loss of consciousness, depressed reflexes, seizures, coma and death
Ketamine	Tachycardia, hypertension, impaired motor function; high doses, respiratory depression
Lysergic acid diethylamide (LSD)	Altered states of perception, hyperthermia, tachycardia, hypertension
Methylenedioxymetamphetamine (MDMA) (group includes ecstasy)	Similar to amphetamines. Mild hallucinogenic effects, impaired memory and learning, hyperthermia, idiosyncratic hyperacute liver failure
Opioids	Pain relief, euphoria, drowsiness, unconsciousness, respiratory depression/arrest
Phencyclidine (PCP)	Panic, aggression, violence, bradycardia, hypotension
Solvents	Stimulants. Headaches, loss of co-ordination, nausea/vomiting, dysrhythmias, sudden death

PROBLEMS ASSOCIATED WITH INTRAVENOUS DRUG ABUSE

Intravenous opioid drug abusers frequently require admission to intensive care. This may be due to the effects of the drugs, trauma occurring while under the influence of drugs, or as a result of medical problems from the side-effects of drug abuse. Common medical problems in this group are shown in Box 9.6.

> **Box 9.6 Problems associated with intravenous drug abuse**
>
> Self-neglect/malnutrition
> HIV/hepatitis
> Venous thrombosis (difficult venous access)
> Arterial thrombosis and limb ischaemia
> Abscess formation
> Endocarditis
> Pneumonia
> Sepsis
> Pancreatitis
> Botulism

It may not be evident on admission that patients are drug abusers, and neither the patient nor the friends or relatives may disclose this. There is a significant risk of such patients being carriers of hepatitis, HIV and other infectious diseases. This highlights the need to use universal precautions at all times when carrying out procedures. (See Universal precautions, p. 19.)

Managing opioid withdrawal

Patients may develop symptoms and signs of drug withdrawal.

- Avoid precipitating withdrawal phenomena by unnecessary discontinuation of drugs.
- Where acute withdrawal is likely, symptoms can generally be controlled by the use of standard ICU sedative regimens.

Occasionally a reformed intravenous opioid drug abuser may want to avoid opioid-based sedative or analgesic regimens to prevent relapse in habit. Consider the use of peripheral, regional or central axial blockade and other analgesic drugs for pain relief. Seek specialist advice from pain management teams.

CHAPTER 10

HAEMATOLOGICAL PROBLEMS

Introduction   246

Anaemia in the
   critically ill   246

Indications for blood
   transfusion   246

Blood products in
   the UK   247

Administration of blood
   products   250

Major haemorrhage   251

Risks and complications
   of blood transfusion   252

Patients who refuse
   transfusion   254

Normal haemostatic
   mechanisms   255

Coagulopathy   258

Thrombocytopenia   262

Disseminated intravascular
   coagulation   263

Purpuric disorders   264

Thrombotic disorders   264

The immunocompromised
   patient   266

INTRODUCTION

Haematological problems are common in the ICU. Most are related to blood loss, the need for large volume blood transfusions and the development of coagulation disorders. Bone marrow failure and immunosuppression are also problems in some patients.

ANAEMIA IN THE CRITICALLY ILL

Anaemia is common in critically ill patients and often necessitates repeated blood transfusion. Anaemia may be the direct result of an underlying disease process, but more commonly is multifactorial. Common factors that may contribute to anaemia are listed in Box 10.1.

Where possible, the underlying causes of anaemia should be addressed. Blood loss, including that from blood sampling, should be minimized.

INDICATIONS FOR BLOOD TRANSFUSION

There has been significant debate about the optimum haemoglobin level for critically ill patients and the level at which transfusions should be instituted (the so-called transfusion threshold). The following are key considerations:

- Oxygen carriage and delivery. The oxygen content of blood is given by $Hb \times SaO_2 \times 1.34$. Raising haemoglobin is an effective way of improving oxygen content and delivery. (See Oxygen delivery and oxygen consumption, p. 68.)
- Myocardial function. Myocardial ischaemia and diastolic dysfunction may occur in the stressed heart when the haematocrit falls below 0.18. In the presence of coronary artery disease, the threshold is 0.24 or higher.

Box 10.1 Factors contributing to anaemia in the critically ill

Repeated blood sampling

Blood loss associated with repeated surgical procedures

Haemorrhage (especially GIT)

Anaemias of chronic disease (e.g. chronic renal failure)

Effects of underlying disease process

Haemolysis (e.g. drugs, antibodies, infection)

Bone marrow suppression

Relative iron/B_{12}/folate deficiencies

- Rheology. In vitro and probably in vivo, blood viscosity is reduced as haematocrit falls below 0.24 and rises above 0.3. This may have implications for perfusion of the microcirculation, particularly in critical illness and following vascular surgery. Recent evidence suggests that both very low and very high haematocrits are associated with impaired tissue perfusion. Haematocrit can be estimated from Hb (g/dL) $\times$ 3/100.
- Immunology. There is some evidence that transfusion induces a degree of immunosuppression, particularly massive transfusion. This is important following any major surgery, and especially so where surgery has been performed for malignant disease.
- Finite risks associated with each individual blood product transfused (see below).

Recent work suggests that restrictive transfusion strategies produce the best outcome in critically ill patients, and that the optimal level in most cases is Hb of 8–10 g/dL. Transfusion thresholds of around 7 g/dL are reasonable in most patients, with an aim to raise the haemoglobin to no more than 10 g/dL. The rate of transfusion will depend on the clinical circumstances, but for many 'routine transfusions' the blood can be given slowly over a number of hours to avoid rapid volume loading effects.

The blood volume of a patient will vary considerably with size and age, but is approximately 80 mL/kg, lean body mass.

BLOOD PRODUCTS IN THE UK

In the UK, blood is donated by unpaid volunteers, who undergo general health screening. Whole blood is collected into a citrate-based anticoagulant solution (chelating calcium to prevent clotting) and then further separated to yield individual blood components such as platelets, fresh frozen plasma (FFP) and cryoprecipitate.

All donations are serologically tested for HIV-1 and HIV-2, hepatitis B and C, syphilis and cytomegalovirus (CMV). CMV-free blood components are used for immunosuppressed patients and those under 1 year of age.

Recently, potential transmission of new variant Creutzfeldt–Jakob disease (vCJD) has become a concern. It is likely that in the near future screening of donors for vCJD will become available. Currently in the UK all blood products have white cells removed (leucodepletion) as a precaution against vCJD transmission (white cell count $< 5 \times 10^6$). Continuing concerns regarding the potential for carriage and transmission of vCJD by the UK blood donor pool has resulted in some plasma products being sourced from outside the UK, principally from the USA.

Despite these and other measures, there remain risks associated with the use of all blood products. Although the most commonly reported major transfusion-related injury results from the wrong blood being transfused into the wrong patient, even when errors such as this are eliminated, there are finite risks associated with infection, immunological and idiosyncratic reactions. Therefore, you should not undertake transfusion of blood products lightly. In many cases, conservative management may be more appropriate. (See Risks and complications of blood transfusion, p. 252.)

The following component blood products are available.

Red cells

Whole blood was traditionally used for the replacement of blood loss. Whole blood is now rarely available. Red cell concentrates are usually used. The plasma component of whole blood is removed by the National Blood Transfusion Service (removes clotting factors and albumin) and the red cells are suspended in an additive solution prior to their issue to hospital transfusion laboratories. The two commonly used additive solutions are:

● citrate, phosphate, dextrose and adenosine (CPDA)
● sodium chloride, adenosine, glucose and mannitol (SAGM).

The blood products potentially available for red cell replacement are shown in Table 10.1.

TABLE 10.1 Red cell products

	Whole blood	Packed red cells	Red cell additive solution
Volume (mL)	470 ± 50	270 ± 50	550 ± 70
Source	Single donor	Single donor	Single donor
Haematocrit (%)	35–45	55–75	50–70
Leucocytes	Depleted	Depleted	Depleted
Additives	CPDA	CPDA	SAGM

Fresh frozen plasma

Fresh frozen plasma (FFP) may be from a single donor or recovered from pooled donors. The volume of units provided therefore varies from 150 to 500 mL. FFP contains both labile and stable factors, including albumin, gamma globulin, fibrinogen and factor VIII. Usually 2–4 units are given when required for coagulopathy (prolonged PT). Plasma products should be ABO compatible.

Recent concerns regarding virus transmission have resulted in treated plasma products becoming available. There are currently two: methylene blue treated and solvent detergent treated. The characteristics of available plasma products are compared in Table 10.2.

Recent reports of procoagulant complications with solvent detergent-treated FFP are thought to be due to relative protein S deficiency. This, together with the problems associated with pooled donors (1000 donors per batch), may limit its widespread use. However, the field is moving forward all the time. There is much current interest in production of a universal (ABO independent) pathogen inactivated plasma that would be safe for use in all blood groups, thereby eliminating the risk of ABO incompatibility and major transfusion reactions.

As with all blood products, the need for fresh frozen plasma should be critically assessed in every case. Although it is well established that fresh frozen plasma corrects coagulopathy and has a self-evident effect on the bleeding, there are no randomized controlled trials showing clinical benefit from the use of fresh frozen plasma. Nevertheless, solvent detergent and methylene blue treated plasma remain licensed in Europe and are an attractive option for patients needing massive or repeated transfusion. (See Major haemorrhage, p. 251.)

Cryoprecipitate

Cryoprecipitate is provided as one to six single donations per pack, suspended in 10–20 mL plasma. It contains fibrinogen and

TABLE 10.2 Fresh frozen plasma products

	Standard FFP	Methylene blue-treated FFP	Solvent detergent-treated FFP
Source	Single donor	Single donor	Pooled donor
Volume (mL)	180–300	235–305	200
Coagulation factor content	Variable	Variable	Constant

factor VIII. It is used to correct coagulopathy where fibrinogen levels are depleted. Six units generally raise fibrinogen levels by approximately 1 g/L.

Platelets

Platelets may be single donor, or pooled (five or six donors). Six units typically raise the platelet count by approximately $10–20 \times 10^9/L$. Platelets should ideally, but not necessarily, be ABO compatible. Platelet transfusion should only be used when absolutely necessary. Apart from all of the other risks of blood transfusion, platelets are kept at room temperature and can rarely give rise to overwhelming bacterial infection due to infusion of infected product. Although this is very rare, it is catastrophic, and is often fatal.

ADMINISTRATION OF BLOOD PRODUCTS

The complications of blood transfusion are discussed below. The biggest cause of major ABO incompatibility reactions is human error. Most commonly these result from failure to follow approved procedures. The following notes are applicable to all blood products.

Requesting blood products

- Ensure that you follow national/locally agreed procedures and guidelines.
- Ensure blood samples are carefully labelled and that the accompanying request forms are accurately completed.
- Ensure that blood products are appropriately prescribed.

Check recipient identity

Before administering any blood product, it is essential that the product is matched to the intended recipient. The product label always states the nature of the contents (e.g. whole blood, FFP), its storage temperature, expiry date and time, ABO and RhD grouping, donation or batch number and details of the patient against whom it has been cross-matched. These details must be verified against the wrist band of the patient who is the intended recipient.

- When possible, ask the patient to confirm his or her identity and that the details on the identification band are correct.
- Ensure that the patient's name and identification number on the wristband match those on the intended blood product.
- Ensure that the ABO blood group, rhesus blood group and unit identification number are all correct.

> ⚠️ In some hospitals, a form accompanies blood products, identifying the units issued; this is intended as a record to be placed in the patient's notes. These forms are not intended to be used as part of the checking procedure, and do not help to ensure that the correct unit of blood is given to the correct patient. The only acceptable checking process is to confirm that the patient details on the product label and those on the patient's wrist band are the same.

TABLE 10.3 Storage and use of blood products

	Red cells	FFP	Cryo-ppt	Platelets
Stored	2–6°C	−30°C	−30°C	22°C on agitators
Shelf life	35 days	1 year	1 year	5 days
Once removed from storage complete transfusion within:	5 h	4 h	4 h	2 h

Administration

Blood products are stored under carefully controlled conditions in the blood bank. Once removed from controlled storage they must be used within set time frames as indicated on the pack, typically as shown in Table 10.3.

Blood should ideally be given through a large cannula (minimum 18 gauge) to avoid haemolysis. Standard giving sets with 170 µm filters are adequate. Microaggregate filters are not necessary and must never be used when giving platelets. If blood is given through the same set as other fluids, calcium-containing solutions should be avoided. Consider the use of a blood warmer.

MAJOR HAEMORRHAGE

A significant risk in managing major haemorrhage is the non-availability of appropriate blood when needed. Clear communication, sending blood samples to the laboratory in a timely fashion and prioritizing preparations (calling help, preparing blood warmers, cell savers and rapid infusion devices) all reduce the risk of disaster.

● Where possible, control the source of the bleeding, for example by direct pressure.

- Ensure adequate vascular access: at least 2×14-gauge peripheral lines or single large-bore cannula such as 8.5-Fr introducer sheath. This need not necessarily be inserted into a central vein; a peripheral vein may well be easier to cannulate in an emergency, and just as adequate.
- Continue background or maintenance fluids to provide free water, glucose and electrolyte requirements.
- Commence initial volume replacement with a crystalloid or simple colloid such as modified gelatin (e.g. Gelofusine or Haemaccel).
- Continue with packed cells to maintain a haematocrit of 0.26–0.32.
- After 5 units of blood, consider changing to whole blood if available and/or giving FFP to minimize the effects of dilutional coagulopathy.
- Recheck FBC, U&Es, clotting and thromboelastogram (TEG) if available.
- Ensure adequate treatment of coagulopathy. In particular, keep the ionized calcium above 0.85 mmol/L. Maintain normothermia with active warming of the patient if necessary.
- After 10 units, recheck clotting. Consider cryoprecipitate, platelets and further FFP (see Coagulopathy below).

The successful management of major haemorrhage usually depends on surgical control of the bleeding. Therefore as soon as significant haemorrhage is identified or suspected inform your consultant and the senior members of the relevant clinical team directly. Notifying the most junior member of other teams, and waiting for him/her to make a decision and refer the matter to more senior members of the team, is likely to waste valuable time. If available, consider the use of a cell saver, to reduce the need for 'bank' blood.

RISKS AND COMPLICATIONS OF BLOOD TRANSFUSION

Complications of blood transfusion include fluid overload, hypothermia, hypocalcaemia, acidosis and dilutional coagulopathy. ARDS and multiple organ failure are also considered to be complications of massive transfusion. Bacterial contamination of blood occurs rarely and is usually fatal (platelet transfusion carries the greatest risk because of the need to store at room temperature).

Recent figures for risk of transmission of viral infection suggest the risk of HIV transmission is around 0.14 per million donor exposures and the risk of hepatitis B and C are a little higher 1.7 and 0.8 per million respectively.

Acute transfusion reactions are relatively uncommon. They include:

- haemolytic (75% due to ABO incompatibility)
- anaphylactic (antibodies to IgA in IgA-deficient patients)
- febrile white cell reactions (antibodies to leucocyte antigens)
- transfusion-related acute lung injury (antibodies to leucocyte antigens)
- urticaria (1–2% of transfusions).

Severe haemolytic reactions due to ABO incompatibility are rare and usually result from the wrong blood being given. Febrile reactions are less common with leucocyte-depleted blood but may still occur.

Management of acute transfusion reactions

Minor febrile / urticarial transfusion reactions may settle following hydrocortisone 100 mg and chlorphenamine 10 mg and it may be possible to cautiously continue the transfusion. Major transfusion reactions require transfusions to be discontinued. Blood bags should be returned to the transfusion laboratory, together with a sample of the patient's blood, for further evaluation. Seek the advice of the haematology department.

Transfusion-related acute lung injury (TRALI)

This is a relatively rare cause of acute lung injury following transfusion of blood or any plasma-containing blood product. It may however be more common than is currently realized (many cases may be labelled as ARDS or pulmonary oedema). Fresh frozen plasma is the most commonly implicated blood product.

Antibodies in the transfused blood product cause activation of the recipient's white cells, leading to an inflammatory response. The onset is typically within a few hours of transfusion and the clinical features are that of non-cardiogenic pulmonary oedema, which may lead on to the development of ARDS. If TRALI is suspected, the blood transfusion service should be advised so that donors can be screened for white cell antibodies. Treatment is supportive, as for any acute lung injury / ARDS. (See acute lung injury, p. 154.)

For more information on serious hazards of transfusion, see www.shotuk.org. SHOT (Serious Hazards Of Transfusion) is an independent professionally led organization that collects information relating to serious adverse transfusion reactions in the UK.

PATIENTS WHO REFUSE TRANSFUSION

Jehovah's Witnesses have strong religious views regarding the acceptability of blood and blood products. Wherever possible, you should clarify the individual's wishes and religious views, which should be respected. Failure to do so may constitute an assault. The Jehovah's Witness patient who requires intensive care may of course be unable to express their wishes and to give or withhold informed consent. In the case of adults, advice may be sought from next of kin or the Jehovah's Witness hospital liaison committee. (See Ethical and legal issues, p. 29, and Death and different cultural views, p. 440.)

The following notes are broad guidelines only, and may not be completely acceptable to all individuals:

- Blood (red cells, whole blood), FFP, platelets may not be given to Jehovah's Witnesses under any circumstances.
- Predonated blood is generally not acceptable.
- Albumin and cryoprecipitate is accepted by some (but not all) Jehovah's Witnesses.
- Factor concentrates: concentrates of specific factors (for example, factor XI, IX and VII) are generally accepted. Seek the advice of your hospital liaison committee.
- Extracorporeal circuits. The majority of Jehovah's Witnesses accept blood that has been passed through an extracorporeal circuit. This allows for cardiac surgery (cardiopulmonary bypass) and for renal dialysis. Intraoperative cell salvage is generally acceptable provided the blood is reinfused immediately, at the time of surgery, and not several hours later on the ICU.
- An individual contract/management plan may be prepared before treatment to clarify treatment options, when the patient is well enough to do this.

Management
- Patients with an anticipated major haemorrhage should receive supplementation of iron and other haematinics preoperatively.
- Erythropoietin (EPO) may be prescribed to stimulate red cell production. Side-effects are uncommon, but include hypertension, headache and stroke. Not all patients respond.

- Minimize any potential blood loss during surgery,
- Consider aggressive hypervolaemic haemodilution to reduce the haematocrit of any blood lost during surgery. Haemoglobin concentrations as low as 5 g/dL may be tolerated (see below).
- Consider techniques such as elective hypotension to further reduce blood loss.
- Avoid unnecessary blood sampling.

Jehovah's Witnesses who develop a coagulation disorder pose a special problem. The use of antifibrinolytic drugs (such as aprotinin) is generally acceptable and should be considered early on. If there is evidence of endogenous heparins (as evidenced by a prolonged APTT), consider giving protamine (see below). Management of the coagulopathy will depend on which clotting factors (if any) the individual is prepared to accept.

Much useful information has come from the management of such patients, with the realization that otherwise reasonably fit patients can survive for long periods with extremely low haemoglobin concentrations. Case reports cite survival down to Hb concentrations of 1–2 g/dL. However, for the older frailer patient with significant comorbidity, the reality is somewhat different and most patients who have a sustained haemoglobin below 5 g/dL will fail to improve and die days/weeks later from multiple organ failure.

NORMAL HAEMOSTATIC MECHANISMS

To understand coagulation disorders you need to understand the mechanisms by which haemostasis is normally achieved. Following injury to a blood vessel, a series of events is initiated:

- Vasoconstriction reduces blood flow in the damaged vessel.
- Factor VII and platelets adhere to exposed tissue factor (TF) in the vessel wall and release a number of mediators, including ADP. More platelets are attracted, which rapidly form a temporary haemostatic platelet plug.
- The coagulation cascade is triggered, which results in the conversion of fibrinogen to fibrin. Cross-linking of fibrin molecules results in conversion of the primary platelet plug to an organized clot.

The classical coagulation cascade is shown in Fig. 10.1. This represents the situation as present in vitro. While it is useful for understanding the serine protease cascade, and for working out in the laboratory the nature of coagulation disorders it does not represent the situation in vivo.

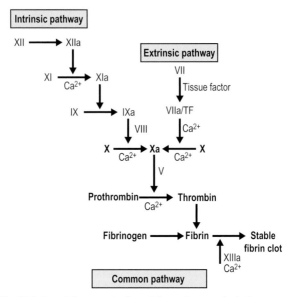

Fig. 10.1 Coagulation cascade. Coagulation pathway as classically described, showing intrinsic, extrinsic and common (shown in bold type) pathways. In-vivo binding of factor VII to exposed tissue factor may be the primary initiating mechanism.

In vivo, it is the interaction between factor VII, platelets and the vessel wall that is pivotal to the coagulation process.

Factor VII forms a complex with tissue factor (TF) on the surface of cells at the site of injury, including platelets. This complex then initiates the coagulation cascade by activating factors X and IX, generating the so-called 'thrombin burst' and accelerating clot formation. This is shown in Fig. 10.2.

The pivotal role of factor VII has led to the development of activated factor VII (VIIa) as a proposed therapy for uncontrolled bleeding. (See Activated factor VII, p. 261.)

There are also mechanisms within the body to prevent clot formation in healthy vessels and to dissolve established clots. These fibrinolytic pathways are shown in Fig. 10.3.

Under normal circumstances, therefore, there is a constant balance maintained between procoagulant mechanisms and anticoagulant mechanisms. If this balance becomes disturbed, bleeding or thrombosis may result.

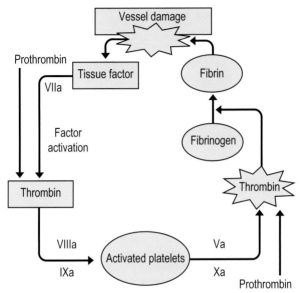

Fig. 10.2 In-vivo clotting mechanism. Note pivotal role of factor VIIIa, platelets and generation of thrombin burst leading to formation of fibrin plug.

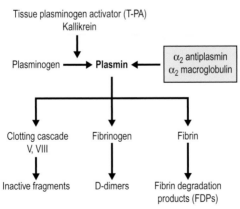

Fig. 10.3 Fibrinolytic pathways. Plasmin is a non-specific proteolytic enzyme that degrades factors V and VIII, fibrinogen and fibrin, and also inhibits both the coagulation cascade and the conversion of fibrinogen to fibrin. α_2-Antiplasmin and α_2-macroglobulin inhibit plasmin.

COAGULOPATHY

The term coagulopathy is generally used in respect of those disorders of haemostasis that produce a bleeding tendency. (Prothrombotic disorders are considered below.)

Causes

Coagulopathy may result from failure of clot formation, failure of clot stabilization or excessive activation of fibrinolysis. Often more than one process is involved, and the early involvement of a haematologist is advisable. Typical causes of coagulopathy are shown in Box 10.2.

In intensive care, acquired causes of coagulopathy are much more common than congenital causes. Many factors may contribute; these are listed below.

- Sepsis may produce bone marrow suppression (thrombocytopenia) and triggers inflammatory cascades, which activate both coagulation and fibrinolysis.
- Reduced gastrointestinal absorption of fat-soluble vitamins (A, D, E, K) leads to reduced manufacture of vitamin K-dependent factors (II, VII, IX, X, protein C).
- Reduced hepatic reticuloendothelial function permits increased circulating levels of endogenous heparinoids (potentiating antithrombin III and inhibiting factors V, X).
- In renal failure uraemia impairs platelet function.
- Massive transfusion and vigorous fluid loading can result in 'dilutional coagulopathy'.
- Citrate anticoagulants may persist in the circulation for some time, chelating calcium and potentially reducing cardiac

---

Box 10.2 Typical causes of coagulopathy

Congenital	Acquired
Haemophilia A (factor VIII)	Acquired/functional factor deficiency
Haemophilia B (factor IX)	Dilutional coagulopathy
Von Willebrand's disease	Thrombocytopenia
Other factor deficiencies	Sepsis
	Hypothermia
	Hepatic dysfunction
	Vitamin K deficiency/malabsorption
	Renal failure
	Drugs

contractility. Additionally, some synthetic colloids may impair platelet function (dextrans, hetastarch in particular).

- Activated fibrinolysis leads to consumptive coagulopathy.
- Effects of heparin given for DVT treatment/prophylaxis, as anticoagulation for extracorporeal circuits, during cardiac/vascular surgery etc.

Patients who require therapeutic anticoagulation for underlying conditions, for example, patients with a mechanical prosthetic heart valve or previous DVT/PE requiring long-term anticoagulation, pose a particular challenge, since continued anticoagulation may lead to risks of bleeding. This may require a balanced judgement about the relative risks and benefits of continuing anticoagulation. Seek appropriate advice, both from your consultant and from a haematologist with an interest in anticoagulation.

Investigations

Basic investigations include platelet count, prothrombin time (PT), activated partial thromboplastin time (APTT), thrombin time (TT), fibrinogen, and fibrinogen breakdown products (FDPs/D dimers). If a specific factor deficiency is considered likely, then individual factor assay may be appropriate. Seek haematological advice. Normal ranges are shown in Table 10.4.

TABLE 10.4 Coagulation tests		
	Normal range	*Significance*
Platelets	$150-450 \times 10^9$/L	See thrombocytopenia below
PT	$12-14$s (INR = PT/control; normal INR = 1)	Extrinsic and common pathway Marker of hepatic dysfunction/ vitamin K deficiency Used to monitor warfarin therapy
APTT	$30-40$s	Intrinsic and common pathway Used to monitor heparin therapy
TT	$10-12$s	Tests conversion of fibrinogen to fibrin Prolonged by heparin/FDPs/D dimers
Fibrinogen	>2g/L	Reduced in dilutional coagulopathy, liver failure, fibrinolysis (DIC)
D dimers	<0.2g/L	Increased in presence of fibrinolysis (DIC)

Thromboelastography (TEG)

While the in-vitro tests listed above can be useful diagnostically to determine the likely cause of a coagulopathy, they test individual aspects of the coagulation process rather than reflect the overall process of clot formation. The thromboelastograph can be used to provide a dynamic test of coagulation and fibrinolysis. This can be used to help identify the need for FFP, cryoprecipitate, platelets or antifibrinolytic therapy. An increasing number of hospitals have access to TEG devices in theatre and some critical care units. If available, you should familiarize yourself with the device and interpretation of the information that it gives you before you have to use it in an emergency situation. There is now a body of evidence to suggest that the management of coagulopathy based on interpretation thromboelastogram and related technologies not only helps in the management of haemostasis, but also reduces the quantities of clotting products required. A typical TEG trace is shown in Fig. 10.4.

Management of coagulopathy

In general, coagulation abnormalities should only be treated if there is active bleeding or when the potential consequences of bleeding may be disastrous.

- Ensure that the patient is adequately resuscitated. Oxygen, i.v. access and adequate volume or blood replacement. Correct hypothermia.
- The commonest cause of bleeding in the postoperative patient is failure of surgical haemostasis. Surgical causes of bleeding must be excluded. Seek surgical advice.
- Other underlying causes of bleeding and coagulopathy should be addressed. Do not forget inherited causes, e.g. the haemophilias, although these are rare.

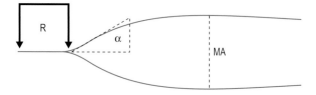

R = Lead time reflects time for activation of clotting cascade
α = Angle reflects rate of clot formation
MA = Maximum amplitude reflects clot strength

Fig. 10.4 Thromboelastogram (TEG) from a normal healthy (non-pregnant) adult.

- Perform basic investigations of haemostasis, as above. The diagnosis should be clear from a combination of history, examination and the results of these tests.
- If the APTT is prolonged, suspect heparinoids or other inhibitors. The laboratory may be able to repeat the APTT in the presence of a heparinase to help distinguish this.
- If heparin is present, but you do not know how much has been given, give protamine 50 mg then repeat the APTT. If you know the dose of heparin given, then protamine 1 mg per 100 units of heparin given should provide adequate reversal.
- If the PT and APTT are prolonged in the absence of exogenous anticoagulants give FFP, which should be administered in 2–4 unit aliquots until PT falls below 20 s. Additionally, if fibrinogen depletion is marked, consider cryoprecipitate 6 units initially.
- If the platelet count is $< 80 \times 10^9/L$, give 4 units of platelets, although more may be required if the count is lower or where the response to transfusion is limited, for example in DIC. In renal failure, platelet function may be abnormal even if platelet numbers are adequate. Desmopressin (DDAVP) 20 µg as a one-off bolus releases peripheral stores of factor VIII:Rag. This increases platelet 'stickiness' and thereby improves function.
- Check the ionized calcium: if below 0.85 mmol/L, this may contribute to coagulopathy. Give 2.5–10 mmol calcium chloride slowly. (See Hypocalcaemia, p. 207.)
- In malabsorption states and liver disease, vitamin K 10 mg can partially correct clotting disorders.

Prothrombin complex concentrate

Patients who have significantly raised INR from absolute or relative warfarin overdose or other causes with significant bleeding can have the coagulation defect rapidly reversed by infusion of prothrombin complex (Beriplex). This is expensive and may carry the risk of overcorrection and a prothombotic tendency. However, it has the attraction of a low infusion volume, and viral safety. Moreover, it does not carry the risk of transfusion-related acute lung injury sometimes encountered with the use of fresh frozen plasma. Although outside current guidelines, prothrombin complex is increasingly used in a number of situations where traditionally fresh frozen plasma has been the mainstay. Seek advice from the Haematology Department.

Activated factor VII (VIIa)

There has been a great deal of interest recently in the role of activated factor VII in the management of coagulopathy and uncontrolled bleeding. Activated factor VII binds to exposed tissue factor on damaged endothelial surfaces and activates the coagulation process, leading to localized fibrin production and clot formation. There is increasing evidence that VIIa is effective in reducing bleeding when other measures have failed. (See Normal haemostatic mechanisms, p. 255.)

THROMBOCYTOPENIA

Thrombocytopenia is a common finding in critically ill patients. Common causes are shown in Box 10.3.

The normal range for platelets is $150–400 \times 10^9/L$. However, a normal platelet count does not necessarily imply normal platelet function. Furthermore, patients with hypersplenism may exhibit a reduced platelet count, but with relatively well-preserved platelet function. Consider a functional test (for example, TEG).

In general terms, significant bleeding secondary to thrombocytopenia is uncommon unless the count is very low. Therefore, do not give prophylactic platelets unless the platelet count is less than $20 \times 10^9/L$. Below this level, there is a risk of spontaneous intracranial haemorrhage. In the presence of active bleeding, it is reasonable to give platelets in order to keep the platelet count above $80–100 \times 10^9/L$. In all cases, attention should be paid to addressing the underlying cause of the thrombocytopenia.

> ⚠ In some cases, thrombocytopenia is associated with increased microvascular thrombotic processes. Under these circumstances, giving platelets may increase the risk of clinically significant thrombosis. Do not give platelets unless there is active bleeding, or the platelet count is less than $20 \times 10^9/L$ and the risk of thrombosis has been excluded (see below).

Box 10.3 Causes of thrombocytopenia

Reduced production	*Increased destruction/sequestration*
Bone marrow failure	Infection
Drugs, toxins	Disseminated intravascular coagulation (DIC)
Viral infections	Mechanical devices (balloon pump/CVVHD)
	Clot/mechanical destruction
	Heparin-induced thrombocytopenia (HIT)
	Immune thrombocytopenia purpura (ITP)
	Thrombotic thrombocytopenia purpura (TTP)
	Sequestration (e.g. splenomegaly)

Heparin-induced thrombocytopenia (HIT)

Heparin-induced thrombocytopenia is an immune-mediated phenomenon which occurs in up to 5% of patients receiving unfractionated heparin and up to 1% of patients receiving low molecular weight heparin. Antibodies to the heparin–platelet complex lead to platelet activation and release of procoagulant mediators, resulting in both thrombocytopenia and major venous and arterial thrombosis. The latter may cause catastrophic limb ischaemia.

Consider the diagnosis if the platelet count falls by more than 50% after exposure to heparin (usually occurs within 4 days), or if thrombosis occurs despite heparinization and / or thrombocytopenia. Thrombosis may be manifest as deep vein thrombosis, pulmonary embolism, arterial thrombosis, thrombotic stroke, or myocardial infarction.

- Send blood for HIT screen (discuss with haematology service).
- Discontinue all heparin, including unfractionated and low molecular weight heparin.
- Avoid platelet transfusion; bleeding is uncommon.
- Consider anticoagulation if necessary with an alternative agent e.g. lepirudin (see BNF).

TTP–HUS

In thrombotic thrombocytopenic purpura (TTP), thrombocytopenia is associated with thrombosis (typically cerebrovascular). In the haemolytic uraemia syndrome (HUS), thrombocytopenia is associated with renal dysfunction.

In adults, TTP and HUS are considered to be different presentations of the same underlying pathological processes. Deficiencies of plasma protease (usually acquired but can be congenital) result in an abnormally large von Willebrand molecule, which activates platelets and causes (microvascular) thrombosis. Depending on the site of this, the clinical picture may be predominantly of renal failure (HUS) or neurological deficit (TTP).

Management is primarily supportive. Do not give platelets. This is associated with increased intravascular thrombosis and a poorer outcome. Fresh frozen plasma (to replace plasma protease) and / or plasma exchange may be of benefit.

DISSEMINATED INTRAVASCULAR COAGULATION

Disseminated intravascular coagulation (DIC) is a complex process arising as a result of generalized activation of the inflammatory cascade. It involves activation of clotting within the microvasculature, with consequent tissue damage. There is a

> **Box 10.4 Causes of purpura**
>
> Thrombocytopenia
> Meningococcal disease (sepsis/meningitis)
> Other causes of severe sepsis
> Henoch–Schönlein purpura
> Vasculitides (e.g. systemic lupus)
> Vitamin C deficiency (rare)

consumptive coagulopathy, where normal clotting fails to take place because of depletion of circulating factors. The process is generally accompanied by activated fibrinolysis, with clot instability. The breakdown products of fibrinogen (D-dimer) and fibrin (FDPs) are in themselves anticoagulant, thus adding an extra level of complexity.

The management of DIC presents a challenge, and early involvement of a haematologist is essential. The principles of management revolve around treating the underlying cause and adequate replacement therapy with FFP, cryoprecipitate and platelets. Some units employ antithrombin III in the treatment of DIC. Seek advice. There is no role for heparinization.

PURPURIC DISORDERS

Purpura are small purple spots in the skin resulting from microvascular haemorrhage. Although these are not always pathological, e.g. 'senile purpura' is secondary to vessel fragility in old age, they should raise suspicion of underlying pathology. Typically, purpura are associated with thrombocytopenia (see above), but they are also seen in other conditions in which there is inflammation or damage to the microvasculature. Important causes are shown in Box 10.4.

A purpuric rash may also be seen distal to a point of venous obstruction or mechanical constriction. For example, it may be seen in the head and neck following hanging or strangulation.

THROMBOTIC DISORDERS

A number of factors predispose to thrombosis in ICU patients (Table 10.5).

Some patients are at particular at risk of thrombosis. These include the pregnant, the obese and those with carcinomatosis, pelvic/hip injuries or surgery, myeloproliferative disease, systemic

---

TABLE 10.5 Factors which predispose to venous thrombosis

Vascular endothelial damage	Trauma/surgery Central venous catheters
Altered blood flow	Vascular disease Immobilization Shock states Central venous catheters Effects of vasoactive drugs
Altered platelet activity and coagulation state	Underlying disease processes Activation of inflammatory cascades Stress response to surgery, trauma, sepsis

---

lupus erythematosus (lupus anticoagulant) and conditions such as
TTP–HUS (see TTP–HUS, p. 263).

There are also some familial disorders that lead to increased
risk of thrombosis, including protein C deficiency, protein S
deficiency and antithrombin III deficiency. If these are suspected,
advice on investigation and management should be sought from a
haematologist.

Venous thrombosis

Despite predisposing factors being common, clinically obvious
venous thrombosis is relatively unusual in ICU patients.
The incidence of venous thrombosis detected by ultrasound
or venography is, however, much higher, and therefore all
patients should receive prophylactic anticoagulation unless
contraindicated. (See DVT prophylaxis, p. 63.)

Peripheral venous thrombosis may present clinically as a tense
swollen painful limb. This may be either a lower or upper limb, the
latter is usually related to subclavian vein cannulation. Unilateral
jugular thrombus is usually clinically unrecognized. Central
venous thrombosis of the IVC or SVC presents with swelling of
the affected area, limbs, trunk or head and neck. Collateral venous
drainage may be apparent (distended superficial veins).

The diagnosis of DVT can usually be made with compression
and Doppler ultrasound, although other imaging (venography,
contrast CT) is required to identify more central clot. The risk of
DVT progressing to pulmonary embolism is significant.

Arterial thrombosis / embolization

Arterial thrombosis/embolization commonly follows vascular
surgery in arteriopathies, but can also be seen following trauma or

accompanying other prothrombotic conditions such as heparin-induced thrombocytopenia (HIT) (see p. 263). Peripheral small vessel occlusion (e.g. trash foot) is common after aortic surgery, but may also accompany other conditions such as bacterial endocarditis and mycotic aneurysm. This usually improves over time. Embolization of a peripheral (limb) artery results in a pale, weak, numb and pulseless limb with loss of Doppler signals. Central arterial thrombosis of the distal aorta also occurs rarely (saddle embolus).

Management of thrombosis

- Treat the underlying cause where appropriate (e.g. plasma exchange for TTP).
- Arterial thrombosis will usually require urgent embolectomy and/or surgical exploration.
- Local infusion of thrombolytic agents may occasionally be an alternative.
- Systemic anticoagulation is usually required either with therapeuatic doses of subcutaneous low molecular weight heparin, e.g. Enoxaprin 150 units/kg/day, or with unfractionated intravenous heparin, typically 5000 unit loading dose followed by an infusion of 18 units/kg/24 h adjusted according to APTT.
- In cases of thrombosis associated with heparin-induced thrombocytopenia, the newer drugs lepirudin and fondaparinux avoid exacerbating HIT and can be administered parenterally, but care is required in appropriate dosing as excessive anticoagulation can be problematic. Unlike heparin or warfarin, they cannot easily be reversed. Seek advice from a haematologist on drug selection, dosage and monitoring.

Local or systemic thrombolysis can be used for venous thrombosis, but is usually reserved for more extensive central clot and pulmonary embolism. Patients with recurrent DVTs/PE may benefit from a temporary (up to 3 weeks) or permanent IVC filter. Do not insert femoral vein catheters if such devices are present. (See Pulmonary embolism, p. 107.)

THE IMMUNOCOMPROMISED PATIENT

All critically ill patients on the intensive care unit should be considered to have some degree of altered immune function (immunocompromise). The causes are multifactorial as shown in Box 10.5.

Some specific patient groups are particularly at risk of relative immunocompromise. These include those with alcoholic

---

Box 10.5 Causes of altered immune function in critically ill patients

Effects of chronic illness

Nutritional depletion

Impaired barrier defences (breaches in skin/impaired cough reflexes/impaired gut perfusion)

Altered liver function

Activation of pro-inflammatory/anti-inflammatory cascades

Bone marrow suppression

Box 10.6 Causes of significant immunocompromise

Cancer chemotherapy

Haematological malignancy

Bone marrow infiltration from any malignant process

Immunosuppressant drugs

HIV infection/AIDS

Chronic illness

Aplastic anaemia (idiosyncratic drug reactions)

---

liver disease and those suffering from malignancy. Such immunocompromise may be difficult to diagnose, as bone marrow function and other measures of response to infection may be apparently normal.

Patients with significant immunocompromise are, however, increasingly common in the ICU. Immune deficiency may be inherited (e.g. severe combined immune deficiency, SCID) or acquired. Most commonly, it is seen in patients with depressed bone marrow function, either as a result of an underlying disease process or as a result of treatment (e.g. following chemotherapy or immunosuppressive treatment following transplantation). Typical causes of significant immunocompromise are shown in Box 10.6.

Most severely immunocompromised patients referred to ICU have an established underlying diagnosis. Referral is usually precipitated either by respiratory failure, febrile neutropenia or sepsis syndrome. Often the time course is short, and the precipitating events may be unclear.

Management
The principles of management are largely the same as for the immunocompetent patient. Resuscitation and stabilization are the initial priorities.

Cross-infection with potentially resistant organisms is a major problem in intensive care, and can be disastrous in the immune-compromised patient. Patients should be barrier nursed in side rooms, ideally with positive pressure airflow, to protect them from further risk of infection. (See Infection control, p. 19.)

Some patients (e.g. those with haematological malignancy or on long-term chemotherapy) will have dedicated long-term venous access (Hickman line, Portacath, etc.). These can be used for resuscitation purposes; however, avoid accessing them for general purposes, to reduce the risk of infection in the catheter. It is often prudent to site a separate central venous catheter for short-term general use.

Baseline blood count including WBC count may give some clue as to the nature and severity of the immunocompromise (neutrophil/lymphocyte count). Temperature and C-reactive protein are useful markers of infection in neutropenic patients. Once the patient is adequately resuscitated, sources of sepsis must be sought. Clinical history and examination may give a strong clue to this. (See Pneumonia in immunocompromised patients, p. 145.)

- Obvious sites of sepsis should be cultured and any abscesses drained.
- Long term venous catheters are a common site of catheter-related sepsis. The infection may be obvious externally (swab entry site), or there may be no external signs of infection despite infected thrombophlebitis and/or catheter associated clot. Consider removal.
- Send blood cultures. Remember previous multiple broad-spectrum antibiotic therapy may mask growth, predispose to resistant organisms, and further increase the risk of fungal infection.
- Send urine and stool cultures.
- Send serology for viral infection (CMV, herpes, EBV, etc.).
- Send *Candida* and *Aspergillus* antigen tests.

Discuss likely or potentially unusual pathogens (e.g. protozoa) with the duty microbiologist and parent team. Suitable culture media should be used (e.g. bottles with antibiotic-binding resins). Alert the microbiology laboratory to this, so they can culture for unusual organisms. Antibiotic therapy is guided by culture results. In the first instance broad-spectrum antibiotics are usually required. Typical regimens are:

- Piperacillin/tazobactam and tobramcycin as first-line agents.
- Imipenem and vancomycin as second-line agents.

- Fluconazole may be added as prophylaxis against fungi.
- Co-trimoxazole may be added as prophylaxis against PCP.

Haematological malignancy

Patients with haematological malignancy are a tremendous diagnostic and therapeutic challenge in the ICU. A frequent problem is neutropenia following marrow ablation and transplantation. Recovery of WBC count may occasionally be hastened by administration of granulocyte–colony stimulating factor (GCSF).

The combination of haematological malignancy and requirement for IPPV carries a high mortality, especially where the pneumonia remains undiagnosed (patients with proven PCP often survive). When renal failure is added to this constellation, the mortality is even higher. As a result of this, some people are reluctant to admit patients with haematological malignancy to intensive care. Blanket policies of this sort are not appropriate and each patient should be considered on their merits. Those who are referred early and those who can be managed on non-invasive forms of respiratory support can do well.

AIDS

Patients known to have AIDS are usually on antiretroviral therapy. If tolerated, highly active antiretroviral therapy (HAART) is associated with maintenance of near normal health for many decades.

Patients with AIDS who develop PCP pneumonia or other intercurrent illness can have a reasonably good prognosis provided multiple organ failure does not supervene. CD4 count is a valuable guide to the likelihood of response to therapy and may give some indication as how advanced the patient is in their disease process. It may also be helpful to consider their viral load, as this is also a useful indicator of disease activity and progression, as well as the risk of infectivity to others. Seek specialist advice.

In a recent study, patients with AIDS showed a similar intensive care unit survival to those without AIDS. Factors predictive of survival included the APACHE score at admission and the CD4 count. Interestingly, HAART therapy does not appear to be a predictor.

Patients newly presenting with a disease characteristic of an immunosuppressed state, and who are subsequently diagnosed as HIV positive during the course of critical care admission, would not normally be commenced on antiretroviral therapy until after discharge from the intensive care unit, or recovery from the acute infective process. This is because acute institution of antiretroviral agents is unlikely significantly to affect the prognosis during the acute illness.

Organ transplant recipients

Solid organ transplant recipients no longer require special protection in the ICU during their perioperative course. The same is probably true should they develop opportunistic infections, surgical sepsis or pneumonia, as their immunosuppression is less severe than those with true immunocompromised states. If necessary, immunosuppression can be withdrawn and patients managed on steroids during an acute illness. Maintenance immunosuppressive therapy can then be reintroduced following recovery or in the event of rejection. Seek advice from the transplant team.

CHAPTER 11

BRAIN INJURY, NEUROLOGICAL AND NEUROMUSCULAR PROBLEMS

Patterns of brain injury   272

Key concepts in brain
  injury   272

Immediate management of
  traumatic brain injury   274

Indications for CT scan   279

Indications for neurosurgical
  referral   280

ICU management of traumatic
  brain injury   281

Common problems in traumatic
  brain injury   284

Monitoring modalities in brain
  injury   288

Outcome following brain
  injury   290

Stroke and intracranial
  haemorrhage   292

Subarachnoid
  haemorrhage   292

Hypoxic brain injury   294

Infection   295

Seizures   296

Brainstem death   297

Neuromuscular conditions   301

Critical illness
  neuromyopathy   304

Neurological deficits
  following ICU   304

PATTERNS OF BRAIN INJURY

The brain is extremely susceptible to injury from a variety of causes, but particularly from the effects of trauma, hypoxia, and hypoperfusion. Typical causes and patterns of brain injury are shown in Table 11.1.

Unlike some other organs, the brain has very limited powers of regeneration. Functional recovery following injury often depends on neuroplasticity (existing pathways/brain regions taking over the functions of the damaged areas) rather than the effect of any regeneration. Key concepts in the management of brain injury are discussed below.

KEY CONCEPTS IN BRAIN INJURY

Following the initial insult, there is little that can be done to reverse the effects of the primary injury and management is largely centred on preventing secondary damage caused by swelling, ischaemia and infarction.

The principles of management are therefore to:

● limit where possible the effect of the primary injury
● identify and treat conditions amenable to surgical intervention

TABLE 11.1 Causes and patterns of brain injury	
Traumatic brain injury	Diffuse swelling
	Diffuse axonal injury
	Acute intracerebral haematoma
	Acute subdural haematoma
	Acute extradural haematoma
	Contusions (bruising)
	Chronic subdural haematoma
Spontaneous haemorrhage	Subarachnoid haemorrhage
	Intracerebral haemorrhage
Cerebrovascular disease (embolic)	Stroke
Infection	Meningitis, encephalitis, abscess
Hypoxic/ischaemic injury	Watershed infarction
	Global infarction
	Hypoxic encephalopathy
Metabolic	Encephalopathy

- identify and treat conditions amenable to medical treatment
- prevent secondary injury.

The prevention of secondary injury is mainly dependent on maintenance of adequate brain perfusion and oxygenation. There are a number of key concepts relating to brain perfusion that underpin the management of the brain-injured patient.

Cerebral blood flow and autoregulation

Cerebral blood flow is normally maintained at a constant level over a wide range of cerebral perfusion pressures, a phenomenon known as autoregulation (Fig. 11.1). In normotensive patients, autoregulation occurs at cerebral perfusion pressures between 50 and 150 mmHg. In previously hypertensive patients, the curve is shifted to the right and autoregulation occurs at a higher blood pressure.

Following significant brain injury, autoregulation is often deranged and cerebral blood flow becomes directly related to cerebral perfusion pressure (CPP).

Cerebral perfusion pressure

Cerebral perfusion pressure is effectively the driving pressure across the cerebral circulation. It is calculated as shown:

Mean cerebral perfusion pressure = mean arterial BP − intracranial pressure
(CPP) (MABP) (1CP)

Central venous pressure is sometimes included in this equation. This is because the cranium behaves as a Starling resistor – so

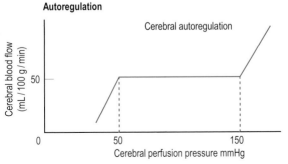

Fig. 11.1 Autoregulation curves.

TABLE 11.2 Typical target values for cerebral perfusion (mmHg)*

Adults	> 60
3–12 years	> 50
< 3 years	> 40

*There is debate about the ideal target values. Some accept lower target values.

where the CVP exceeds the ICP, the CVP becomes the effective downstream pressure and should be used to calculate CPP.

Inadequate CPP results in inadequate cerebral blood flow and the maintenance of an adequate CPP is therefore crucial. However, there is debate about what constitutes an adequate CPP and what the target values for therapy should be. Typical target values are shown in Table 11.2.

Intracranial compliance

The skull can be conceptually considered as a rigid box containing the brain, CSF and blood. If the volume of one of these components is increased, e.g. by cerebral oedema, then the volume of the others must be reduced. Initially, CSF is displaced into the spinal canal, followed by a reduction in blood volume. Eventually, when no further compensation is possible, the ICP will rise rapidly, impairing cerebral perfusion. If the pressure is not relieved, the brain itself may become displaced, leading to so-called herniation or coning. (See Control of intracranial pressure, p. 288.)

In the presence of reduced intracranial compliance, the cerebral blood volume is an important determinant of ICP. If the cerebral circulation becomes vasodilated, cerebral blood volume increases and ICP may increase. Hypercapnia and hypoxia both cause cerebral vasodilatation and should be avoided. Brain-injured patients are normally ventilated to a $PaCO_2$ of 4–4.5 kPa. Hyperventilation to a lower $PaCO_2$ than this should be avoided, as there is a risk of significant cerebral vasoconstriction and ischaemia.

IMMEDIATE MANAGEMENT OF TRAUMATIC BRAIN INJURY

The following notes relate to the management of traumatic brain injury. The principles apply equally well to the management of other forms of brain injury.

Depending on local policy, you may be required to assist with the management of head-injured patients in the resuscitation room. You should be familiar with Advanced Trauma Life Support (ATLS) protocols as well as the acute management of the brain-injured patient. (See Trauma, p. 309.)

Primary survey

The initial assessment includes:

- A Airway (with cervical spine control)
- B Breathing
- C Circulation
- D Disability (neurological assessment).

Airway (with cervical spine control)

The maintenance of a clear airway and the prevention of hypoxia and hypercapnia are paramount. Indications for intubation and ventilation are shown in Box 11.1.

Intubation/ventilation of brain-injured patients

(See Practical procedures: Intubation of the trachea, p. 398.)

Laryngoscopy and tracheal intubation are a major stimulus and may produce a significant elevation in blood pressure and ICP. Adequate anaesthesia and muscle relaxation must be provided in order to blunt this response and avoid potential worsening of the brain injury.

Establish intravenous access. Give volume loading, particularly if there is haemorrhage and other injuries. Blood, colloid or

---

Box 11.1 Indications for intubation and ventilation of brain-injured patient

GCS less than 8 or falling rapidly

Hypoxia

Hypercapnia ($PaCO_2 > 6.5$ kPa), or hypocapnia ($PaCO_2 < 3.0$ kPa)

Inability to protect the airway

Significant facial injuries and bleeding (swelling may make intubation very difficult if delayed)

Seizures

Major injuries elsewhere, especially chest injuries

Evidence of shock state (tachycardia, low BP, acidosis, etc.)

A restless patient who requires transfer to CT

Any patient with a significant brain injury requiring interhospital transfer

Requirement for anaesthesia and surgery for other injuries

crystalloid is used as appropriate. If possible, establish direct arterial pressure monitoring.

- Check all intubation equipment, breathing circuits, ventilators and suction, etc. Monitoring should be available for BP, ECG, SaO_2 and $ETCO_2$.
- Note the baseline GCS score and pupil size for reference. The pupils are the principal clinical monitor of the brain following anaesthesia and paralysis.
- Assume there is cervical spine injury until proved otherwise. A second person should provide in-line immobilization of the neck. (It may be useful to use a bougie/airway exchange catheter/video laryngoscope to facilitate intubation without extending the neck.)
- Assume the stomach is full and perform a rapid sequence induction. Preoxygenate with 100% oxygen. Ask a trained assistant to apply cricoid pressure. Use etomidate if the BP is low, otherwise thiopentone or propofol are suitable induction agents. Suxamethonium is used to provide muscle relaxation (unless absolutely contraindicated, see p. 43).

 Suxamethonium causes a transient rise in intracranial pressure. However, in the context of the multiply-injured patient with brain injury, securing the airway rapidly and safely is essential. Suxamethonium is usually the drug of choice.

- Opioid, e.g. fentanyl 100 μg increments or remifentanil by infusion, $0.1\,\mu g\,kg^{-1}\,min^{-1}$ can be used to help block the hypertensive response to intubation.
- Intubate the patient and pass an orogastric tube to drain stomach contents.

Endotracheal and gastric tubes should be inserted via the oral route in the first instance. This is because in the presence of a base-of-skull fracture, there is a risk of these tubes entering the cranium if placed nasally. Only change to nasotracheal/nasogastric tubes once base-of-skull fractures have been excluded.

- Ventilate to normocapnia or moderate hypocapnia ($PaCO_2$ 4–4.5 kPa). Significant hypocapnia is associated with cerebral vasoconstriction and reduced cerebral perfusion. This may potentially cause cerebral ischaemia and worsen brain injury.

- Monitor the SaO_2 and $ETCO_2$. Measure direct arterial blood pressure and blood gases as soon as possible. Maintain adequate cerebral perfusion pressure with fluids and vasoactive drugs (see below).
- Maintain sedation with benzodiazepines, propofol and opioids. During the early resuscitation and stabilization phase continue paralysis with a cardiovascularly stable non-depolarizing muscle relaxant.

Circulation

It is vital to maintain adequate cerebral perfusion pressure in brain-injured patients:

- Give colloid or normal saline to restore circulating volume. Avoid hyponatraemic fluids as these worsen outcome.
- Give blood if Hb low and correct any coagulopathy.
- Consider inotropes / vasopressors early to maintain blood pressure.
- Boluses of hypertonic saline (3–7.5%) may be valuable to maintain perfusion / circulating volume and limit cerebral oedema formation. Follow local protocols or seek advice.
- Exclude other sites of bleeding.

(See Intensive care management below.)

Neurological assessment

Neurological assessment requires serial documentation of conscious level, pupillary signs, lateralizing limb signs (suggesting space-occupying lesion), tone and posture. Fundal haemorrhages, papilloedema, CSF rhinorrhea / otorrhoea and bleeding from the ear should be documented.

Conscious level

The simplest assessment of conscious level utilizes a four-point scale:

- **A** <u>A</u>lert
- **V** Responds to <u>V</u>ocal stimuli
- **P** Responds to <u>P</u>ainful stimuli
- **U** <u>U</u>nresponsive.

This score is insufficiently sensitive for neurological assessment of the brain-injured patient and is only used during A&E resuscitation to give a broad indication of conscious level. Response to pain only represents a significant decrease in conscious level equivalent to a GCS score of 8 or less.

The Glasgow Coma Scale

The Glasgow Coma Scale (GCS), shown in Table 11.3, is a more comprehensive neurological assessment, which is universally used to describe conscious level and has prognostic value. It should be performed as soon as the patient is stabilized. It is repeated throughout the resuscitation process to identify any deterioration in the patient's condition, which may suggest expanding intracerebral haematoma or brain swelling.

Pupils

Pupillary size and response to light (direct and consensual) should be documented regularly. Any asymmetry greater than 1 mm or a change in response to light must be assumed to be due to the effects of an intracranial space-occupying lesion causing compression of the ipsilateral third nerve. Urgent CT scan of the brain is required. Bilateral, dilated and unresponsive pupils in the context of a brain injury and in the absence of mydriatic agents is a grave sign.

Reassessment and secondary survey

Having completed a primary survey and stabilized the patient, the patient should be reassessed before moving on to secondary survey. Traumatic brain injury may be an isolated injury, but

---

TABLE 11.3 Glasgow Coma Scale (GCS)

Eye opening	Spontaneously	4
	To speech	3
	To pain	2
	None	1
Best verbal response	Orientated	5
	Confused	4
	Inappropriate words	3
	Incomprehensible sounds	2
	None	1
Best motor response (arms)	Obeys commands	6
	Localization to pain	5
	Normal flexion to pain	4
	Spastic flexion to pain	3
	Extension to pain	2
	None	1

Maximum score 15. Minimum score 3. (A modified GCS is used for children under 5 years)

this should never be assumed. The care of the brain injury must proceed alongside the continuing re-evaluation and resuscitation of the other injuries according to ATLS protocols. In particular, remember:

- cervical spine injury (immobilize, X-ray lateral cervical spine, CT spine)
- cardiothoracic trauma (CXR, CT ± drains)
- abdominal injuries (diagnostic peritoneal lavage, US, CT, laparotomy)
- pelvic fractures (X-ray, early external fixation)
- splint limb injuries (assess neurovascular integrity).

Which injury should take priority?

In the multiply-injured patient with a brain injury priorities must be decided. The following are important considerations:

- Many brain injuries do not require neurosurgical intervention.
- Any brain injury will be worsened by significant hypoxia or hypotension.

Any injury that compromises the airway, breathing or circulation takes priority. In particular, life-threatening bleeding from the chest or abdomen requires immediate surgical intervention and should not be delayed by CT head scan or neurosurgery. In exceptional cases, blind burr holes or craniotomy can be performed simultaneously with other surgery, and a CT scan performed before transfer to ICU.

INDICATIONS FOR CT SCAN

Plain skull X-rays may be useful in the initial evaluation of patients with mild head injuries, as the presence of a skull fracture greatly increases the risk of subsequent intracerebral haematoma. In the more severely head-injured patient, however, CT scans are required to:

- confirm the diagnosis, e.g. haematoma, brain injury, subarachnoid bleed, tumour, skull fractures
- identify space-occupying lesions
- direct surgery to the site of injury.

CT scan should not be delayed by taking plain X-rays. Indications for CT scan are shown in Table 11.4.

TABLE 11.4 Indications for CT scan

All patients with moderate/severe injury plus any of the following:	GCS < 13 Neurological signs Inability to assess conscious level, e.g. due to anaesthetic drugs
Any patient with mild injury plus any of the following:	High-risk mechanism of injury GCS < 15 for more than 2 h Skull fracture Vomiting Age > 60 years*

*High risk patient group for occult intracranial injury

Following CT scan and depending upon other injuries, options for the further management of the patient can be decided. These may include:

- CT normal or minimal changes only: stop sedative drugs; allow the patient to wake up and reassess neurological state.
- CT diffuse or non-operable injury (e.g. diffusely swollen brain): admit patient to ICU for further management, including monitoring of ICP.
- CT space-occupying lesion with a mass effect: requires urgent neurosurgical referral and craniotomy.

> ⚠ **CT scans require skilled interpretation. Do not make clinical decisions until senior experienced staff have reviewed them. Minor subarachnoid bleeding, mild cerebral oedema, early cerebral infarction, pituitary lesions and brainstem lesions are all easily missed.**

INDICATIONS FOR NEUROSURGICAL REFERRAL

The facilities available for dealing with the head-injured patient vary. Hospitals may have no CT scanner, a CT scanner but no neurosurgery, or all facilities. The decision to transfer a patient will therefore be influenced not only by the patient's condition, but also by the local availability of resources. Indications for referral are summarized in Box 11.2.

Identification of a vacant ICU bed space should not delay transfer of patients, who require an urgent CT scan or craniotomy for evacuation of a haematoma. Most neurosurgical units try to

---

Box 11.2 Indications for referral to neurosurgical centre

CT scan indicated but not available locally

CT scan shows intracranial haemorrhage/midline shift

CT scan suggests diffuse axonal injury

CT scan suggests raised intracranial pressure/hydrocephalus

GCS < 15 for more than 24 h

GCS deteriorates 2 points or more

GCS < 9

Base-of-skull fracture or compound skull fracture

---

adopt an open admission policy, taking all seriously injured patients who have not had a CT scan and those who require operative intervention, regardless of the availability of ICU beds. Once appropriate interventions have been performed, any delay in finding an intensive care bed will not place the patient at further significant risk. Patients can if necessary be transferred back to the referring hospital once the need for further intervention has been excluded.

Indications for less urgent transfer include:

- isolated depressed skull fractures with no neurological deficit
- isolated CSF leak
- patients with lesser injuries who fail to improve neurologically over time.

ICU MANAGEMENT OF TRAUMATIC BRAIN INJURY

The ICU management of brain injury is based upon maintenance of adequate cerebral perfusion and oxygenation in order to prevent secondary brain damage. Limitation of cerebral oedema and surges in ICP may help to prevent brain herniation. Other general principles of management are the same as for any patient:

- Use tracheal intubation and assisted ventilation to maintain adequate oxygenation and normocapnia, or mild hypocapnia ($PaCO_2$ 4–4.5 kPa).
- Maintain adequate sedation and analgesia. Paralysis is usually required in the early phases of treatment but should only be continued in unstable patients, those with raised intracranial pressure or when required to enable satisfactory ventilation.
- Nurse the patient 15–20° head-up to ensure adequate venous drainage. Avoid tight tapes to secure endotracheal tube, which may occlude jugular veins.

- Establish monitoring. Arterial blood pressure and CVP, urinary catheter, NG tube. If possible avoid internal jugular routes of cannulation (except for jugular bulb cannula). Insertion difficulties may impair cerebral venous drainage and also risk carotid injury. Use ultrasound guidance in all cases to avoid arterial puncture and other complications. The femoral route has some advantages, avoiding the need for head-down tilt during insertion.

- Give maintenance fluids as 0.9% saline (plus K^+) initially. In the past maintenance fluids were restricted, but maintenance of cerebral perfusion is now considered paramount. Hyponatraemia and hyperglycaemia worsen outcome and should be avoided. Hypertonic saline (3–7.5%) have been used as boluses. Follow local protocols.

- Prevent a rise in temperature. Give regular paracetamol and use surface cooling (tepid sponges, fans, cool air blankets. There may be some benefit from mild hypothermia 35.5–36.5°C.

- Stress ulcer prophylaxis. Commence enteral feeding as soon as practicable. Otherwise an H_2 antagonist or proton pump inhibitor should be prescribed.

- There is no indication for routine use of prophylactic anticonvulsants.

There is little evidence that specific regimens designed to produce cerebral protection, e.g. the use of barbiturates, or steroids, alter the outcome of brain-injured patients. Hypothermia is known to produce cerebral protection in some settings, e.g. near drowning, but studies of induced hypothermia in traumatic brain injury have failed to show any benefit beyond that afforded by maintaining normothermia (i.e. preventing pyrexia). (See Management of patients post-cardiac arrest, p. 109.)

Maintenance of cerebral perfusion pressure (CPP)

Maintain the CPP above 60 mmHg in adult patients. It may need to be even higher in elderly hypertensive patients (normal autoregulation curve shifted to the right). Similarly CPP may need to be higher if there is evidence of cerebral vasospasm (e.g. in subarachnoid haemorrhage) or inadequate perfusion (e.g. low SjO_2). (See Jugular venous bulb oxygen saturation, p. 259.)

- Titrate fluid therapy according to CVP. If there is no improvement or if the patient is haemodynamically unstable, consider the use of advanced haemodynamic monitoring devices (optimize cardiac output, stroke volume, vascular resistance etc.).

- After adequate fluid resuscitation, if CPP remains low, use vasopressors, e.g. noradrenaline (norepinephrine) or phenylephrine to increase mean arterial pressure and improve CPP.
- Adrenaline (epinephrine) may be used if invasive monitoring indicates that the primary reason for a low MAP is low CO.
- The use of progressively higher doses of vasopressors in order to maintain a target CPP may produce subendocardial myocardial ischaemia and other end-organ damage. If increasingly higher doses are required, seek advice.

Control of intracranial pressure (ICP)

The measurement of ICP is now routine practice in the management of head injury. It may also be used in other conditions where there is likely to be raised ICP, e.g. the management of metabolic conditions such as liver failure. It is used to give an indication of increasing cerebral oedema, the re-accumulation of haematoma, and to calculate CPP.

Normal ICP is less than 10 mmHg and a sustained pressure higher than 20 mmHg is associated with poorer outcomes. If ICP is greater than 20–30 mmHg then intervention may be necessary, particularly in the first 24–48 h following injury. Table 11.5 provides a checklist of causes of a raised ICP. Exclude measurement errors and avoidable rises before starting treatment.

TABLE 11.5 Checklist for management of raised ICP

Problem	Action
Accuracy of measurement	Reposition, flush and recalibrate device.
Inadequate sedation or paralysis	Give a bolus of sedation, analgesia and/or relaxants. Increase infusion rates.
Hypoxia or hypercapnia	Check Et CO_2/blood gases. Adjust FiO_2 and/or ventilation as necessary.
Inadequate CPP	Consider additional i.v. fluids. Increase vasopressors/inotropes.
Impaired venous drainage from head and neck	Head turned (occluding neck veins). Endotracheal tube tapes too tight. Nurse 15–20° head up.
Seizures	May be masked by muscle relaxants. Check CFM trace or EEG. Treat appropriately.
Pyrexia	Give antipyretics. Consider surface cooling.

If all factors are optimized, exclude the development or re-accumulation of haematoma. Consider repeat CT scan to exclude evolving intracranial pathology (e.g. expanding haematoma) and seek neurosurgical opinion. Correct any coagulation defects. Other measures to control ICP include the following.

1st line

- Mannitol 0.5 g/kg over 20 min, and/or furosemide (frusemide) 0.5 mg/kg. Any benefit tends to be temporary.
- Hypertonic saline infusion/boluses (3–7.5% saline). Follow local protocols or seek advice.
- Moderate hyperventilation. Do not reduce $PaCO_2$ to less than 4 kPa. Lower levels may result in excessive cerebral vasoconstriction and may produce areas of ischaemia. Any benefits will tend to disappear over a few hours.
- CSF drainage via external ventricular drain.
- Ensure that adequate CPP is maintained at all times. If there is no response to simple measures, consider further increasing CPP. The benefit of this may not be immediate and may take a few hours.

2nd line

- Thiopental (thiopentone) infusion. 15 mg/kg 1st hour, 8 mg/kg 2nd hour, 5 mg/kg/h thereafter. The aim is to achieve burst suppression on CFM monitoring. The disadvantage of this approach is that the time taken for thiopental to wear off once the infusion is stopped delays the ability to clinically assess the patient. Monitor levels over time.
- Decompressive craniotomy. Removal of bone flap and lobectomy.
- Induced hypothermia.
- Aggressive hyperventilation to $PaCO_2 < 3$ kPa. See note above.

COMMON PROBLEMS IN TRAUMATIC BRAIN INJURY

Cardiovascular instability

Haemodynamic instability is common and may be seen in association with neurogenic pulmonary oedema (see below). The importance of an adequate cerebral perfusion pressure has already been stressed. Hypotension may be due to a combination of factors. You should exclude causes such as hypovolaemia, pneumothorax and sepsis. All patients should have direct arterial pressure and CVP monitoring. In complex cases, consider other monitoring devices to guide fluids, inotropes and vasopressor therapy, as for any shock state.

Dilated pupil

Sudden increases in pupil size, particularly if unilateral and non-reactive to light, may be due to stretching of the 3rd cranial nerve and may herald brainstem herniation. This is an indication for an urgent repeat CT scan. Dilated pupils may reflect underlying seizure activity. Bilateral persistent fixed dilated pupils are an ominous sign, suggesting impending brain death, but should not be considered in isolation.

Seizures

Generalized or focal seizures are common with brain injury from any cause. In the complicated ICU patient the distinction between focal and generalized seizures is indistinct and usually of little relevance. Continued seizure activity increases the oxygen requirement of the brain and worsens brain injury, therefore seizures should be treated promptly

Acutely brain injured patients at risk of repeated seizures will usually be ventilated. The use of muscle relaxants blocks the peripheral manifestations of seizure activity making clinical detection more difficult. Seizure activity may be accompanied by changes in blood pressure/heart rate and pupils but these signs are unreliable.

Cerebral function monitors (CFM) or cerebral function analysing monitors (CFAM) are frequently used to detect abnormal seizure activity in paralysed patients. The simplest of these displays two channels, base line activity (to detect artifacts) and global cerebral electrical activity. Seizures are indicated by an abrupt elevation of the cerebral activity level. A saw tooth pattern is typical of recurrent short seizures.

More advanced CFAMs display the electrical activity of each cerebral hemisphere separately and have multiple channels able to display separately the various frequencies that make up global cerebral activity (alpha, beta, theta delta activity). You should seek advice on the interpretation of the output of these monitors.

If in doubt about the presence or absence of seizure activity in the paralysed patient request a formal EEG. Alternatively, there is usually little harm in temporarily reducing/stopping muscle relaxants to assess seizure activity; ensure adequate doses of sedative/analgesic drugs first!

Exclude any treatable precipitating cause such as hypoxia, hypercapnia, hyperthermia or electrolyte disturbance.

1st line treatment

- Intravenous benzodiazepines, e.g. diazepam 5–10 mg or clonazepam as necessary. Large cumulative doses may be needed. Midazolam is also effective.
- Intravenous phenytoin. Loading dose 15 mg/kg. Give 300 mg loading dose over 1 h and then 1200 mg over next 24 h. Daily dose 300 mg thereafter. Measure levels over time. Phenytoin may cause disturbances of cardiac rhythm in some patients.
- Intravenous propofol, bolus followed by infusion 200–400 mg/h may also be effective.

2nd line treatment

- If seizure activity is not controlled, then additional anticonvulsant agents such as clonazepam, sodium valproate, phenobarbital, clormethiazole, paraldehyde or magnesium may be required. Seek expert advice and check dose regimens in BNF.
- Consider thiopental (thiopentone) bolus 500 mg over 5 min, followed by infusion 2.5–5 g daily. Check levels over time.

Prophylactic anticonvulsants may be given to at-risk patients; for example, patients with significant contusions on CT or documented seizures after injury. Phenytoin is the usual drug as it does not produce significant sedation (see doses above).

Diabetes insipidus (DI)

Neurogenic DI results from failure of the posterior pituitary to produce antidiuretic hormone (ADH). It may result from either localized damage to the pituitary/hypothalamic area or from diffuse brain injury/brain death. It is manifest as excessive urine output due to inability to concentrate the urine. Untreated, this results in progressive dehydration and hypernatraemia.

DI should be considered if urine outputs persist at greater than 300–400 mL/h in the absence of diuretics. Other causes of excessive urine output include excretion of resuscitation fluids and use of mannitol or other diuretics.

- To confirm the diagnosis, check urine/plasma osmolality. Normal plasma osmolality is 286 mosmol/L.

If increased >310 mosmol/L then urine should be highly
concentrated. In this context urine osmolality <500 mosmol/L
implies DI.

- Give DDAVP 1–2 μg i.v. as required.
- Replace urinary losses with 5% dextrose with added K⁺.

 **If left untreated, patients with DI develop rapid and
progressive dehydration and hypernatraemia. Avoid
rapid correction, which may lead to acute cerebral
oedema. (See Hypernatraemia, p. 202.)**

Poor gas exchange

Respiratory problems are very common in the presence of brain
injury and are often a reason for initial ICU admission or delayed
discharge. The precise mechanisms are multifactorial, but may
include inadequate cough and gag reflexes, pulmonary aspiration,
chest infection (particularly staphylococcal), pulmonary capillary
leak and depressed immune function. (See Hospital acquired
pneumonia, p. 143.)

Many patients with severe brain injury require a tracheostomy
to facilitate airway management for short-to-medium term care.
Neurological function is typically assessed 48–72 h post-injury if
the patient is stable enough to awake and assess. If the patient is
thought to have a survivable injury but is obtunded consider
early tracheostomy to avoid the scenario of repeated extubation
and reintubation and then subsequent tracheostomy. Tracheostomy
protects the airway, is more comfortable for the patient, allows
early reduction in sedative and analgesic drugs, aids nutrition and
mobilization, and allows easier weaning of ventilatory support. If
survival from the brain injury is uncertain or the patient remains
unstable (e.g. raised ICP, critical oxygenation), then it may be
prudent to delay tracheostomy until the situation is clearer.

Neurogenic pulmonary oedema

Pulmonary oedema is a well-recognized complication of
brain injury. In its severest form, it is characterized by
extreme cardiovascular instability with profuse pink frothy
pulmonary oedema. Simplistically, it is thought to result from a
catecholamine surge caused by a rapid rise in ICP. This results in
an acute increase in left ventricular afterload and left ventricular
dysfunction, increased pulmonary vascular volume (blood
returned from peripheries) pulmonary hypertension and increased

permeability of pulmonary vascular endothelium, all of which may contribute to the development of oedema.

The management of acute neurogenic pulmonary oedema is supportive with IPPV, high FiO_2 and PEEP. Diuretics are not usually effective and the volume of fluid leaking into the alveoli and out of the lung may lead to marked hypovolaemia. Cardiac instability will often require advanced haemodynamic monitoring, inotropes/vasopressor therapy. The pulmonary oedema usually settles over time but may produce an acute lung injury leading to ARDS. (See Acute lung injury, p. 154.)

Cerebrospinal fluid (CSF) leaks

Clear or bloodstained fluid from nose or ear may represent a CSF leak, which is a feature of injuries to the frontal sinus and base of skull. CSF tests positive for glucose on test strips. In the past, antibiotic prophylaxis was thought to be necessary, but most centres have stopped this practice. It is usual to wait about 10 days to see if the leak will cease spontaneously, if not then craniotomy and placement of a dural patch may be required.

The irritable brain-injured patient

Irritability and restlessness are common in patients with minor brain injury or in the recovery phase of more severe injuries. In the latter, there will often be severe movement disorders in the form of extensor spasms. Despite the theoretical risks of masking neurological signs it is often necessary to give sedatives (benzodiazepines) and major tranquillizers (chlorpromazine/haloperidol) to such patients to allow nursing care and prevent further injury. Large doses of drugs may be required. The patient with extensor spasms will generally benefit from a tracheostomy to prevent biting on the endotracheal tube and airway obstruction.

Consider nursing such patients on a mattress on the floor to avoid them falling out of bed (cot sides do not always prevent this and increase the height of the fall!). NG tubes tend to be repeatedly pulled out by such patients. Feeding gastrostomy/jejunostomy may be required in the longer term.

MONITORING MODALITIES IN BRAIN INJURY

You may encounter a number of monitoring modalities that are currently either routinely used or under evaluation in brain injury. Most are intended to provide additional information regarding

perfusion, oxygen delivery and oxygen consumption in the brain.
The majority of these techniques are limited either by technical
difficulties or by inability to detect small, critically ischaemic areas
within the brain. The overall outcome benefit is still debated.

Intracranial pressure monitoring

Routine in most centres. Intracranial pressure can be monitored
using an intraventricular catheter (measures CSF pressure and
allows drainage of CSF) or via transducers placed in the subdural
space or in brain parenchyma. Various devices are available,
typically consisting of a micro-pressure transducer on the end of
a flexible wire. These can be inserted on the intensive care unit via
a small burr hole and are usually placed on the side most affected,
as indicated by surgery/CT scan. (See Management of traumatic
brain injury above.)

Jugular bulb oxygen saturation (SjO₂)

Measuring the saturation in venous blood from the brain gives
an indication of the adequacy of oxygen delivery and utilization
by the brain. The normal range is 55–75%. Changes are more
valuable than isolated values and reflect global/regional perfusion
and oxygenation.

A low SjO_2 implies inadequate oxygen delivery. Consider
measures to improve cerebral blood flow, in particular raising
CPP. If the saturation is high then the brain is either hyperaemic
or failing to extract oxygen. Barbiturates may be helpful to control
ICP in the presence of hyperaemia. In brain death, the saturation
may approach 100% as the brain ceases to extract oxygen.

> ⚠ **Jugular bulb lactate–oxygen index, may be
> helpful in distinguishing critically perfused brain.**
> $LO_i = AVDL/AVDO_2$ **(AV difference in lactate/AV
> difference in oxygen content.) If this is used in your unit, seek
> advice on calculation and interpretation.**

Near infrared spectroscopy

This technique uses light absorption to measure brain tissue
oxygenation. Light of a particular wavelength is passed through
the skull and the absorption by brain cytochrome aa3 (representing
the terminal step of the mitochondrial electron transport chain) is
detected. The technique is limited by the depth to which the incident
light is able to penetrate effectively. Changes probably reflect
perfusion/oxygen delivery in superficial areas of the brain only.

Brain tissue PO$_2$

Brain tissue PO$_2$ can be measured directly using a miniaturized electrode placed within or on the surface of the brain through a cranial burr hole. It is usually combined with an ICP device.

Brain tissue microdialysis

A microdialysis catheter is placed into brain parenchyma through a small cranial burr hole. Fluid is passed through the catheter and allowed to equilibrate with brain tissue interstitial fluid. This is then aspirated and analysis of the chemical content of the fluid retrieved provides an indication of local tissue perfusion and oxygenation. Except in a few specialized neurosurgical units, this technique remains largely a research tool.

Cerebral activity

The traditional approach to monitoring of cerebral activity in brain-injured patients who are sedated and paralysed has been based on the use of cerebral function monitors (CFM) and cerebral function analysing monitors (CFAM) and intermittent EEG. These are limited either by the amount of clinically useful information they provide, difficulty in interpretation or their intermittent nature. Newer approaches to monitoring cerebral activity aim to provide real time, clinically relevant assessment of cerebral activity.

Compressed spectral array provides a way of continuously monitoring and displaying the EEG signal in a simple, easily interpretable, bedside monitor. It is likely to replace traditional CFAM as the standard monitor of cerebral activity in brain injury.

Bispectral index (BIS®) uses a proprietary algorithm to produce a single numerical value indicative of conscious level. Its primary role is as a guide to depth of anaesthesia during surgical procedures. It is not formally validated for use in a head injury, and gives only a general guide as to the conscious level.

A number of advanced neurophysiological imaging techniques are available in specialist centres, including functional magnetic resonance imaging, SPECT scanning, PET scanning and xenon CT. At present, these are primarily diagnostic and research tools, although they are likely to become more routine in future clinical practice.

OUTCOME FOLLOWING BRAIN INJURY

Following severe brain injury, patients typically require tracheal intubation, assisted ventilation and sedation/paralysis. Cerebral perfusion pressure and other parameters are optimized for a period of 48–72 h in the hope of minimizing secondary brain injury. If after this they remain unstable, have raised ICP or other ongoing system failure, further time will be required to allow for the patient's condition to improve. Otherwise, a decision is usually made to stop sedatives and to allow patients to waken, so that their neurological status can be assessed.

If such patients respond purposefully to commands, move both sides normally and are haemodynamically stable, a trial of weaning and extubation can be commenced. If, however, they fail to waken, to obey commands, have a hemiparesis, abnormal flexion or extensor posturing, then rapid weaning and extubation is unlikely to be successful. Consideration should be given to tracheostomy as an aid to weaning.

Once weaned from mechanical ventilation the neurologically damaged patient can usually be managed on a high dependency unit. Tube feeding will usually be required initially via a fine bore nasogastric tube or gastrostomy (PEG). Neurological improvement may occur over time and long-term rehabilitation is important.

Outcome following brain injury depends on a number of factors, including the mechanism and severity of the initial injury, subsequent episodes of hypotension, hypoxia or hypercapnia, adequacy of resuscitation, and the presence of other injuries. Age is important, young patients have a substantially better outcome than elderly patients for a given injury. In particular, young children may make a good recovery from an apparently devastating injury. There is a wide spectrum from mild to devastating injury. The Glasgow Outcome Scale (Table 11.6) can be used to classify outcomes.

It is relatively easy to predict outcomes at either end of the spectrum but not in between. The passage of time (weeks/months) is essential to assess potential for recovery. Clinicians learn from experience that it is often impossible to predict longer-term outcome in any individual patient. Furthermore, even apparently

TABLE 11.6 Glasgow Outcome Scale for brain-injured patients

Description	Classification
Return to pre-injury levels of function	Good recovery
Neurological deficit but self-caring	Moderately disabled
Unable to self care	Severely disabled
No higher mental function	Vegetative
Dead	

good physical recovery may mask subtle underlying cognitive deficits or psychological impairment and these problems may be manifest even after apparently trivial injuries.

STROKE AND INTRACRANIAL HAEMORRHAGE

The sudden onset of acute neurological deficit associated with cerebral vascular occlusion/haemorrhage is commonly referred to as a stroke. There have been significant improvements in the care of patients with stroke in recent years. Increasingly stroke patients will now receive an urgent CT scan to determine the nature of the injury and dictate subsequent treatment. Those with occlusive disease may receive thrombolysis if presenting early enough. Those with haemorrhage are likely to be managed conservatively in the first instance. A recent international study showed no overall benefit from surgical intervention in spontaneous intracerebral haemorrhage, although there is some evidence that early haemostatic treatment might improve outcome. Subarachnoid haemorrhage is distinct in that there is an established benefit in early surgical or radiological intervention (see below).

Patients may require intensive care following a stroke to protect the airway, support ventilation or because of complications of treatment. It can sometimes be difficult to know how aggressive intensive care management should be, in this predominantly elderly group of patients who often have significant co-morbidity. As with most situations, unless palliative care is obviously the most appropriate option, it is better to instigate intensive care and then revaluate the situation later. The outcome will depend upon the site and nature of the stroke (infarct or haemorrhage), the patient's neurological state and conscious level, age and coexisting medical problems.

SUBARACHNOID HAEMORRHAGE

Patients present with sudden onset of headache, neurological deficit and collapse. Subarachnoid haemorrhage is confirmed by CT scan and/or lumbar puncture. The site and appearance of bleeding may suggest an aneurysm or arteriovenous malformation. There are associations with other diseases, e.g. atheromatous vascular disease, polycystic kidney disease, collagen/connective tissue disease and other congenital malformations.

Management and outcome is determined by grading. Two common grading systems are shown in Table 11.7 and Table 11.8. Grading is difficult once the patient is sedated/ventilated. Rebleeding or vasospasm may rapidly worsen neurological state.

TABLE 11.7 Hunt and Hess grading system for subarachnoid haemorrhage

Description	Grade
Unruptured aneurysm	0
Asymptomatic, minimal headache or nuchal rigidity	1
Moderate headache or nuchal rigidity	2
No neurological deficit except cranial nerves. Drowsiness, confusion or mild focal deficit	3
Stupor, hemiparesis	4
Deep coma, decerebrate rigidity, moribund appearance	5

TABLE 11.8 World Federation of Neurological Surgeons scale

Glasgow Coma Scale	Motor deficit	Grade
15	No	1
13–14	No	2
13–14	Yes	3
7–12	Yes or no	4
3–6	Yes or no	5

Management

For patients with lower grades of bleed, there is established benefit in early angiography and embolization or clipping of aneurysm to reduce the risk of rebleeding and further neurological insult.

Patients with significant subarachnoid bleeds and large intracerebral haematomas may require emergency, surgical evacuation of the haematoma. Intraventricular drainage may be used to decompress the brain and treat hydrocephalus. These patients will require intensive care support.

Definitive management is either by embolization of the aneurysm under radiological control or surgical clipping depending on the nature of the lesion. Timing depends upon the patient's age (increasing risk of cerebrovascular disease and cerebral infarction) preoperative status and the perceived risk of rebleeding. Early intervention reduces the risk of rebleeding and of intercurrent medical problems, but where surgical intervention is required is technically more difficult and is associated with an increased risk of cerebral vascular spasm. Delayed intervention (10–14 days post-bleed) is technically easier and carries less risk of vasospasm, but increases the risk of bleeding in the intervening period.

ICU management

Patients with spontaneous subarachnoid haemorrhage (SAH) frequently require intensive care, either early at presentation, after surgery or some time later due to respiratory or other complications.

The ICU management of SAH is essentially no different from other causes of brain injury. Cerebral vasospasm may occur. The exact mechanism by which this occurs is unclear but it can result in areas of ischaemic infarction. It is diagnosed by angiography or transcranial Doppler. Management is centred on prevention.

- Maintenance of cerebral perfusion pressure using fluids and vasopressors is crucial. Aim for mean systemic pressure of 90–100 mmHg. It is not usual to monitor ICP. Vasopressor therapy is usually used and may be required for up to 3 weeks.
- The Ca^{2+} channel blocker nimodipine has been shown to improve neurological outcome. Its effect is thought to be independent of any anti-vasospasm action. Its systemic vasodilator effects may worsen CPP and require vasopressor therapy. It is available in oral and i.v. preparations.
- Cardiac dysrhythmias are common in SAH. These do not usually require treatment.

Typically many patients are managed in an HDU/ward area. More severe cases may need a period of ventilation in ICU, followed by a period of weaning and tracheostomy.

HYPOXIC BRAIN INJURY

Hypoxic brain injury is most commonly seen following prolonged resuscitation from cardiac arrest. Other causes include:

- profound hypotension/hypoxaemia from any cause
- prolonged seizures
- carbon monoxide poisoning
- attempted strangulation or hanging
- near drowning.

Patients who are resuscitated following cardiac arrest are usually referred for intensive care because of a failure to regain consciousness, haemodynamic instability or inadequate respiratory effort. There is little evidence that a period of elective ventilation, or the use of so-called cerebral protection agents (e.g. barbiturates/steroids), affect neurological outcome. Recent guidelines however, support the provision of moderate hypothermia in the management of the post-arrest situation, and this requires a period of artificial ventilation. Limited trials have shown encouraging results, but the optimum duration or degree of cooling is not yet known.

The emphasis should be on prevention of secondary insults.

- Ventilate for 12–24 h, with minimal sedation where possible, then reassess neurological state. If the patient begins to get agitated then short-acting agents, e.g. propofol, allow subsequent periodic reassessment of neurology.
- Purposeful or semi-purposeful movements are a good sign and usually herald recovery. Absence of respiratory effort, myoclonic jerking and fixed dilated pupils usually indicate severe hypoxic damage and a poor long-term outlook.

(See Management of patients following cardiac arrest, p. 109.)

Outcome

The prediction of long-term outcome after hypoxic brain injury is difficult. If the patient does not awaken, longer-term management will depend upon the patient's background health, age, previous wishes (advance directives, etc.). The patient's relatives and family need to be kept aware of the situation and their wishes must also be considered. Unless a consensus is reached regarding withdrawal of active management, the patient should be stabilized, weaned from IPPV, usually via a tracheostomy, established on enteral feeding and transferred for ward-based care awaiting neurological change over time. If the patient does not improve over time and all parties agree that further treatment is futile, then it is reasonable to wean from assisted ventilation, extubate the trachea, and await events. (See Treatment limitation decisions, p. 430.)

Following cardiac arrest, a proportion of patients enter a vegetative or near vegetative state. The duration of such a state is often difficult to predict. In some cases it is permanent, whereas in a very small minority of cases, meaningful recovery has been described after months or years. Such patients need assessment by a neurologist with an interest in rehabilitation.

INFECTION

Meningitis

It is unusual for adults to require intensive care when meningitis is the primary presenting diagnosis. In the case serious enough to warrant intensive care it is advisable to perform CT scan prior to lumbar puncture to exclude cerebral oedema and the potential risk of coning after lumbar puncture. If lumbar puncture is contraindicated, empirical antibiotic therapy is then started. Steroids have been shown to reduce longer-term neurological sequelae in both adults and children presenting with *Haemophilus*, pneumococcal and recently meningococcal meningitis and should be given on presentation.

Occasionally more severe cases develop secondary hydrocephalus and may benefit from intraventricular CSF drainage; therefore, perform a CT scan in patients who deteriorate or who fail to improve over time.

Encephalitis

As for meningitis, it is unusual for adults to require intensive care. Occasionally encephalitis needs to be considered as a diagnosis of exclusion in cases of coma. There are characteristic EEG changes with herpes encephalitis. A brain biopsy may be indicated to confirm the diagnosis. Start aciclovir and broad-spectrum antibiotics (cefotaxime and clarithromycin) until diagnosis is proved/disproved.

(See Empirical antibiotic therapy, p. 336.)

Brain abscess

This is an occasional cause of ICU admission. Look for embolic sources of infection, e.g. endocarditis, and local sources, e.g. middle ear infection. Check tuberculosis status. Immune-suppressed patients (e.g. HIV) may present with unusual CNS abscesses/meningitis, e.g. toxoplasmosis and cryptosporidiosis. Large abscesses require surgical drainage. Seek neurosurgical advice.

SEIZURES

Seizures are common in the critically ill, either as a presenting diagnosis of epilepsy or as a secondary complication of other disorders. Some of the more common predisposing factors are listed in Box 11.3.

Status epilepticus

Status epilepticus can be defined as seizures lasting longer than 30 min, or so frequently that no recovery occurs between attacks. Patients are at risk of brain injury, cerebral oedema, hypoxia and aspiration. Typically, intensive care referral occurs when first-line

---

Box 11.3 Conditions predisposing to seizure activity

Worsening of existing seizure disorder

Alcohol or other drug withdrawal

Drug overdose, e.g. tricyclic antidepressants

Brain injury

Brain abscess or tumour

Metabolic, e.g. hypoglycaemia/hypomagnesaemia

Hypoxia

---

drug treatment has failed and the patient becomes increasingly obtunded due to the effects of ongoing seizures and sedative drug accumulation. If untreated, patients may suffer further complications from immobility, hypothermia, hyperthermia and rhabdomyolysis.

Occasionally patients will present with convincing pseudo-seizures as part of a Münchausen-type syndrome. If there is doubt as to whether jerky movements or loss of consciousness represent a true seizure, request an EEG.

Management

Most cases severe enough to require admission to ICU will need a period of tracheal intubation and assisted ventilation. Consider CT scanning and/or lumbar puncture to exclude treatable disorders. Correct any metabolic abnormality or derangement of body temperature. For first line anticonvulsant therapy, consider the following, then seek specialist advice:

● Intravenous benzodiazepines, e.g. diazepam 5–10 mg or clonazepam as necessary. Large cumulative doses may be needed. Midazolam and propofol are also effective.
● Intravenous phenytoin. Loading dose 15 mg/kg. Give 300 mg loading dose over 1 h and then 1200 mg over next 24 h. Daily dose 300 mg thereafter. Measure levels over time. Phenytoin may cause disturbances of cardiac rhythm in some patients.

BRAINSTEM DEATH

Brainstem death is caused by irreversible damage to the brainstem, which is the control centre for the autonomic functions of the brain. Its description in 1959 followed the introduction of assisted ventilation in brain-injured patients. Criteria for the diagnosis of brainstem death were first proposed in the UK in 1976 and an updated code of practice for the diagnosis and confirmation of death (including brainstem death) has recently been produced by the Academy of Medical Royal Colleges (*A Code of Practice for the Diagnosis and Confirmation of Death*, 2008).

It is usually clear from clinical bedside observations when brainstem death is impending or has occurred. The typical features of brainstem herniation are tachycardia and hypertension, followed by bradycardia, hypotension and pupil dilatation. A lack of response to endotracheal suctioning, turning and mouth care, with fixed dilated pupils, suggests the diagnosis of actual or impending brainstem death. All are performed routinely during nursing care. Formal brainstem death tests are then used to confirm that brainstem death has already occurred. It looks unprofessional to do formal tests and then find that the patient is not brain dead after all!

Preconditions

Before brainstem tests are performed, there are a number of preconditions that must be satisfied in order to exclude potentially reversible causes of brainstem dysfunction. These are shown in Box 11.4.

Active measures to maintain blood pressure, temperature and normal electrolytes may be required if the patient is to fulfil preconditions, and to be potentially suitable for organ donation. This may require fluids, inotropes, vasopressors and DDAVP in the hours prior to tests (often overnight). Replacement of the large urine volumes seen with diabetes insipidus with isotonic saline or synthetic colloid solutions will lead to progressive hypernatraemia. Use DDAVP and fluid replacement with dextrose solutions (with added K^+) to avoid this. (See Diabetes insipidus, p. 286, Practicalities of donor management, p. 438.)

Before performing tests ensure that all preconditions are satisfied. Always confirm the integrity of the neuromuscular junction and exclude the effects of muscle relaxants by use of a

---

Box 11.4 Preconditions to performing brainstem death tests

Known cause of brain damage, e.g. trauma, intracerebral haemorrhage, hypoxia

Absence of neuromuscular blocking drugs

Absence of any residual CNS depressant drugs

Normothermia (core temperature > 35.5°C)

Normal metabolic and endocrine state

No significant electrolyte or blood glucose disturbance

nerve stimulator (see p. 43). Scrutinize the drug chart and intensive care chart to ensure that sufficient time has elapsed for any centrally acting drugs to have been metabolized and eliminated. Beware of active metabolites, which may have long half-lives. If in doubt, drug levels can be measured. Check the patient's core temperature and recent biochemistry results.

 The preconditions for the diagnosis of brainstem death are absolutely fundamental to the process and must be satisfied before consideration of the diagnosis.

Conduct of brainstem death tests

In the UK, the tests are carried out by two doctors who are 5 years post-registration. At least one these must be a consultant who should have been responsible for the patient during the admission and neither should be associated with the transplant services. The tests should be performed together and each doctor should satisfy themselves of the results. The tests should be repeated at a suitable interval to confirm the findings. Following the completion of the second set of tests, brainstem death is confirmed.

Occasionally families will ask to observe the tests being done. This is acceptable providing that staff have taken the time to explain the process and they understand the nature of the tests including spinal reflexes. The whole process of testing, counselling the family and explaining the concept of brain death and organ donation is, of necessity, time consuming.

Most hospitals will have pre-printed documentation for brainstem death tests and organ donation. The tests required are listed in Table 11.9.

TABLE 11.9 Brainstem death tests	
Test	*Brainstem function (cranial nerves)*
Pupil light reflex	II , III
Corneal reflex	V, VII
Caloric tests	VIII, IV, VI, III
Gag reflex	IX, X
Tracheal suction	X
Response to pain (see text below)	Sensory afferents; motor efferents
Apnoea tests	Respiratory centre

Response to pain

Deep pain is produced peripherally by pressure on sensitive points such as the nail beds and centrally by pressure over the supraorbital nerves, while observing for a response within the cranial nerve distribution. Peripheral non-purposeful movements in response to peripheral pain represent spinal reflexes, and are not indicative of brainstem function. Simplistically these reflect the loss of descending control over the spinal cord from higher centres and may become exaggerated over time. Relatives and attending staff should be warned of these and their significance explained.

Apnoea test

The patient is preoxygenated with 100% O_2, and then disconnected from the ventilator and connected to a breathing circuit with high flow 100% O_2. If the lungs are healthy, oxygenation is maintained and the $PaCO_2$ rises gradually. The $PaCO_2$ must be allowed to rise to a level at which the patient could be expected to breathe ($PaCO_2$ of 6.6 kPa for a previously healthy patient, higher in patients with chronic lung disease and CO_2 retention). The rise in CO_2 usually takes about 10 min. If pulmonary function is poor, there is a risk of profound hypoxia and cardiac arrest during apnoea testing. In such cases ventilate slowly with 100% oxygen and added CO_2, or add a dead space into the circuit, then briefly disconnect the ventilator to look for respiratory movement.

Completion of tests

Following completion of the second set of brainstem tests, brainstem death is confirmed and the patient can be declared legally dead. Although two sets of tests are performed, the time of death is taken to be the time of the completion of the first set of tests. (In this respect, the second set of tests are confirming the original findings of brainstem death.) The death should be reported to the coroner if this is required (see Reporting deaths to the coroner, p. 436).

Do not use the terms pass or fail in relation to brainstem death tests. This creates confusion. Brainstem death is either confirmed or not confirmed.

Following confirmation of brainstem death, arrangements may be made to retrieve organs for transplantation if consent has been obtained. (See Organ donation, p. 437.) Alternatively ventilation may be withdrawn. The family should be offered the opportunity to sit with the patient and allowed time for distant relatives to visit. At the time of ventilator disconnection they may choose to stay with the patient. Alternatively, some prefer to say their farewells before the event and leave or visit later.

Residual brainstem function

If, during brainstem testing, residual brainstem function is demonstrated (usually residual cough or respiratory effort), ventilatory support should be continued and the situation reassessed. Assuming catastrophic brain injury has occurred, residual brainstem activity will usually disappear over 24–48 h and then repeat brainstem tests can be performed to confirm brainstem death. Alternatively, further discussions may be held with the family to consider withdrawal of active treatment in anticipation of death according to conventionally accepted criteria. (See Withdrawal of treatment, p. 431.)

Management of catastrophic brain injury

Some patients, despite suffering an apparently catastrophic and presumed fatal brain injury, retain some residual brainstem function. They cannot be declared brainstem dead, yet appear to have no prospect of meaningful survival. Honest discussions with the family regarding the benefits versus burdens of continuation or withdrawal of treatment should take place, so that decisions can be reached over a period of time that are in the best interests of the patient. If a consensus is reached that further active management is inappropriate, then treatment should be withdrawn. Such patients may be suitable for consideration as asystolic or non-beating heart organ donors. (See Non-heart beating organ donation, p. 439.)

NEUROMUSCULAR CONDITIONS

Both acute and chronic neuromuscular conditions are important in intensive care practice. The characteristics of the various conditions vary in detail and many patients will never have a definitive diagnosis made. However, you should consider all such patients to be at risk from the following:

- Incipient respiratory failure. Commonly follows chest infections or major surgery.
- Bulbar palsy leading to recurrent pulmonary aspiration.
- Autonomic neuropathy leading to cardiovascular instability. Bradycardias, tachycardias, hypertension or hypotension may all occur.

- Cardiomyopathy. There is a risk of arrhythmias and sudden death.
- Marked sensitivity to muscle relaxants. There may be long lasting weakness after non-depolarizing drugs. Massive K^+ release after suxamethonium is well recognized even before clinical manifestations are seen, and is thought to be caused by extrajunctional acetylcholine receptors. Avoid using it!

Although increasingly patients with neuromuscular disorders are managed in the community with non-invasive forms of respiratory support, they may require intensive care either as part of their first presentation or for subsequent intercurrent illness. Occasionally patients who have difficulty with weaning from assisted ventilation may be found to have a previously undiagnosed neuromuscular disease. Treatment is primarily supportive, with assisted ventilation, (invasive/non-invasive), tracheostomy to aid weaning, physiotherapy etc.

> ⚠ **Patients with neuromuscular disease may be profoundly weak but usually retain a normal conscious level. If ventilator-dependent, they may be unable to move or show any sign of distress. (The only means of communication may be by blinking the eyelids.) It should be assumed that they are conscious until proved otherwise. Ensure adequate levels of sedation/analgesia.**

Muscular dystrophies

Increasing numbers of patients with inherited neuromuscular disease are surviving into young adulthood. Many of these will require nocturnal CPAP or non-invasive ventilatory support. They frequently require intensive care admission for intercurrent chest infection. In many cases, however, there is a gradual decline in respiratory function, cough reflex and general condition over time. There may come a point, therefore, at which further intensive care admission is no longer appropriate. This may lead to difficult discussions with the patient and their relatives/carers. Always seek senior advice.

Myasthenia gravis

This autoimmune disease results from antibodies to the cholinergic receptors in the neuromuscular junction. The mainstay of treatment is with anticholinesterase drugs, which increase the level of acetylcholine available at the cholinergic receptors.

Deterioration, increasing muscle weakness and subsequent respiratory failure may result from intercurrent disease, surgery or

overdosage of anticholinesterase drugs (cholinergic crisis).
The short-acting anticholinesterase edrophonium may be given to test whether muscle function can be improved ('Tensilon test').
In practice, by the time myasthenic patients require intensive care it is often difficult to distinguish a cholinergic crisis from other causes of muscle fatigue.

Acute exacerbations are treated by increases in anticholinergic drugs, steroids and plasma exchange. Azathioprine, cyclophosphamide and thymectomy are useful treatments in the longer term.

Guillain–Barré syndrome

This condition of ascending muscle paralysis usually follows an intercurrent illness. The early use of intravenous immunoglobulin and plasmapheresis may reduce the need for assisted ventilation. Patients who require assisted ventilation may take weeks or months to recover, and recovery is not always complete. Autonomic disturbances and neuropathic pain are common. A variant of this condition, known as Miller Fisher syndrome, predominantly affects the cranial nerves. Treatment options include plasmapheresis, immunoglobulins and steroids. Plasmapheresis is generally arranged through the regional transfusion service.

Tetanus

This is rare in the UK, due to successful immunization programmes. It is, however, a major problem abroad. The toxins produced by the bacteria *Clostridium tetani* disrupt normal neuromuscular control and produce severe spasms and autonomic disturbances. The management is supportive, with wound debridement, antibiotics, immunoglobulins, control of autonomic dysfunction and muscle spasms. Baclofen (systemically and intrathecally) has been used for muscle relaxation with variable effectiveness. Severe cases may require protracted sedation and assisted ventilation. Seek specialist advice.

Botulism

This is rare in the UK but occasional outbreaks have been associated with contaminated packaged food. Toxin produced by *Clostridium botulinum* blocks cholinergic receptors. Nausea and vomiting are followed by blurred vision, laryngeal and pharyngeal paralysis and generalized paralysis. Tachycardia, urinary retention and constipation occur. Treatment is largely supportive. Seek specialist advice.

⚠ **Occasional cases of tetanus and botulism have been seen in recent years, in association with drug abuse, in particular, by drug abusers who self inject, using intramuscular, subcutaneous, or "skin popping" techniques, rather than intravenous injection. Treatment is as above. (See Problems associated with intravenous drug abuse, p. 243).**

CRITICAL ILLNESS NEUROMYOPATHY

As more and more critically ill patients survive, increasing numbers of patients are developing residual neuromuscular problems: the so-called 'critical illness neuromyopathy'. The exact aetiology is unclear but severe sepsis, prolonged immobility, poor nutritional status, neuromuscular blocking drugs and elderly medically unfit patients are all considered risk factors. Typically, it is first noticed when a critically ill patient is in the recovery phase of illness and is unable to move limbs. It is important to recognize the diagnosis and appreciate that the patient may be completely awake but unable to move. Craniofacial movements are often relatively spared and the patient's only means of communication or response may be to blink.

It is important to rule out other causes of weakness like cervical cord problems. Neurological examination usually reveals a flaccid paralysis. EMG indicates a mixed picture of neuropathy and myopathy. Biopsy, although not routine, shows axonal degeneration with preservation of myelin sheaths. The condition usually improves over weeks or months but recovery may be incomplete and neuropathic pain is common.

NEUROLOGICAL DEFICITS FOLLOWING ICU

Occasionally as patients recover on ICU it becomes clear that they have sustained a new isolated neurological deficit. This may range from a mild, peripheral neuropraxia resulting from pressure on a peripheral nerve to significant central deficits such as bulbar palsies (difficulty swallowing) or profound hemiplegia. Where there is likely to be a remedial cause, investigation including imaging and intervention (surgery/thrombolysis etc.) should be expedited. In most cases, however, intervention is inappropriate. Peripheral nerve injuries will usually recover. More significant central deficits may or may not improve over time. Management is supportive. Tracheostomy may be appropriate to enable suctioning or to aid weaning. Imaging can be undertaken at intervals to aid prognosis.

CHAPTER 12

TRAUMA

Introduction 306

Primary survey 306

Exposure and secondary survey 308

Intensive care management 309

Head, face and neck injuries 310

Spinal cord injuries 311

Thoracic injuries 313

Abdominal injuries 316

Skeletal injuries 317

Fat embolism 318

Peripheral compartment syndromes 319

Rhabdomyolysis 320

Burns 320

Electrocution 322

Near drowning 323

Outcome following trauma 324

INTRODUCTION

The successful management of major trauma requires early
identification and treatment of life-threatening injuries followed
by systematic evaluation and treatment of all other injuries. Best
outcomes are achieved by a coordinated team approach and
protocol-based management.

Depending upon local policy, you may be called to assist in the
initial resuscitation of major trauma victims. Although an A&E
doctor or trauma surgeon will generally lead trauma resuscitation,
you should be familiar with advanced trauma life support
protocols.

PRIMARY SURVEY

The purpose of the primary survey is to identify and begin the
treatment of any immediately life-threatening injuries. These
include:

- airway obstruction
- tension pneumothorax
- cardiac tamponade
- massive haemorrhage.

The principal elements of the primary survey are A, B, C and D,
as follows.

(A) Airway (with cervical spine control)
Assess the adequacy of the airway. Clear the upper airway with
suction and simple airway manoeuvres and provide 100% oxygen
using a mask with reservoir bag.

If necessary, secure the airway by intubation or
cricothyroidotomy, depending on the clinical situation and degree
of urgency. (See Spinal cord injury, p. 311.)

> ⚠️ The cervical spine should be assumed to be unstable
> and must be protected at all times. Use in-line
> immobilization during airway manoeuvres. A cervical
> collar should be applied and sandbags and tape used to prevent
> unnecessary movement of the cervical spine.

(B) Breathing
Support ventilation if necessary. Expose the chest and examine
for adequacy of respiration. Identify and treat life-threatening

conditions such as flail chest, open wounds, tension pneumothorax or massive haemothorax.

(C) Circulation

- Stop major haemorrhage by direct pressure.
- Assess the adequacy of circulation; in particular, pulse rate, BP, and capillary refill.
- Insert two 14-gauge peripheral intravenous cannulae. If this is not possible, then cannulate the internal jugular or femoral vein, or consider peripheral venous cut-down (e.g. saphenous vein). In ATLS doctrine, CVP lines are used for monitoring and not for resuscitation purposes. Adapt practice dependent on local skills, kit and expertise.
- Send blood for cross-matching.
- Commence fluid resuscitation with 2–3 L of crystalloid. If there is an ongoing fluid requirement, continue with blood/blood products. Colloids remain controversial in this setting, with growing evidence they may contribute to increased bleeding. Fully cross-matched blood is preferable but group-specific, or non-cross-matched O negative can be used, depending upon circumstances.

> ⚠ **Evidence suggests that following trauma, early over aggressive fluid resuscitation may worsen outcome. Where surgical haemostasis cannot be immediately achieved, the goal of fluid resuscitation should be to only restore the circulating volume sufficiently to achieve a blood pressure compatible with critical organ perfusion (see below).**

- If volume loading does not restore perfusion, consider an adrenaline (epinephrine) infusion.

(D) Disability (neurological assessment)

- Assess conscious level, pupil size and note any obvious neurological deficit. A deteriorating Glasgow Coma Score, or a GCS of 8 or below, is an indication for intubation and ventilation. (See Immediate management of brain injury, p. 274.)

Reassessment

- Reassess A, B, C and D to ensure continued stability and appropriate response to treatment before moving on to the secondary survey.

Box 12.1 Investigations and monitoring

Routine investigations	Monitoring
FBC	ECG
U&Es, glucose	Blood pressure (non-invasive or invasive)
Arterial blood gases	Pulse oximeter
(Pregnancy test)	CVP
ECG	Urine output
Lateral cervical spine X-ray	
Chest X-ray	
Pelvic X-ray	
Urine (stick test)	

EXPOSURE AND SECONDARY SURVEY

Once the initial survey is complete and the patient is stabilized, ensure that appropriate monitoring is established and that necessary investigations have been organized (Box 12.1).

Ensure that an adequate medical history has been obtained. At a minimum, this should include the patient's past medical history, medications, allergies, time of last meal and the mechanism of injury. The mechanism of injury is particularly important in providing important clues as to the likely injuries that may have been sustained.

● Completely expose the patient, while at the same time taking steps to avoid hypothermia.
● Systematically examine the patient from head to toe, looking for other injuries.
● Log roll the patient to examine the back and spine, and perform rectal and vaginal examinations.
● A urinary catheter and nasogastric tube may be inserted if there are no contraindications.

Following resuscitation, stabilization and re-evaluation of the patient, further management can be planned. This may include immediate surgery for life-threatening injuries, or further investigations such as ultrasound or CT scan.

Ultrasound is increasingly used to identify free fluid (blood) in the peritoneal, pleural and pericardial spaces. In this context, its value is in identifying a problem (e.g. peritoneal fluid) rather than the definitive diagnosis (e.g. ruptured spleen). There is much current interest in the use of 'focused' ultrasound examinations in trauma, which are easily learned and reliably performed by non-specialist medical staff (e.g. the 'FAST' scan) (Trauma Ultrasonography. The FAST and Beyond. http://www.trauma.org/archive/radiology/FASTintro.html).

Many larger centres also now routinely perform CT scanning of chest, abdomen, head and spine in all patients with a significant history of major trauma. With modern fast scan times such approaches are increasingly seen to optimize care in these vulnerable patients; occult injuries are often found.

Blunt versus penetrating trauma

Blunt and penetrating trauma produce different patterns of injury. Blunt trauma is associated with significant soft-tissue injury and haemorrhage into tissues and body cavities. In penetrating trauma, tissue injury may be quite localized and haemorrhage may be tamponaded by clot or the presence of a foreign object. There is ongoing debate about resuscitation strategies in the two groups.

Aggressive intravenous fluid resuscitation with blood, colloid or crystalloid may raise blood pressure, disturb blood clots and restart bleeding. There is some evidence, particularly in penetrating trauma, that restrictive fluid strategies, which limit the volume of resuscitation fluid given until surgical control of bleeding can be achieved, are associated with better outcomes. Similar considerations may apply in other surgical situations, such as leaking aortic aneurysm.

INTENSIVE CARE MANAGEMENT

Patients with multiple injuries frequently require transfer to an ICU after initial resuscitation, stabilization and surgery. Care of the multiply injured patient is essentially no different to care of any other ICU patient. Multiple trauma is by its nature a multisystem disorder, rather than a collection of isolated injuries. Treatment is generally supportive, with appropriate intervention for problems as they are identified.

Multiple organ failure

Multiple organ failure is common after massive trauma. Typically patients develop a systemic inflammatory response syndrome (SIRS), 24–48 h after apparently adequate resuscitation, which then progresses to multiple organ failure. Tissue damage, activation of the immune system and massive blood transfusion are all implicated but exact mechanisms are still not fully understood. Treatment is largely supportive. Possible sources of any ongoing inflammatory response, including necrotic tissue and foci of infection, must be excluded. (See Multiple organ failure, p. 329, and SIRS, p. 326.)

The management of specific groups of injuries is discussed below.

HEAD, FACE AND NECK INJURIES

Head injury
(See Traumatic brain injury, p. 274.)

Facial injury
In the unconscious or obtunded patient the airway should be secured early by intubation. With time, swelling may make subsequent reintubation or airway manipulation impossible. In severe injuries consideration should be given to early tracheostomy. In the presence of facial or base-of-skull fractures, avoid nasal intubation or nasogastric tubes as these may pass into the cranium. Use the oral route.

Heavy bleeding from facial injuries should not be underestimated. Bleeding from the nose may require nasal packing to tamponade bleeding. Seek ENT/maxillofacial surgical advice. Injuries to the jaw often require internal fixation and jaw wiring. Do not be afraid to cut the wires in the event of airway problems. When extubating these patients, ensure they are awake and have full return of protective reflexes before removing the endotracheal tube.

Broken or dislodged teeth may be aspirated. These are usually visible on X-ray, but are not usually densely radio-opaque unless there are amalgam filling present. Careful scrutiny of films is required and a lateral film may help to confirm position (note position of NG tube to delineate the oesophagus). Rigid bronchoscopy may be required for the location and removal of radiolucent teeth/fragments. (See Airway obstruction, pp. 138, 309.)

Cervical spine injury
(See Spinal cord injury, below.)

Cervical soft-tissue injury
Direct injury to soft tissues of the neck can result in airway compromise, due either to haematoma/tissue swelling causing

compression of the airway or to direct injury to the larynx or trachea. Secure the airway by early intubation and seek expert surgical help. Vascular injuries in the neck may compromise the cerebral circulation. Dissection of the carotid arteries by blunt injury from seatbelts or other trauma is rare but easily missed. Bleeding may track down into the chest, resulting in haemothorax or haemomediastinum and rarely cardiac tamponade. Carotid dissection can be identified using ultrasonography, CT scan or angiography.

SPINAL CORD INJURIES

Spinal cord injury may occur as a result of trauma, vertebral collapse, infection, tumours, infarcts and other pathologies. The classic features of complete spinal cord injury are total loss of motor and sensory function below the level of the injury. (In the acute setting, the apparent level of the injury may be higher than actual due to inflammation and oedema around the site of injury.) A number of patterns of incomplete injuries are also recognized (Table 12.1).

In all cases of significant trauma, assume that the spine (cervic, thoracic or lumbar) is injured until proven otherwise and immobilize it as part of initial resuscitation. Signs suggestive of spinal cord injury in an unconscious patient are given in Box 12.2.

TABLE 12.1 Patterns of spinal cord injury

Complete cord injury	Total paralysis and loss of sensation below level of injury
Cord hemisection, Brown–Séquard syndrome	Ipsilateral paralysis and contralateral loss of sensation below level of lesion
Central cord syndrome	Greater motor loss in upper limbs than lower. Variable sensory loss below level of lesion
Anterior cord syndrome	Paralysis, loss of pain/temperature sensation below level of lesion Proprioception and vibration preserved

> **Box 12.2 Signs suggestive of spinal cord injury in an unconscious patient**
>
> Diaphragmatic pattern of breathing
>
> Unexplained hypotension/bradycardia
>
> Absence of response to pain (below level of lesion)
>
> Flaccid paralysis/areflexia
>
> Reduced anal tone
>
> Urinary retention
>
> Priapism

Management

- Follow advanced trauma life support protocols (see p. 306).
- Immobilize the spine to prevent secondary damage. Use a cervical collar, sandbags and tape for cervical spine, plus spinal board. (Log roll with inline stabilization to control head and neck movement.)

 X-rays of the spine do not exclude instability resulting from ligament injury. Spinal cord damage can only be fully excluded by clinical examination in an awake, co-operative patient. Therefore, even if X-rays are normal, you should maintain immobilization until the spine can be assessed clinically. CT or MRI can give further information.

- Establish i.v. access. Give volume load to support the blood pressure.
- Sympathetic interruption from cord injury will produce hypotension and bradycardia, depending upon the level of cord injury. Vasopressors/inotropes may be required to maintain the circulation. Exclude haemorrhage from other injuries (e.g. in the 'silent' denervated abdomen).
- Tracheal intubation and assisted ventilation may be required for respiratory insufficiency or to facilitate surgery. Consider awake fibreoptic intubation using local anaesthesia. Alternatively, intubate the anaesthetized patient with inline immobilization of the neck. The use of a bougie and McCoy laryngoscope or video laryngoscopes limit the need to extend the neck.

 Suxamethonium can be used in the first few hours after injury. Avoid after 24 h because of the potential for massive K^+ release. (See Suxamethonium, p. 43.)

- Gastric stasis is common: pass a nasogastric/orogastric tube.
- Urinary retention is common (and is an important cause of spinal hyperreflexia). Pass a urinary catheter.
- High-dose steroids (methylprednisolone), if given early, may have beneficial effects in spinal injury.
- Discuss the management with the local spinal injuries unit or spinal surgeon. The indications for early spinal decompression and surgical stabilization are controversial. Transfer to a spinal injury unit only after exclusion and stabilization of other injuries in a general/neurosurgical unit.

Respiratory complications are the leading cause of death following cervical cord injury. Marked changes in respiratory physiology/mechanics occur and recovery can be prolonged as a result of impaired ventilation and cough reflexes. This leads to predictable difficulties weaning from artificial ventilation. Early tracheostomy may be of benefit. Those with injuries at a level to effect the phrenic nerve (C3, 4, 5) may remain ventilator-dependent in the long term.

THORACIC INJURIES

Pneumothorax

All traumatic pneumothoraces should be drained. (See Practical procedures, p. 416.)

Massive air leaks may require bronchoscopy to exclude bronchial rupture. Bronchial rupture should be suspected in the presence of deceleration injury, mediastinal widening, haemoptysis, first rib or clavicular fractures. An urgent thoracic surgical opinion should be sought, as surgical repair is usually required.

Haemothorax

This requires early drainage. Once clot becomes well established it becomes difficult to drain and thoracotomy may be required later. Initial drainage > 600 mL or continuing drainage >150 mL/h needs urgent surgical referral. Before attempting drainage of massive haemothorax, ensure good venous access, as decompression of a vascular tear can sometimes occur, resulting in massive haemorrhage. A large drain (28–32 Fr) will generally be required to drain blood effectively.

Rib fractures

These are significant because of the potential for injury to the underlying viscera. Elderly patients with brittle ribs may have impressive rib fractures with little underlying injury. Conversely, younger patients with more flexible ribs may have severe visceral injury without obvious fractures.

- Apical rib fractures are associated with injury to great vessels.
- Mid-zone rib fractures are associated with pulmonary contusions.
- Basal rib fractures are associated with abdominal visceral injury (liver, spleen, kidneys).

Simple rib fractures without major visceral injury can often be managed conservatively. Adequate analgesia is essential, consider patient-controlled analgesia ± NSAIDs, continuous thoracic epidural, or paravertebral block. Supplemental oxygen, CPAP and physiotherapy are useful.

In the presence of a significant flail segment and underlying pulmonary contusions, IPPV is generally required and should be instituted early before exhaustion and significant hypoxia develop. Typically assisted ventilation will be required for 7–10 days in such cases. Severe life-threatening ARDS may develop.

There is little place for surgical fixation of the rib cage. Assisted ventilation (IPPV and PEEP) will usually restore reasonable alignment of a distorted rib cage over a few days. Occasional patients require thoracic or plastic surgical intervention for debridement of contaminated wounds, reconstruction of missing part of chest wall or protruding rib(s).

Mediastinal injury

Rapid deceleration injuries can result in injury to the mediastinal contents; in particular, traumatic transection of the aorta or other great vessels. Many patients with such injuries will die before reaching hospital, but some develop a contained rupture that is at risk of massive rebleeding at any time, hours or even days ahead. The typical finding is that of a widened mediastinum on CXR. Typical features are shown in Fig. 12.1.

Investigations include aortic angiography and spiral CT scan. Transoesophageal echocardiography may have a role but does not provide all the information required for surgery. Not all cases of bleeding into the mediastinum will require surgery. Smaller venous bleeds may be managed conservatively. Always seek advice.

The management of great vessel injury is increasingly by radiological stenting rather than open surgery, where such facilities exist. Refer the patient to cardiothoracic surgeons, vascular surgeons, or vascular interventional radiologists. Immediate management includes controlled hypotension (e.g. GTN or esmolol infusion).

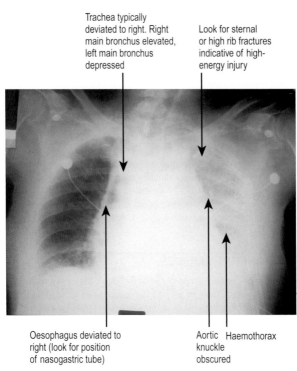

Trachea typically deviated to right. Right main bronchus elevated, left main bronchus depressed

Look for sternal or high rib fractures indicative of high-energy injury

Oesophagus deviated to right (look for position of nasogastric tube)

Aortic knuckle obscured

Haemothorax

Fig. 12.1 Chest X-ray appearances of possible mediastinal haematoma (widened mediastinum).

Cardiac contusions

Blunt trauma to the anterior chest wall can result in injuries to the myocardium, coronary arteries, valves and other related structures. The presence of a fractured sternum should raise suspicion. Typically myocardial contusions may result in dysrhythmias and ischaemic injury patterns on ECG. These are often transient and not significant but dysrhythmias may require appropriate intervention. Rarely, injury to the anterior descending coronary artery may lead to myocardial infarction. Perform serial 12-lead ECGs and send blood for troponin. Echocardiography can indicate dyskinesia suggestive of myocardial contusion, valvular damage, and pericardial effusions. Transthoracic views may be sufficient, but have poor sensitivity for detecting aortic dissection or root injury. A transoesophageal echo or CT angiogram (where available) are valuable for excluding these diagnoses. Seek specialist advice.

Ruptured diaphragm

Blunt trauma to the abdomen may cause the diaphragm to rupture. This usually occurs on the left, due to the protection afforded by the liver on the right. The diagnosis is suggested by abdominal visceral gas shadows in the chest. Check the position of the NG tube as a marker of stomach position. Surgical repair is indicated via the chest or abdomen. Occasional patients have a missed ruptured diaphragm and present later with strangulation of hernia contents. Rupture of the diaphragm may also occasionally be a long-standing, incidental finding. In these situations do not confuse X-ray appearances of viscera in the chest with pleural fluid/gas collections needing a chest drain!

ABDOMINAL INJURIES

Any intra-abdominal structure can be damaged. Major visceral injury may be obvious, but more minor injuries such as mesenteric tears are easily missed. Pain, guarding, distension, and presence or absence of bowel sounds cannot be reliably elicited in the unconscious, sedated and ventilated patient. If previously unrecognized injury or continued intra-abdominal bleeding is suspected, seek immediate surgical opinion. Investigations including ultrasound and CT scan may be helpful, but all can potentially miss significant injuries. If doubt remains, laparotomy should be considered.

Ruptured spleen

Surgeons increasingly try to preserve the spleen following injury and there is a place for conservative management of more minor injuries to the spleen. Patients following splenectomy tend to show initial raised white count in the postoperative period. Following splenectomy there is greatly increased risk of life-threatening infection (particularly pneumococcal). Patients require long-term prophylaxis with penicillin (2 years minimum) and immunization against *Pneumococcus*, *Meningococcus*, and *Haemophilus influenzae* in the convalescent phase. (See BNF and local guidelines.)

Ruptured liver

Where possible, liver trauma is managed conservatively. Post-traumatic liver haemorrhage is often amenable to radiological intervention (embolization). Where laparotomy is unavoidable, surgeons may pack the liver bed and close the abdomen, with the aim of returning to theatre after 48 h. If haemodynamically stable, patients with liver rupture should be transferred to a specialist unit.

Abdominal compartment syndrome

If intra-abdominal pressure rises above venous pressure (e.g. as a result of intra-abdominal haemorrhage) then perfusion to the abdominal organs is impaired. The first indication may be a falling urine output in the presence of an increasingly tense and quiet abdomen. Intra-abdominal pressure can be measured by connecting the urinary catheter to a pressure transducer. Intra-abdominal pressures above 20 mmHg, together with evidence of end organ dysfunction, are suggestive of abdominal compartment syndrome. The management is surgical exploration (see p. 174).

Patients may bleed torrentially when the abdomen is opened and become haemodynamically unstable following visceral reperfusion. In some cases, it may be necessary to leave the abdomen 'open' after decompression. Closure may be achieved either after a few days, when the cause of the abdominal distension has subsided, or much later after the primary defect has closed by granulation. Abdominal distension can impede diaphragmatic function and make weaning from ventilation difficult (see Weaning, p. 135).

SKELETAL INJURIES

Pelvic injuries

Pelvic injuries can result in major blood loss. Unstable pelvic injuries are managed by early external fixation, which is typically performed in A&E. This helps to reduce bleeding and ultimately allows for earlier mobilization.

Urethral injury should be considered in all cases of pelvic injury. Suspect if there is bleeding from the urethral meatus or an abnormal rectal examination. Do not attempt urethral catheterization. Seek help from urologists. Diagnosis is by urethrogram, which can be performed in A&E. Contrast is injected via the urethra, looking for extravasation on X-ray. Management is by suprapubic catheter, with definitive repair at a later date.

Long bone injuries

Look for obvious limb deformity and check for neurovascular integrity. Early reduction of deformity and splinting reduces bleeding and pain. (See also Fat embolism, Compartment syndrome and Rhabdomyolysis below.)

The timing of internal fixation of significant long bone fractures in the face of other multiple injuries is controversial. In principle, early fixation is ideal. There is some evidence, however, that fixation may have adverse effects on ICP and may also worsen acute lung injury/ARDS. Furthermore, it is pointless spending 8–12 h in theatre undertaking extensive orthopaedic instrumentation when the patient stands little chance of survival. In unstable patients and those with significant head injury, fixation may therefore be better delayed. As a result, there has been much study in recent years of the best timing for definitive orthopaedic surgery. The evidence seems to favour either immediate or delayed as 'safe', with intermediate time points carrying a higher risk of the 'second hit' phenomenon.

FAT EMBOLISM

Fat embolism classically presents with dyspnoea, hypoxaemia, petechial rash and acute confusional state following long bone fracture or orthopaedic instrumentation. The signs are non-specific and can be caused by pneumonia, sepsis and other complications of trauma and surgery. The mechanisms by which fat embolism occurs are not clear. The simplest explanation is embolization of fat from long bone marrow into the circulation, and then to the lungs and other organs. This does not explain how fat droplets cross the lungs into the systemic circulation to produce CNS effects, nor why most patients do not develop the condition despite the common presence of fat droplets in the circulation after long bone injury. Although operative intervention may precipitate fat embolism, trauma studies suggest that early orthopaedic fixation of fractures reduces the overall incidence of clinically significant fat embolism.

Investigations

The diagnosis is often one of exclusion. Fat droplets may be seen in retinal vessels, sputum or urine: none of these findings is specific for the condition. CT scan of the brain is usually normal or shows mild diffuse cerebral oedema; MRI scans show areas of microinfarction in severe cases.

Treatment

Management is essentially supportive. Respiratory insufficiency may progress to severe ARDS. The CNS signs usually settle over time but occasional patients develop severe brain injury, with long-term damage or even death.

PERIPHERAL COMPARTMENT SYNDROMES

After initial resuscitation, injured areas often become swollen. Swelling of soft tissues where muscle groups are restricted by fascial layers may result in increased pressure inside the compartments. This restricts blood flow to and from the muscles, which become ischaemic. If left untreated, necrosis, rhabdomyolysis and late ischaemic contractures may develop. This is well recognized in the calf or forearm, but can also occur in the upper arm, thigh, buttocks and in other areas.

Compartment syndrome may be caused by any process that leads to soft-tissue swelling, including infection, haemorrhage or ischaemia. Typical causes are shown in Box 12.3.

Diagnosis relies upon clinical suspicion. Look for swollen, tense and painful muscles (particularly on extension) in the calf and forearm. Remember pain may be masked by epidural/regional anaesthetic blocks. Pulses may be absent but are not invariably so. Diagnosis is confirmed by measurement of compartmental pressure, obtained by insertion of a 21-gauge (green) needle connected to a flush device and pressure transducer (as for any intravascular monitoring). It should be appreciated that there are multiple compartments in each limb so measurement requires knowledge of the appropriate anatomy (seek advice). Pressures greater than 30 mmHg are an indication for fasciotomy and debridement of dead muscle. This can be performed in the ICU. Wounds are left open, and closed subsequently when swelling subsides. Seek surgical advice.

Box 12.3 Typical causes of peripheral compartment syndrome

Forearm fracture

Lower limb fracture

Vascular injury (including surgery)

Reperfusion injury

Pressure from any cause (including crush injury/coma)

Local infection

Local haemorrhage

RHABDOMYOLYSIS

This classically occurs after lower limb crush injury, but can occur following injuries to any muscle group or even from necrotic muscle in surgical wounds. It may follow a missed compartment syndrome. It also occurs with prolonged immobility, e.g. following drug overdosage, epilepsy or head injury. Muscle breakdown (rhabdomyolysis) releases toxic products into the circulation. These produce a systemic inflammatory response syndrome, which may progress to multiple organ failure. In addition, myoglobin specifically precipitates in renal tubules and causes ARF.

Management

The management involves prevention, recognition of the problem and supportive care. Measure creatinine kinase (CK), which is usually greater than 5000 units, and urinary myoglobin (rapidly disappears after a few hours). Exclude and treat compartment syndromes and excise dead muscle (amputation may be required).

Myoglobinuria

Fluid loading and diuretics help maintain urine output. An alkaline diuresis may prevent myoglobin precipitation in the renal tubules. Replace the hourly urine output + 50 mL with alternating hours of 1.4% bicarbonate solution and 5% dextrose. In addition give 0.5 g/kg mannitol. Measure serial urine pH, and aim to keep in alkaline range. Continue this regimen until resolution of myoglobinuria. (See Forced alkaline diuresis, p. 232.)

Should renal failure occur, supportive treatment is required. Once renal failure is established, the course typically follows that of ATN, with gradual complete recovery of renal function. (See Indications for renal replacement therapy, p. 140.)

BURNS

Patients with extensive burn injuries (>20% body surface area) are usually managed in regional burns centres. You may, however, be called to help in the initial resuscitation of a burns victim or may be required to manage the patient in the general ICU because of other coexisting problems. A typical chart for the assessment of burn area is shown in Fig. 12.2.

Resuscitation

The basic principles of resuscitation of the burn victim are the same as for any other patient. The main problems relate to the

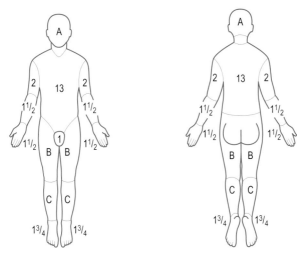

Relative percentage of body surface area affected by growth

Area	Age 0	1	5	10	15	Adult
A=$\frac{1}{2}$ of head	$9\frac{1}{2}$	$8\frac{1}{2}$	$6\frac{1}{2}$	$5\frac{1}{2}$	$4\frac{1}{2}$	$3\frac{1}{2}$
B=$\frac{1}{2}$ of one thigh	$2\frac{3}{4}$	$3\frac{1}{4}$	4	$4\frac{1}{2}$	$4\frac{1}{2}$	$4\frac{3}{4}$
C=$\frac{1}{2}$ of one leg	$2\frac{1}{2}$	$2\frac{1}{2}$	$2\frac{3}{4}$	3	$3\frac{1}{4}$	$3\frac{1}{2}$

Fig. 12.2 Assessment of burns – Lund and Browder charts.

potential for thermal injuries to the airway, large fluid losses and potential for infection.

- Give humidified oxygen by face mask. If there are extensive facial burns, or any evidence of thermal injury to the airway, the airway should be secured by endotracheal intubation. This should be performed electively before oedema and swelling make intubation impossible.
- Establish i.v. access. Where possible, avoid siting cannulae through burned skin, to reduce the risk of infection. (Ultrasound is helpful to guide central venous cannulation if burns are extensive.)
- Give i.v. analgesia and commence fluid resuscitation.

The fluid requirements depend on the size of the burn. This is estimated from the rule of nines or from burns charts. A number of regimens are described for fluid replacement based on either crystalloid or colloid infusion. Examples are shown in Box 12.4.

Box 12.4 Examples of fluid regimens for the resuscitation of burns victims

Mount Vernon formula	Parkland formula
4.5% albumin	Ringer lactate
Volume (mL) = 0.5 × weight (kg) × % burn	Volume (mL) = 4 × weight (kg) × % burns
Over six consecutive periods of 4, 4, 4, 6, 6 and 12 h each	Given over 24 h

Follow local protocols and/or seek advice. It is important to realize that such formulae are a guide only and frequently underestimate fluid requirements, particularly if there are other injuries present. The aim of fluid resuscitation is to restore plasma and extracellular volumes and thus adequate tissue and organ perfusion. Urine output and core–peripheral temperature gradient provide a guide. Many burns units avoid central cannulation because of the risk of infection; however, CVP monitoring or other haemodynamic monitoring may be required.

- Monitor electrolytes and haemoglobin/haematocrit.
- Blood may be required to maintain Hb > 8 g/dL.
- Circumferential burns may require emergency incision (escharotomy).
- Burns should be covered in sterile drapes or plastic film to reduce infection and fluid loss.
- Major burns may cause SIRS (see p. 326).

Smoke inhalation
Smoke inhalation is common in fires occurring in an enclosed environment, such as house fires. Patients may or may not have accompanying burns. Significant smoke inhalation frequently leads to acute lung injury (see p. 154).

Carbon monoxide and cyanide poisoning
Smoke inhalation may be accompanied by the effects of carbon monoxide and cyanide poisoning (see p. 239).

ELECTROCUTION

Electrocution may occur from the domestic mains supply, from high-tension power supplies or occasionally from a lightning strike. Effects depend upon current strength and duration. These include:

- Tachydysrhythmias, particularly ventricular tachycardia, ventricular fibrillation.

- Asystole.
- Respiratory arrest secondary to prolonged contraction of the diaphragm.
- External burns and internal tissue destruction, rhabdomyolysis.
- Other trauma, e.g. from being thrown clear.

Management is largely supportive:

- Ensure adequate airway and ventilation.
- Appropriate fluid resuscitation for burns and other injuries.
- Manage dysrhythmias appropriately. Check ECG, cardiac enzymes and troponin.
- Early surgical debridement of burns and fasciotomy for compartment syndrome. (See Peripheral compartment syndrome, p. 319.)
- Management of other injuries as appropriate

NEAR DROWNING

There is little practical difference between the effects of fresh water and salt water drowning. The problems associated are similar in each case. These include:

- hypothermia
- dysrhythmia
- aspiration/acute lung injury
- trauma
- hypoxic brain injury.

Management
- Ensure adequate airway and ventilation.
- Establish invasive cardiovascular monitoring (arterial line and CVP) and support circulation as necessary.
- Treat any dysrhythmias. Actively rewarm and correct electrolyte disturbances.
- If evidence of aspiration on CXR, consider broad-spectrum antibiotics (seek microbiological advice). Otherwise await cultures.
- Manage acute lung injury as appropriate.
- Look for and manage other injuries as appropriate.

The degree of hypoxic brain injury is the main factor in quality of outcome following near drowning. Severe hypothermia can, however, provide significant brain protection, particularly in children, and therefore it can be difficult to predict outcomes.

Good outcomes can occasionally be achieved despite prolonged periods of immersion and prolonged cardiac arrest. (See also Hypothermia, p. 226)

OUTCOME FOLLOWING TRAUMA

The outcome following major trauma is critically dependent on the site of trauma. Significant brain or spinal cord injury greatly increases the risk of disability and death. There is clear relationship between increasing number and severity of injuries and death. Age is an important independent variable. The mortality curve starts to accelerate after the age of about 50–55 such that in old age there is a significant morbidity and mortality even following relatively minor trauma.

A number of scoring systems have been described in trauma.

Injury Severity Score (ISS)

An anatomical scoring system is based on six body areas. For each area of the body (head and neck; face; chest; abdomen; extremity; skin) an abbreviated injury score (AIS) from 1 to 6 is assigned (1 = minor injury; 5 = severe injury; 6 = unsurvivable injury). The abbreviated injury scores for the three worst affected body areas are squared and added together to give the ISS. [Any injury which is deemed unsurvivable (AIS of 6) is assigned an ISS of 75.] The ISS scores range from 0 to 75 and correlate linearly with outcome.

Revised Trauma Score (RTS)

RTS is a physiological scoring system based on the Glasgow Coma Scale, systolic blood pressure and respiratory rate and scored from the first set of observations recorded from the patient. Values range from 0 to 7.8408 (0 = low probability of survival; 7.8408 = high probability of survival). RTS correlates well with outcome.

Trauma Score—Injury Severity Score (TRISS)

TRISS combines the ISS (anatomical scoring system), RTS (physiological scoring system) together with the patient's age, to predict the probability of surviving either blunt or penetrating trauma.

(See also Prediction of outcome, p. 7, and APACHE score, p. 8.)

CHAPTER 13

INFECTION AND INFLAMMATION

Infection 326

Systemic inflammatory response syndrome (SIRS) 326

Definitions 327

Distinguishing infection 328

Sepsis care bundles 329

Septic shock 331

Investigation of unexplained sepsis 334

Empirical antibiotic therapy 336

Source control 336

Problem organisms 336

Catheter-related sepsis 340

Infective endocarditis 341

Necrotizing fasciitis 342

Meningococcal sepsis 342

Notifiable infectious diseases 345

INFECTION

Infection is common in the ICU and may be the primary cause of a patient's admission, or may occur as a secondary phenomenon in patients who are already critically ill and whose normal barriers to infection are impaired. Factors that predispose to infection in critically ill patients are shown in Box 13.1. (See also Infection control, p. 19)

Box 13.1 Factors predisposing to infection in critical illness

Chronic disease states

Effects of acute illness

Effects of sedative and analgesic agents (suppressed cough reflex, GI stasis, etc.)

Endotracheal tube

Vascular catheters, urinary catheters and drains

Increased gastric pH

Poor nutrition and impaired tissue healing

Immune suppressive effects of drugs

Increased risk of cross-infection

Prolonged broad spectrum antibiotics selecting out resistant and other organisms

---

It has been claimed that infection is responsible for up to a quarter of all deaths in intensive care. Early identification of developing infection, drainage / removal of septic foci and the instigation of appropriate antibiotic therapy are therefore vital.

SYSTEMIC INFLAMMATORY RESPONSE SYNDROME (SIRS)

Typical signs of infection in critically ill patients include pyrexia, tachycardia, hyperventilation (failure to wean), non-specific deterioration in overall condition and a change in inflammatory markers (rising CRP, rising or suppressed white cell count). These changes are not specific, however, and similar changes may be produced by any inflammatory process, such as those produced by endotoxaemia, ischaemia reperfusion syndromes, liver failure and pancreatitis.

It is now recognized that many processes (including infection) may trigger activation of endothelial cells, white cells, platelets and other cells, leading to the release of proinflammatory mediators, including platelet-activating factor (PAF), tumour necrosis factor (TNFα), interleukins, chemokines and other inflammatory mediators. These have effects such as increased vascular permeability (capillary leak), vasodilatation, sequestration of neutrophils, platelet adhesion and activation of complement systems. Simultaneous activation of the coagulation and fibrinolytic pathways may lead to disseminated intravascular coagulation (DIC) and failure of the microcirculation. Indeed, in sepsis, the coagulation and inflammatory pathways are inextricably linked and mutually activated.

The consequent systemic inflammatory response may range from relatively mild with minimal sequelae, to severe, resulting in multiple organ dysfunction, multiple organ failure and death.

DEFINITIONS

The common definitions for sepsis, systemic inflammatory response syndrome (SIRS) and multiorgan dysfunction syndrome (MODS) were established in the early 1990s in a consensus statement from the American College of Chest Physicians and the Society of Critical Care Medicine. Although these definitions are of limited value clinically, they have been used as a means to standardize many clinical trials and have become a standard, internationally recognized nomenclature. These definitions are as follows:

Systemic inflammatory response syndrome (SIRS)

The systemic inflammatory response syndrome can be said to exist when two of the criteria listed in Box 13.2 are present, in the absence of a documented infection.

Sepsis

Features of SIRS, together with a documented infection. The infection may be bacterial, viral, fungal, parasitic or other

---

Box 13.2 Definition of SIRS

Requires the presence of two or more of the following features:

Temperature $> 38°C$ or $< 36°C$

Heart rate > 90 beats/min

Respiratory rate > 20 breaths/min or $PaCO_2 < 4.3$ kPa

White blood count $> 12\,000$ cells/mm^3 or < 4000 cells/mm^3 or presence of $> 10\%$ immature neutrophils

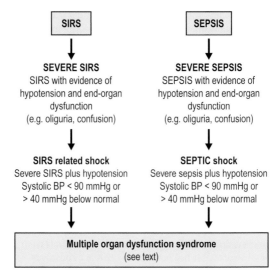

Fig. 13.1 SIRS and sepsis of increasing severity.

organism. Difficulty may sometimes arise in patients with positive cultures in distinguishing between clinically insignificant colonization and true infection (see below).

Both SIRS and sepsis may vary in severity from mild to severe, and both may progress to multiorgan dysfunction. Parallel definitions may be used, as shown in Fig. 13.1.

Multiorgan dysfunction syndrome (MODS)

MODS is described as abnormal function of more than one organ such that normal homeostasis cannot be maintained without intervention. In this context 'organ' can be taken to include the respiratory, cardiovascular and gastrointestinal systems, kidneys, liver, brain (altered conscious level), bone marrow and immune systems. MODS may respond to general supportive measures and resolution of the underlying condition, or may progress to established multiple organ failure.

DISTINGUISHING INFECTION

In view of the similarities in the clinical picture produced by SIRS and sepsis (above), the problem may arise as how to distinguish infection. C-reactive protein (CRP) is a commonly used marker of infection but is not specific. Procalcitonin is an alternative marker that is thought to be more specific for infection, but is not yet widely available.

In general, infection is only confirmed when a positive microscopy or culture result is obtained from a normally sterile body space. Repeated samples are often required. (See investigation of unexplained sepsis, p. 334.) The time taken to obtain microbiological results varies with the particular sample type and the technique used to process it. Techniques for confirming infection, and potentially identifying the causative organism, include:

- microscopy and staining (4 h)
- cultures (24–48 h)
- conventional PCR (48 h)
- antigen tests, antibody titres, e.g. diagnosis of fungal infection esp. *Candida, Aspergillus* (24–48 h).

Rapid screening tests

There has been considerable interest recently in the development of systems for the more rapid identification and diagnosis of infection and a number of proprietary diagnostic systems are now coming to the market. Typical of these is the 'Septifast' system. A rapid diagnosis is made using PCR, screening against a panel of common infective organisms. Claims made for this technology are that its enables the rapid detection of the majority of pathogens causing infection in critical care within a few hours. In principle this should enable earlier targeted antibiotic therapy, with the potential for improvement in outcomes.

As yet the technology is not widely available, as it is costly, not fully automated, and is extremely demanding of laboratory technician time. Another drawback is that it does not, at present, provide information on antibiotic sensitivity. Accurate subtyping and sensitivity can only be provided following full cultures, which may take a further 24–48 h, therefore immediate antibiotic choice is based upon the microbiologist's 'best guess'. These technologies are, however, in their infancy, and further advances are likely. (See investigation of unexplained sepsis below.)

SEPSIS CARE BUNDLES

Recent international consensus guidelines on the management of sepsis in critical care have been widely adopted (Table 13.1).

TABLE 13.1 Guidelines for initial treatment of sepsis. Adapted from surviving sepsis campaign[1]

Initial resuscitation	Resuscitation goals
Begin resuscitation immediately in patients with hypotension or elevated serum lactate >4 mmol/L, do not delay pending ICU admission	CVP 8–12 mmHg Mean arterial pressure > 65 mmHg Urine output >0.5 mL kg⁻¹ h⁻¹ Central venous (SVC) oxygen saturation > 70% or mixed venous > 65%
Diagnosis Obtain appropriate cultures before starting antibiotics provided this does not significantly delay antimicrobial administration	Obtain two or more blood cultures (BC) One or more BCs should be percutaneous One BC from each vascular access device in place > 48 h Culture other sites as clinically indicated Perform imaging studies promptly to confirm any source of infection
Antibiotic therapy Begin intravenous antibiotics as early as possible and always within the first hour of recognizing severe sepsis and septic shock	Use broad-spectrum antibiotics, one or more agents active against likely pathogens and with good penetration into presumed site of infection Reassess antimicrobial regimen daily to optimize efficacy, prevent resistance, avoid toxicity, and minimize costs Duration of therapy typically limited to 7–10 days; longer if response is slow or there are undrainable foci of infection or immunological deficiencies Stop antimicrobial therapy if cause is found to be non-infectious
Source identification and control A specific anatomic site of infection should be established as rapidly as possible and within first 6 h of presentation (see below).	Formally evaluate patient for a focus of infection amenable to source control measures, e.g. abscess drainage, tissue debridement Implement source control measures as soon as possible following successful initial resuscitation (exception: infected pancreatic necrosis, where evidence suggests that surgical intervention is best delayed) Choose source control measure with maximum efficacy and minimal physiologic upset Remove intravascular access devices if potentially infected

[1]Dellinger RP et al. 2008 Surviving Sepsis Campaign: International guidelines for management of severe sepsis and septic shock. *Crit Care Med* **36:** 296–327 [published correction appears in *Crit Care Med* **36:** 1394–1396].

While much of the evidence is low level (based on expert opinion), the recommendations also include some high level evidence, the document as a whole forms a rational and coherent approach to the management of the patient with sepsis. Central to these sepsis care bundles is the need for early effective resuscitation, early effective antibiotic therapy and source control, and where possible, the use of an appropriate 'biological response modifier'. Currently, activated protein C, (drotrecogin alpha), is the only such agent available (see Septic shock below). The key recommendations are summarized in Table 13.1.

SEPTIC SHOCK

The clinical features are those of SIRS, with significant hypotension and end-organ dysfunction (see above). Initially patients may have a hyperdynamic circulation, with an elevated cardiac output (CO) and reduced systemic vascular resistance (so-called 'warm septic shock'). At this stage patients exhibit warm peripheries, flushing and visible cardiac pulsation. This may rapidly progress, however, to 'cold septic shock' with reduced CO and cold, poorly perfused peripheries. This is frequently accompanied by marked metabolic acidosis.

The first imperatives are resuscitation and stabilization. This is followed by investigation of the underlying source of sepsis. The third stage involves management of specific underlying problems and complications.

Resuscitation and stabilization

- Give high flow oxygen.
- Consider the need for intubation and ventilation.
- Secure venous access. (Take blood for culture and give i.v. antibiotics as appropriate.)
- Give i.v. fluid challenge.

If end-organ failure is compromising respiration (respiratory failure, severe confusion, etc.), early consideration should be given to securing the airway and instituting artificial ventilation. There is a risk, however, that the drugs used to facilitate intubation may cause circulatory collapse. (See Intubation, p. 398.) Therefore, where ventilation is not required immediately, it is often wiser to institute fluid resuscitation prior to attempting intubation and to insert an arterial line to provide accurate blood pressure monitoring. If peripheral arterial cannulation is not feasible, consider femoral or brachial artery.

Patients with sepsis and septic shock are often grossly hypovolaemic because of vasodilatation and capillary permeability changes leading to third-space fluid loss. This situation may well be exacerbated by pyrexia and fluid loss related to any underlying pathology. Vigorous fluid resuscitation may therefore be required. There is controversy over whether colloid or crystalloid solutions are most appropriate. You should follow local guidelines.

- Give 2–3 L fluid as initial resuscitation volume (0.9% saline or colloid).
- Establish invasive monitoring, arterial line and CVP. Consider cardiac output monitoring, central venous saturation monitoring (see p. 74).
- Optimize volume loading. Initially aim for a CVP 8–12 mmHg depending on patient's condition and response, (10–15 mmHg in a ventilated patient). Above this level, it is unlikely that additional fluid loading will produce any further increase in left ventricular stroke volume index.
- If there is evidence of significant myocardial depression (low MAP with high CVP; low CI or SVI where monitoring is available), consider addition of an inotrope e.g. dobutamine/adrenaline (epinephrine) to support cardiac output. (See Cardiovascular system, p. 82.)
- Maintain adequate tissue perfusion pressure (MAP ≥ 65 mmHg). If MAP remains low despite adequate volume loading and cardiac output, add a vasoconstrictor, e.g. noradrenaline (norepinephrine).

Therapeutic end points involve adequate clinical organ and tissue perfusion, e.g. warm pink peripheries, adequate urine output, mentally alert (if not sedated). Ensure all relevant microbiological investigations have been sent and appropriate antibiotics started. In cases of refractory shock:

- If significant metabolic acidosis, pH < 7.1, consider bicarbonate.
- If serum ionized calcium <0.8 mmol/L, consider IV calcium chloride/gluconate.
- Vasopressin infusion at physiological replacement doses. Vasopressin levels can become rapidly depleted in septic shock. Consider vasopressin as a second line vasopressor treatment. (See Optimizing perfusion pressure, p. 85.)
- Functional adrenal insufficiency – low (physiological NOT pharmacological) dose steroid supplementation may be helpful, e.g. 25–50 mg hydrocortisone TDS. Seek advice and follow your local policy.

Role of haemofiltration in sepsis

There is anecdotal evidence that the clinical condition of some patients with septic shock may improve significantly when haemofiltration is commenced. This effect is independent of improvements in acid–base status and is possibly due to the removal of proinflammatory mediators. However, recent clinical trials in this area are conflicting and further trials are on-going. Seek local advice.

Role of anti-inflammatory agents

There has been a great deal of research over recent years on the use of agents to block or modulate the effects of proinflammatory mediators in the inflammatory cascade, in the hope of reducing the inflammatory response to sepsis and improving outcome. Clinical trials of anti-endotoxin antibodies, anti-TNFα antibodies and anti-PAF receptor antibodies have failed to show any benefit.

Activated protein C

A multinational trial of recombinant human activated protein C (PROWESS Trial) reported an overall 6% reduction in mortality in patients with severe sepsis. Activated protein C is now licensed and available for use in the UK. Uncertainty remains about the most effective duration of treatment. It appears to show greatest benefit in patients with a high APACHE score and does not benefit those with a score <20 or children. Therapy with activated protein C does carry an increased risk of bleeding and many patients will have relative or absolute contraindications to its use. Patients with intracranial haemorrhage, recent stroke and multiple trauma fall into this category. Post-surgical patients should be considered on the balance of risks. Recent experience suggests that in many situations the overall balance of risks may still favour its use, and it is currently recommended as part of the Surviving Sepsis Care Bundle. At the time of writing, however, a further large multinational study testing the efficacy of the product is underway. Follow local protocols and seek senior advice.

Complications

The specific complications and pattern of organ dysfunction varies from patient to patient. Many patients require renal support, some may develop prolonged GI tract failure, and a large proportion develop ARDS or coagulopathy. Some develop multiple organ dysfunction and multiple organ failure. Specific supportive measures for each system are required (see relevant sections).

Prognosis

Overall, the mortality from severe sepsis with shock remains high, ranging from 30 to 70% in various studies. Best results are likely to be obtained by early recognition, effective resuscitation, timely source control and overall attention to detail.

INVESTIGATION OF UNEXPLAINED SEPSIS

Any patient in the ICU with unexplained 'sepsis' or rising markers of infection should have a thorough examination to identify possible sources. Appropriate microbiological samples should be obtained prior to the institution of antibiotic therapy. These should ideally include 'clean stab' blood cultures from a peripheral vein (in addition to cultures from any existing cannulae), sputum or BAL for microscopy and culture. Urine and any drain fluids should also be cultured. Additional investigations will be guided by the clinical picture (Table 13.2). It is important to repeat blood cultures and other microbiological investigations regularly to help make a diagnosis and to facilitate antibiotic de-escalation. (See also Distinguishing infection above.)

Imaging in sepsis

Where the source of infection is not immediately obvious, radiological imaging (abdominal ultrasound, CT) may help locate the focus of infection. Potential sites of occult infection include the chest, and abdomen. Spinal or paraspinal abscesses are easily missed, particularly in the patient who already has chronic back or other skeletal problems and can be identified by CT or MRI. Any collections identified should be sampled, cultured and drained.

Infective endocarditis

Always consider the possibility of infective endocarditis, particularly in the case of on-going positive blood cultures or cultures with no evident primary source. Transoesophageal echocardiography is the investigation of choice. (See Endocarditis below.)

Intra-abdominal sepsis

Intra-abdominal causes of sepsis account for a significant number of cases of unexplained sepsis. Abdominal ultrasound and CT scan are likely to be the most valuable investigation. If pus or abscesses are confirmed, these should be drained and cultured. In the absence of an identifiable cause of sepsis, and in the face of a deteriorating clinical picture, laparotomy may be warranted.

TABLE 13.2 Investigation of unexplained sepsis	
Potential source	*Investigation*
Catheter-related	Blood cultures from catheters/peripheral stab. Request differential cultures Change indwelling vascular catheters and culture tips
Embolic	Serial blood cultures Precordial or transoesophageal echocardiography
Chest	CXR Tracheal aspirates for culture Bronchoscopy + BAL Tap and culture pleural fluid CT scan
Abdomen and pelvis	Amylase Culture drain fluids (fresh samples) Tap and culture ascites Plain abdominal X-ray Abdominal and pelvic ultrasound/CT scan Laparotomy
Urinary tract	Urine microscopy and culture Plain abdominal film/ultrasound/CT renal tract
Wounds/soft tissues	Pus/tissue/swabs for culture Re-exploration
CNS	CT scan/MRI scan for spine and soft tissues Lumbar puncture
Joints	X-ray/ultrasound/CT scan Needle aspiration
Sinuses	X-ray/ultrasound/CT scan

Seek senior advice and a surgical opinion. (See Acalculous cholecystitis, p. 176, and Pancreatitis, p. 181.)

Pyrexia of unknown origin

If the cause of sepsis is not apparent, consider investigation for other causes of pyrexia. Pyrexia of unknown origin may be associated with myocardial infarction, autoimmune inflammatory processes (autoantibodies and vasculitic screen), malignancy, drugs and rare infectious diseases. Seek advice.

EMPIRICAL ANTIBIOTIC THERAPY

In many cases of sepsis antibiotics are started on an empirical basis before the results of cultures and/or the sensitivity of organisms are known.

Although early appropriate antibiotic therapy is one of the few evidence-based interventions leading to improved outcome in sepsis and septic shock, prolonged use of broad-spectrum antibiotics can lead to the emergence of resistant organisms. It can also lead to the suppression of normal gut flora and has been implicated in a outbreaks of potentially lethal infections from organisms such as *Clostridium difficile* and MRSA. Antibiotics should be used sensibly, with due regard to their adverse effects, as well as the benefits. It is important to have a coherent policy for both antibiotic use and early de-escalation of therapy.

Table 13.3 provides a guide to empirical antibiotic therapy. You should, however, always follow your hospital antibiotic policy and/or ask advice from your hospital microbiologist.

SOURCE CONTROL

Wherever possible the source of an infection should be eradicated. If catheter-related sepsis is suspected remove existing arterial and venous lines and send the tips for culture (see Catheter-related sepsis below). Obvious collections of pus should be drained and cultured and potentially infected wounds derided. Ensure appropriate specimens are sent to the lab. Potential means of source control are listed in Table 13.4.

PROBLEM ORGANISMS

GRAM-POSITIVE ORGANISMS

Methicillin-resistant *Staphylococcus aureus* (MRSA)

Colonization of skin and wounds with MRSA is increasingly common. Patients are usually isolated in side rooms and barrier nursed to prevent cross-infection. Eradication can be difficult and antibiotic treatment (of colonization) is often pointless. The patient's flora generally changes over time as their condition improves. If treatment is required, vancomycin, linezolid or teicoplanin are usually the antibiotics of choice. Seek microbiology advice.

TABLE 13.3 Empirical first-line antibiotic therapy

Source	Common pathogens	Suggested antibiotic
Community-acquired pneumonia Including possible atypical pneumonia	Strep. pneumoniae H. influenzae Staphylococcus aureus Legionella Mycoplasma Chlamydia Coxiella	Cefuroxime or coamoxiclav (coamoxiclav lower risk of C. difficile in elderly) Cefuroxime or coamoxiclav and clarithromycin
Hospital-acquired pneumonia	Strep. pneumoniae H. influenzae Staph. aureus* Enterobacteria	Early (<5 days) as for community acquired (above) Late (>5 days) piperacillin + tazobac-tam, or ciprofloxacin/ ceftazidime/ carbapenem
Intra-abdominal sepsis	Staphylococci Enterobacteria Anaerobes	Cefuroxime and metronidazole
Pelvic infection	Anaerobes Enterobacteria	Cefuroxime and metronidazole or carbapenem, plus doxycline
Urinary tract	Escherichia coli Proteus species Klebsiella species	Cefuroxime or gentamicin
Wound infection	Staph. aureus* Streptococci Enterobacteria	Amoxicillin, and flucloxacillin (add metronidazole for traumatic wounds)
Necrotizing fasciitis	Mixed synergistic flora If group A streptococcus	Ceftazidime, gentamicin and metronidazole Benzylpenicillin + clin-damycin
i.v. line sepsis (remove line)	Staph. aureus* Coag. neg. staph.* Streptococci Enterococci Gram-neg. species Yeasts	Flucloxacillin and ceftazidime, amphotericin or fungin
Meningitis	Neisseria meningitidis Strep. pneumoniae H. influenzae	Cefotaxime

*If MRSA or Coag. neg. staph. possible, consider vancomycin or teicoplanin (see below)

TABLE 13.4 Potential means of source control

IV catheter related infection	Remove
Chest	Drain pleural collections
Abdomen	Drain collections/surgical intervention
Soft tissues	Drain and debride infected collections
CNS	Drain collections, remove infected shunts
Uterus	Remove infected products of conception
Urinary tract	Relieve obstruction/drain
Joints	Aspirate and wash out

Coagulase-negative staphylococci

Coagulase-negative staphylococci (e.g. *Staph. epidermidis*) are part of the normal skin flora. They adhere to plastic devices and commonly colonize indwelling central venous lines. They may cause systemic infection and are often multiply resistant to antibiotics. If suspected, remove or change indwelling lines and discuss with a microbiologist. Community-acquired strains may be sensitive to flucloxacillin but vancomycin or teicoplanin is often required.

Enterococci and vancomycin-resistant enterococci (VRE)

Enterococci are part of the normal flora of the GI tract and female genital tract, but in ICU patients they may be responsible for bacteraemia, endocarditis, urinary tract and wound infections. They are usually sensitive to ampicillin or a combination of ampicillin and aminoglycoside but there is increasing incidence of antibiotic resistance. Vancomycin-resistant enterococci are an increasing concern.

Clostridium difficile

This is an anaerobic Gram-positive bacillus that is the main cause of antibiotic-associated 'pseudomembranous colitis', following broad-spectrum antibiotics. Presents with profuse diarrhoea (may be blood-stained). *Clostridium difficile* toxin can be identified in stools. Treatment is with oral (or i.v.) metronidazole or vancomycin. Occasional patients who do not respond to antibiotics may need a colectomy.

Importantly, *Clostridium difficile* is a spore-forming organism. This means that, unlike many other infections, rapid hand disinfection with alcohol or similar substances is ineffective. Therefore, patients suffering from *Clostridium difficile* infection should be effectively barrier nursed. Hand washing with soap and water is essential before and after contact with such patients and before contact with subsequent patients. Because of its ease of transmission, all patients who develop *Clostridium difficile* should be viewed as a potential risk to other patients, and may indeed have developed their own infection as a result of cross-contamination. Rigorous hand washing and infection control measures are vital to prevent cross-infection. (See also p.171.)

GRAM-NEGATIVE ORGANISMS

Escherichia coli, *Klebsiella* sp. and coliforms

These Gram-negative bacteria are normal commensals in the gastrointestinal tract but are a significant cause of infection on the ICU. They typically infect the respiratory tract, urinary tract and wounds, and may lead to bacteraemia, septicaemia and septic shock. Cephalosporins can be used as first-line treatment, but again there is increasing antibiotic resistance. Seek advice.

Pseudomonas species

The overall incidence of *Pseudomonas* infection in ICUs seems to be declining; however, it remains a serious problem, particularly affecting the respiratory tract. Antibiotic resistance is widespread, but aminoglycosides, ceftazidime, imipenem and ciprofloxacin are useful agents.

Acinetobacter species

This organism is widespread in the environment and is increasingly recognized as an important pathogen in ICU patients, particularly causing respiratory tract and wound infection and occasionally bacteraemia. They are often multiply resistant to antibiotics.

FUNGAL INFECTIONS

Fungal infection on the ICU is increasingly recognized, particularly among patients who are immune compromised and who have received multiple courses of broad-spectrum antibiotics. *Candida albicans* is the most common species. Diagnosis is difficult, but the presence of *Candida* at more than one site (e.g. oral, genital, wounds) should raise suspicion of systemic candidiasis. Positive blood cultures, or isolation from body cavities or deeper seated infections, e.g. abdominal drains, is diagnostic of systemic candidiasis. Fungi grow poorly in conventional blood culture bottles, and serological markers (e.g. *Candida*, *Aspergillus* antigen and antibody tests) may be helpful, although this may not distinguish colonization from infection. Empirical treatment with antifungals may be appropriate. There are a number of conventional and newly introduced agents. Standard treatments include liposomal amphotericin and azoles such as fluconazole. Newer agents include itraconazole caspafungin, micafungin and anidulafungin. Resistance patterns of fungal infection change rapidly. Seek microbiological advice.

CATHETER-RELATED SEPSIS

Catheter-related sepsis is a common problem on the ICU and should be considered in all patients with suspected sepsis in whom vascular catheters have been in place for more than 48 h.

Following catheter insertion, thrombus forms around the puncture site of the vessel and may propagate along the length of the catheter. This provides an excellent culture medium for bacteria, which may rapidly colonize all catheters either via the puncture site in the skin or following bacteraemia. In addition, catheters may be colonized by bacteria introduced via the access ports when the catheter is used, for example to administer drugs.

Colonization is common and does not necessarily warrant removal of the catheter or treatment. Infection is difficult to diagnose. Cultures taken through the catheter do not distinguish between colonization, infection and unrelated bacteraemia. Brush specimens taken from the lumen of the line are semiquantitative and can suggest infection. Alternatively, paired cultures can be taken from the suspect catheter and from a peripheral vein (clean stab), and the shorter time taken for development of positive cultures from the catheter used to suggest the presence of catheter-related infection.

If there is a strong suspicion of catheter-related sepsis the catheter should be removed and the tip cut off (sterile scissors) and sent for culture. In most cases, the diagnosis is made retrospectively after removal of the suspect catheter, positive tip culture and resolution of the clinical condition.

Established clot in central veins may get infected to and lead to septic thrombophlebitis. It may take a number of days to clear the infection even though the original catheters have been removed.

- Ideally catheters should be replaced at a new clean puncture site.
- Ideally there should be a 'line-free' interval between removing and replacing catheters but this is often impractical.
- If necessary, provided the entry site is not obviously infected, catheters can be changed over a guide wire at the same site. This should only be considered when a clean puncture site is not available or is high risk.
- The risk of line-related sepsis increases with the number of days for which lines have been present. It is unclear whether this risk is reduced by routine or 'protocol' line changes (see p. 386).
- The risk varies significantly according to the site of cannulation (groin > jugular > subclavian).

INFECTIVE ENDOCARDITIS

Patients with valvular heart disease or prosthetic heart valves, intravenous drug abusers and patients with long term indwelling central venous catheters are at risk of infective endocarditis. Immune compromise may be an additional risk factor in the ICU patient.

Subacute bacterial endocarditis is a chronic form of the condition with insidious onset. Acute bacterial endocarditis (e.g. i.v. drug abusers) can lead to heart failure (disruption of normal valvular function) widespread embolic infection/infarction, and the rapid development of septic shock and multiorgan failure.

Clinical vigilance for signs and symptoms of endocarditis is important. The diagnosis should be suspected in any patient with persistent fever, unexplained positive blood cultures (characteristic organisms) and the onset of new or changing heart murmurs. Murmurs may be difficult to detect in a ventilated ICU patient. Other stigmata of endocarditis include Roth spots (retinal haemorrhages), splinter haemorrhages, Osler's nodes (fingers), and Janeway lesions (palms). Transthoracic echocardiography is useful in patients who have developed valve dysfunction or who have a gross valvular lesion such as regurgitation or incompetence. Smaller valve lesions can however be difficult to detect using transthoracic echo, particularly when the patient is artificially ventilated (poor echo window). Transoesophageal echo (TOE) is the imaging of choice which may identify vegetations or abscess formation around the valves.

Once a diagnosis of infective endocarditis is made, specialist endocarditis teams are usually involved in the ongoing management of the patient. Typically these comprise a microbiologist, cardiologist and a specialist in infectious diseases. Treatment is by high dose antibiotics and treatment may have to be extremely prolonged. Cardiac surgery is the treatment of last resort, and is often associated with a poor prognosis, especially in patients who have already been significantly debilitated by a period of critical illness. Despite optimum care, the mortality of patients who develop multi-system failure from acute endocarditis remains high.

NECROTIZING FASCIITIS

This is a rapidly spreading soft-tissue infection, which can affect any part of the body. It frequently follows minor trauma, but the aetiology is not fully understood. Typically, the affected area is indurate and discoloured. Laboratory findings and other diagnostic tests may be useful, but the diagnosis is primarily clinical.

Multiple organisms have been implicated. Commonly it is caused by a synergistic infection with a mixture of Gram-negative and anaerobic organisms (e.g. *Bacteroides* species, *Clostridium* species and anaerobic streptococci) or by infection with group A streptococcus alone. Infection spreads along fascial planes, causing necrosis of skin and subcutaneous tissues. Muscle layers are usually spared. The infection may spread rapidly and can be fatal within a few hours. Treatment is by urgent and extensive surgical excision of infected and necrotic tissue together with appropriate antibiotics. Seek microbiological advice. (See Empirical antibiotic therapy, p. 336.)

MENINGOCOCCAL SEPSIS

Neisseria meningitidis is a Gram-negative organism, which approximately 10% of the population carry as a nasal commensal. It causes a spectrum of illness from meningitis (without systemic sepsis) to severe septicaemia resulting in multiple organ failure, limb loss and death within a few hours.

Although meningococcal sepsis is more common in paediatric intensive care, occasional cases occur in young adults. It can be a devastating illness resulting in death within a few hours. Always seek senior help.

Diagnosis

Early symptoms of systemic infection include fever (often >40°C), arthralgia, myalgia, headache and vomiting. The diagnosis of meningococcal sepsis is made on the basis of the typical non-blanching purpuric rash together with evidence of hypotension, tachycardia and poor perfusion.

> ⚠ **The diagnosis of meningococcal sepsis is based on clinical signs. Life-saving antibiotic treatment (cefotaxime or benzylpenicillin) and resuscitation should be commenced immediately on suspicion. This must not be delayed by investigations.**

Management

- Antibiotics should be given as soon as the diagnosis is suspected.
- Give high-flow oxygen by face mask. May require intubation and ventilation. Beware of cardiovascular collapse!
- Establish i.v. access. Give fluids, crystalloid/colloid, to support the circulation. Large volumes are usually required to maintain blood pressure and improve peripheral circulation.
- Establish invasive arterial blood pressure and haemodynamic monitoring CVP/pulmonary artery catheter or alternative.
- Commence inotropes as required. Typically adrenaline (epinephrine) is first-line.
- Peripheral and digital ischaemia. If blood pressure is adequate consider epoprostenol (prostacyclin) infusion $5–10\,ng\,kg^{-1}\,min^{-1}$. This improves microvascular perfusion and may reduce risks of digital ischaemia.
- Coagulopathy and DIC are common. Send coagulation screen. Avoid giving FFP, platelets and cryoprecipitate unless there is active bleeding as these may increase the tendency to microvascular thrombosis and worsen digital ischaemia.
- Hypocalcaemia is common. Consider calcium bolus and possible calcium infusion.
- Metabolic acidosis is normal. This will improve as the patient's condition improves. Do not give bicarbonate unless extreme (pH < 7.1) or inotropes ineffective.
- There is no evidence for the routine use of steroids in meningococcal shock but if adrenal insufficiency is suspected then replacement steroid therapy is appropriate. (This is in contrast to meningococcal meningitis in which recent evidence

suggests that steroids may be of benefit. See Meningitis, p. 295.) Waterhouse–Friderichsen syndrome (adrenal haemorrhage/infarction) is rare and is usually a post-mortem finding.

● Activated protein C may have a specific beneficial role in meningococcal sepsis in reducing the microvascular thrombosis and tissue ischaemia but numbers in adults are insufficient to prove benefit and studies in children have not shown benefit. (See Activated protein C, p. 333.)

There is increasing use of haemofiltration and plasma exchange in meningococcal sepsis to remove endotoxin, cytokines and other factors, in an attempt to improve overall survival and also to reduce the incidence of sequelae such as digital ischaemia. The benefits of these treatments are as yet not proven. You should seek senior advice.

Microbiological diagnosis

Although treatment is based on clinical suspicion, it is helpful to attempt to establish a microbiological diagnosis. Blood should be sent for culture and polymerase chain reaction (PCR). Skin lesions should be scraped onto a glass slide for microscopy and sent for culture. Seek microbiological advice.

Antibiotics

Meningococcus is usually sensitive to benzylpenicillin in the UK; however, other severe infections, most notably pneumococcal sepsis, may occasionally produce a similar clinical picture and purpuric rash, so high-dose cefotaxime is the first-line agent of choice. When meningococcal disease is confirmed later and the sensitivities are known, benzylpenicillin may be substituted. Neither of these antibiotics eradicates nasal carriage of meningococcus, and the patient should receive rifampicin or ciprofloxacin for this purpose during the recovery phase. (See Prophylaxis below.)

Prophylaxis

Most cases of meningococcal disease are sporadic and 'outbreaks' of infection are rare. However, the index patient, direct family contacts and other close contacts require prophylactic treatment with rifampicin (or ciprofloxacin) to abolish nasal carriage of meningococcus. This is organized by the public health department and the case should be reported to them as soon as possible. (See Notifiable infectious diseases below.)

It is not normally considered necessary for the medical or nursing staff involved in the care of these patients to receive prophylaxis, unless direct contamination has occurred.

Box 13.3 Notifiable infectious diseases in the UK

Common	Uncommon
Acute encephalitis	Acute poliomyelitis
Food poisoning	Anthrax
Leptospirosis	Cholera
Measles	Diphtheria
Meningitis	Dysentery
Meningococcal septicaemia	Malaria
Mumps	Paratyphoid fever
Ophthalmia neonatorum	Plague
Rubella	Rabies
Scarlet fever	Relapsing fever
Tetanus	Smallpox
Tuberculosis	Severe acute respiratory syndrome (SARS)
Viral hepatitis	Yellow fever
Whooping cough	Typhoid fever
	Typhus fever
	Viral haemorrhagic fever

NOTIFIABLE INFECTIOUS DISEASES

In the UK there is a statutory duty to report a number of infectious diseases to the public health services. This is either to enable disease surveillance or because of the broad risk posed to contacts or the public generally. Notifiable infectious diseases are shown in Box 13.3.

CHAPTER 14

POSTOPERATIVE
AND OBSTETRIC
PATIENTS

**Peri-operative
  optimization**   348

**Stress response to surgery
  and critical illness**   348

**Postoperative
  analgesia**   349

**ICU management of the
  postoperative patient**   357

**Postoperative
  haemorrhage**   359

**Anaphylactoid
  reactions**   361

**Malignant
  hyperpyrexia**   363

Obstetric patients   364

**Pre-eclampsia /
  eclampsia**   365

**Peripartum
  haemorrhage**   366

HELLP syndrome   366

**Pregnancy-related
  heart failure**   367

PERI-OPERATIVE OPTIMIZATION

There is ongoing interest in so-called 'peri-operative optimization' of cardiovascular variables in order to minimize the physiological disturbances and stress responses caused by surgery. In some centres, patients may be admitted to ICU or HDU preoperatively, invasive haemodynamic monitoring instituted, and fluids and inotropes used judiciously to optimize stroke volume. The process is similar to that described previously in Chapter 4. (See Optimization of cardiovascular system, p. 78.) There is some evidence that peri-operative optimization reduces peri-operative complications and reduces the need for unplanned ICU admission (or length of ICU stay) after major surgery.

 This is a complex area. Some patients with ischaemic heart disease, for example, may benefit from β-blockade to protect the myocardium, rather than being driven with inotropes. Seek advice and follow local protocols.

STRESS RESPONSE TO SURGERY AND CRITICAL ILLNESS

The local and systemic inflammatory responses to tissue injury and illness vary between patients, and may vary from mild pyrexia to systemic inflammatory response syndrome (SIRS), multiple organ failure and death. The clinical magnitude of this response depends in part on the extent of the injury, although other factors, including infection, immune status, genetic predisposition and physiological reserve, are also important. In addition to these inflammatory responses, which are mediated by cytokines, there are a number of physiological hormonal and metabolic responses to injury and critical illness, which are collectively known as the stress response. (See SIRS, p. 326.)

Hormonal responses

The secretion of the pituitary hormones antidiuretic hormone (ADH), adrenocorticotrophin (ACTH) and growth hormone (GH) is increased. ADH causes salt and water retention and also has vasopressor activity. ACTH leads to increased secretion of adrenal corticosteroids, cortisol and aldosterone, which further lead to salt and water retention. Growth hormone has a hyperglycaemic effect, but this effect is variable.

There is a generalized increase in sympathetic activity and the adrenal secretion of catecholamines adrenaline (epinephrine) and noradrenaline (norepinephrine) is increased. These have predictable cardiovascular effects. Adrenaline also has metabolic effects, most notably hyperglycaemia. Increased production of renin from the kidney leads to activation of the renin–angiotensin–aldosterone pathway. Angiotensin II is a potent vasoconstrictor that increases blood pressure, while aldosterone increases renal salt and water retention.

Metabolic effects

The primary metabolic effects of the stress response are those of salt and water retention and increased catabolism. Salt and water retention is multifactorial in origin. The degree of water retention may exceed that of sodium retention, such that hyponatraemia is common.

The catabolic effects of catecholamines, steroids and growth hormone include increased glycogenolysis and gluconeogenesis, resulting in hyperglycaemia. Endogenous insulin production is increased in response, but an insulin infusion is often required to control the blood sugar. Fat and protein are broken down to provide energy substrates for tissue repair.

Role of the stress response

The stress response has evolved to provide survival advantages following severe injury or during critical illness. There is evidence that those that fail to mount an appropriate physiological response to critical illness have a poor outcome despite maximal support (e.g. elderly patients following trauma, burns or apparently minor head injury). At times, however, the stress responses can be detrimental. For example, exaggerated cardiovascular responses can lead to myocardial ischaemia and impaired tissue perfusion. Increased salt and water retention can lead to oliguria. Extreme catabolic responses can lead to severe wasting. For these reasons, there has been a great deal of interest in attempting to reduce the stress response.

The most important factors in reducing the stress response are ensuring good quality anaesthesia and peri-operative care, where possible preventing or minimizing tissue injury (e.g. laparoscopic surgery), careful fluid resuscitation, and good postoperative pain relief. (See Postoperative analgesia below.)

POSTOPERATIVE ANALGESIA

Patient-controlled analgesia (PCAS)

These techniques are extensively used to provide analgesia particularly in postoperative patients. Typically the patient will be established on such a device prior to transfer to a general ward.

> **Box 14.1 Typical PCAS regimen**
>
> 50 mg morphine in 50 mL 0.9% saline
> 1 mg bolus
> 5-min lockout time
> No background infusion

Although not intended for operation by nurses, they have been used safely and conveniently in this way in an ICU setting.

Care should be taken in setting devices up; a dedicated intravenous catheter or non-return valve should be used. There have been a number of problems due to excessive background dosing, surges of morphine on unblocking i.v. lines, and siphoning of contents under gravity from syringes. Avoid background infusions if possible. Position syringe drivers below the level of the patient to avoid siphoning, and use antireflux valves on giving sets. A typical PCAS regimen is shown in Box 14.1.

Regional blockade

An increasing number of patients undergoing major surgery have analgesia provided by the epidural and spinal route. These techniques may also be used to relieve pain from trauma (e.g. fractured ribs) and ischaemic limbs.

Potential advantages include the avoidance of centrally acting sedative analgesic drugs, resulting in a more awake, cooperative and pain-free patient, who is better able to cough and clear airway secretions. In addition, in patients with ischaemic limbs, neuroaxial blockade (which includes sympathetic blockade) may provide both analgesia and improvement in perfusion of the ischaemic limb.

Detailed description of epidural techniques is beyond the scope of this book. When a patient is admitted with an epidural catheter in situ, you should make sure that you confirm the analgesic regimen with the responsible anaesthetist. Local anaesthetic and opioid drugs may be used alone or in combination. If opioid drugs are administered, additional systemic opioids should be administered with care because of the risk of respiratory depression. Typical regimens are shown in Table 14.1.

If breakthrough pain occurs and the patient is otherwise stable, give a 5–10 mL bolus of the epidural solution and then increase the infusion rate. This is normally effective within 10–15 min. Beware of hypotension.

 Do not prescribe or administer epidural drugs if you are not familiar with epidural techniques. Seek help.

TABLE 14.1 Typical postoperative epidural infusion regimens

Agent	Rate	Comment
Bupivicaine 0.1–0.15%	8–15 mL/h	
Bupivicaine 0.1–0.15% plus fentanyl 2 µg/mL	8–15 mL/h	No concomitant systemic opioids to be given

Box 14.2 Complications of epidural blockade

Local anaesthetics	Opioids
Potential local anaesthetic toxicity	Itching
Hypotension (sympathetic blockade)	CNS depression including apnoea
Muscle weakness (including respiration)	Urinary retention
Bradycardia (block > T4 level)	Nausea and vomiting
Urine retention	
Complete or high spinal block (cardiovascular collapse, respiratory paralysis, loss of consciousness)	

Complications of epidural blockade

The potential complications of epidural blockade are shown in Box 14.2.

- Hypotension usually responds to fluid loading (500 mL colloid) and reducing the rate of epidural infusion. If significant hypotension develops, reduce or stop infusion and consider the use of a vasopressor infusion.
- Significant muscle weakness can usually be avoided by the use of low concentrations of local anaesthetic drugs for postoperative analgesia (as opposed to that required for surgery). If significant motor block develops, consider reducing the infusion rate and/or concentration of local anaesthetic.
- If the block is too high (e.g. involving arms), reduce the rate of infusion and/or the concentration of local anaesthetic. If respiratory muscle weakness occurs, ventilation may be necessary until the effects of the local anaesthetic wear off.
- At the doses used, the addition of opioids to epidural infusion may significantly improve analgesia without significant increase in the side-effect profile. Nausea and itching may be helped by low-dose naloxone without loss of analgesia. CNS depression may require ventilation.

- Analgesia produced by regional blockade may mask the pain associated with the onset of lower limb complications such as compartment syndrome following trauma or limb surgery. Check distal limbs regularly for evidence of infection, pressure injuries and compartment syndrome.
- Epidural techniques carry a small but serious risk of epidural haematoma or abscess formation, which if unrecognized, can lead to spinal cord compression and paralysis. In routine practice this risk is very small. In ICU patients, however, the risk may be higher because of the effects of coagulopathy and sepsis. The magnitude of this risk is unquantifiable, although overall it remains very low.

> ⚠ **The use low concentration local anaesthetic agents in epidurals is intended to provide adequate analgesia whilst minimizing the risk of significant motor blockade. If profound motor block develops in a patient with a postoperative epidural, suspect possible spinal cord compression. Seek urgent advice.**

Intrathecal drug adminstration

Be sure to understand the difference between epidural and intrathecal catheters. An epidural catheter is placed in the 'epidural space'. This is a potential space deep to the ligamentum flavum but outside the layers of the dura. An intrathecal catheter is placed through the dura and arachnoid mater, and lies within the subarachnoid space, i.e. in the cerebrospinal fluid. An intrathecal catheter may be used for CSF drainage and pressure monitoring following neurosurgery, spinal surgery or thoracic aortic aneurysm repairs, and occasionally for intrathecal drug administration (rarely, continuous spinal anaesthesia).

> ⚠ **Do not give drugs by the intrathecal route unless you have been specifically trained to do so. There have been a number of cases where incorrect drugs administered by this route have caused catastrophic and permanent neurological damage and death.**

Common postoperative problems

Problems in the immediate postoperative period may include the effects of prolonged surgery, massive fluid/blood loss, sepsis, tissue ischaemia/reperfusion, delayed recovery from anaesthesia and the effects of the stress response to surgery and trauma.

Effects of prolonged surgery

Anaesthesia and surgery may be prolonged because of the extensive nature of the procedure or because of technical complexity. Problems may include hypothermia, atelectasis, dehydration and fluid loss, anaesthetic drug accumulation, and the effects of pressure, including the development of compartment syndromes. This phenomenon has re-emerged recently following prolonged robotic surgery. (See Hypothermia, p. 224, and Peripheral compartment syndromes, p. 319.)

Delayed recovery of consciousness

The causes of delayed recovery of consciousness following anaesthesia are often multifactorial. It may be impossible to determine initially which is the predominant problem. Factors that may contribute are shown in Box 14.3.

Most patients with delayed recovery of consciousness require a period of supportive care on ICU. A CT scan of the brain and EEG may be helpful to exclude significant intracranial pathology. In most cases the problem will resolve gradually over hours or days.

Prolonged neuromuscular block

Muscle relaxants are used extensively in anaesthesia to facilitate tracheal intubation, provide relaxation for surgical procedures, and allow lighter planes of general anaesthesia. In the ICU, patients are usually left to clear muscle relaxants without use of reversal agents. Following anaesthesia, the recovery of neuromuscular function is often hastened by the use of anticholinesterase drugs (e.g. neostigmine). These increase the concentration of acetylcholine at the neuromuscular junction and reverse the effects of non-depolarizing neuromuscular blocking drugs (competitive antagonists at the acetylcholine receptor).

Box 14.3 Factors that may contribute to delayed recovery from anaesthesia

Residual effects of anaesthetic drugs

Hypoxia

Hypercarbia

Hypotension

Hypoglycaemia

Metabolic encephalopathy

Hypothermia

TIA/CVA

They are used in combination with glycopyrrolate, which reduces the undesirable (muscarinic) effects of acetylcholine. Typical doses are:

- neostigmine 2.5 mg + glycopyrrolate 0.5 mg.

Problems relating to residual neuromuscular blockade have become less common since the introduction of newer shorter-acting drugs such as atracurium. Occasionally, however, there may be delayed recovery of neuromuscular function. Factors that may contribute to this are shown in Box 14.4.

Patients with partial residual neuromuscular blockade typically exhibit jerky movements and make poor respiratory effort. Supra-maximal stimulation with a nerve stimulator may reveal fade on 'train of four' confirming residual neuromuscular blockade. (See Monitoring neuromuscular blockade, p. 43.)

- Give oxygen. Support ventilation if necessary.
- If the patient has some neuromuscular function it may be appropriate to administer a first or second dose of reversal agent (usually neostigmine and glycopyrrolate) and then reassess the situation.
- If this fails to improve the situation or if there is minimal neuromuscular function, the patient should be resedated, re-intubated and ventilated until return of neuromuscular function. Remember to explain to the patient what is happening. He or she may be paralysed, in pain and aware of the surroundings, but unable to communicate.

Cholinesterase deficiency

Hereditary cholinesterase deficiency (1:3000 population) is a specific cause of delayed recovery of neuromuscular function resulting from the delayed metabolism of suxamethonium (and mivacurium). Muscle function usually returns in 2–6 h. FFP

Box 14.4 Factors contributing to delayed recovery neuromuscular blockade

Elderly, frail, medically unfit patients

Relative overdose

Renal or liver dysfunction

Underlying neuromuscular disease

Effects of ether drugs (e.g. aminoglycosides)

Electrolyte abnormalities

Hypothermia

Cholinesterase deficiency

can be given to replete cholinesterase and hasten the return of motor power, but is not usually necessary. Send blood to regional centre for identification of the particular pattern of cholinesterase deficiency. (See Suxamethonium, p. 43.)

Airway obstruction

This is common in the immediate postoperative period while patients are still in the recovery room and before full return of consciousness. This is usually transient, not severe, and readily managed by support of the chin, jaw thrust or the use of an artificial airway (e.g. oral or nasal airway).

More severe or prolonged cases, or those with associated respiratory depression, may require intubation and ventilation.

Following surgical procedures in the neck (e.g. thyroidectomy), postoperative bleeding into the tissues of the neck may occasionally produce airway obstruction by direct compression. In an emergency, you should open the surgical wound and decompress the bleeding to relieve pressure on the airway. The wound can then be formally explored by a surgeon in order to achieve haemostasis. If this fails to relieve the problem the patient will require intubation.

Patients with a fractured mandible frequently have their jaws wired together to ensure correct dental occlusion while the fracture heals. These patients should only be extubated once full consciousness and respiratory effort has returned. They are often admitted to intensive care in the immediate postoperative period for observation and monitoring. If airway obstruction occurs (e.g. due to vomiting), you should cut the wires to gain access to the airway and manage the situation as appropriate. (See Airway obstruction, p. 138.)

Respiratory insufficiency

Postoperative respiratory insufficiency may be predictable in patients with pre-existing respiratory disease and this may be an indication for elective postoperative ventilation. In other patients it may arise for a number of reasons, and the problem is often multifactorial. Typical causes are shown in Box 14.5.

Many of these problems are resolved by a short period of ventilation in the ICU combined with simple corrective measures. (See also Respiratory failure, p. 118.)

Cardiovascular instability

Cardiovascular instability may arise due to pre-existing cardiovascular disease, from the predictable effects of the surgery,

Box 14.5 Common causes of postoperative respiratory insufficiency

Residual effects of anaesthetic drugs

Residual effects of neuromuscular blockade

Airway obstruction

Bronchospasm

Pre-existing respiratory disease

Pulmonary collapse/consolidation

Pneumothorax

Pulmonary oedema

Cardiovascular instability

Sepsis

Hypothermia

Box 14.6 Causes of postoperative CVS instability

Pre-existing CVS disease

Myocardial ischaemia/infarction

Myocardial depression (effects of drugs/sepsis, etc.)

Fluid losses and bleeding

Fluid overload

Effects of drugs

Effects of epidural/spinal anaesthesia

Sepsis

Effects of tissue ischaemia and reperfusion

Hypothermia

particularly when large fluid losses are expected, or as a result of untoward cardiovascular events. Typical causes are shown in Box 14.6. Many of these problems are solved by simple attention to details of fluid balance as the patient warms up after surgery. More difficult cases may require full invasive monitoring and cardiovascular support. (See Optimizing haemodynamic status, p. 78.)

Oliguria

Oliguria in the postoperative patient is often multifactorial, with cardiovascular instability, hypovolaemia and the stress response to surgery all contributing. This often improves with fluid loading as the patient rewarms and haemodynamic stability improves. (See Oliguria, p. 188, and Stress response to surgery and critical illness, p. 348.)

ICU MANAGEMENT OF THE POSTOPERATIVE PATIENT

Patients are frequently admitted to ICU following prolonged or complex surgery for a period of monitoring, ventilation, cardiovascular support and stabilization, prior to discharge to a high-dependency area or ward. Admission to the ICU may be planned, because of pre-existing disease and/or the nature of the surgery, or may be unplanned as a result of unexpected difficulties in the peri-operative period or the emergency nature of the surgery.

The postoperative admission of patients to intensive care allows for:

- controlled recovery from the effects of anaesthesia and surgery
- a period of rewarming
- optimization of respiratory function and controlled weaning from ventilation
- optimization of cardiovascular function
- monitoring of other organ function, e.g. renal output
- adequate analgesia.

When an elective postoperative patient is admitted to the ICU you should be sure that the management plan is agreed with the referring anaesthetist and surgeon.

A typical approach is given below:

- Continue ventilation.
- Maintain sedation and analgesia by infusion using short-acting drugs such as propofol and alfentanil. Muscle relaxants are generally discontinued unless there is an indication to continue them.
- Assess the patient fully and decide on priorities for management. Send blood for FBC, clotting screen, U&Es and arterial blood gases. Correct abnormalities as necessary.
- Rewarm patient using warm-air blanket if necessary. As temperature increases, the peripheral circulation will open up (reduction in core–peripheral temperature gradient). Give fluid (colloid or blood) as necessary to maintain adequate circulating volume.
- Metabolic acidosis usually improves as the patient rewarms and circulation improves. Persistent metabolic acidosis usually indicates either inadequate fluid resuscitation, bleeding or ongoing tissue ischaemia (e.g. gut) requiring further investigation.
- Any inotropes/vasopressors can be gradually reduced as the patient's condition improves.

The aim is to achieve a warm, cardiovascular stable patient, requiring minimal inotropic support, with minimal fluid/blood requirements, adequate urine output and satisfactory arterial blood gases.

Depending on the premorbid condition of the patient and the nature of the surgery, this can often be achieved over 6–24 h. Sedation can then be reduced and the patient woken up and extubated as appropriate. Good analgesia should be maintained by appropriate use of opioids, anti-inflammatory agents, paracetamol and/or regional blockade.

Where appropriate, you should keep the attending family updated as regards to the patient's condition. If any peri-operative problems have arisen, they should be offered the opportunity to talk to the responsible surgeon or anaesthetist.

Aortic aneurysm repair

Following elective aortic aneurysm repair, patients can generally be allowed to warm up and are extubated after a few hours, as described above. Emergency aneurysm repairs may be more unstable and the management will depend upon individual circumstances.

Control of blood pressure is important. This should be maintained at a level which is normal for the patient to ensure adequate perfusion of vital organs, in particular the kidneys. At the same time significant hypertension should be controlled to prevent undue strain on both the myocardium and the vascular anastomosis. This may require use of nifedipine or GTN infusion, especially during the phase of emergence from sedation.

Renal dysfunction is common, particularly after suprarenal cross-clamping of the aorta. Spinal cord ischaemia and lower limb paralysis may also occur. Persistent ischaemia of the lower limbs despite optimization of haemodynamic status may require embolectomy or re-exploration of the graft. Persistent or worsening metabolic acidosis may indicate gut ischaemia. Seek surgical opinion.

Free tissue transfer (free flap)

The management of patients following free tissue transfer is similar to that described above. In addition, however, the adequate perfusion and survival of the graft is paramount.

The normal mechanisms that control blood flow in tissues are compromised in grafted tissue. The circulation to the graft is essentially passive and depends predominantly on the flow through the feeding vessels. Aggressive fluid therapy should be used to maintain the patient's circulating volume. This should be balanced, however, against the deleterious effects of increased oedema in the graft, caused by increased endothelial permeability resulting from reperfusion injury and the absence of lymphatic drainage. Fluid management is guided by CVP, urine output and core–peripheral temperature gradient. The usual response to any deterioration in these parameters should be to give further fluid.

At the same time the denervated vessels of the graft are highly sensitive to circulating catecholamines (endogenous or exogenous). Adequate analgesia is therefore essential. The patient should be kept as warm as possible and inotropes/vasopressor agents should be avoided except in extremis. Inodilators such as dopexamine may be of value in improving graft blood flow and survival. Seek advice.

If despite these measures graft perfusion appears impaired (dusky/congested/swollen), call the surgical team immediately. The vascular pedicles and vascular anastomoses may need surgical exploration.

Transplants

Transplantation is a special case of free tissue transfer. The principles are similar to those described above, with particular management issues depending on the particular organ involved. Follow local protocols.

POSTOPERATIVE HAEMORRHAGE

A common problem seen on the intensive care unit is postoperative surgical bleeding. Most commonly this is easily recognized and treated by the surgical team. Occasionally however, unexpected occult bleeding may occur. Depending on the patient's age, physiological reserve and site of bleeding presenting features may range from the very subtle to the very obvious. Typical features of occult bleeding are:

- Gradual decline in haemoglobin
- Persistent/worsening acidosis
- Oliguria
- Unexplained hypotension and/or tachycardia. (May be late features in young patients with good physiological reserve.)

None of these signs is specific, and other potential complications (for example, sepsis) may present similarly. Acidosis and hypotension are common after prolonged/emergency surgery, particularly as patients rewarm and vasodilatation leads to relative hypovolaemia.

Tachycardia may occur in response to pain, while postoperative analgesic agents given to relive pain may lead to hypotension. (At the same time, analgesic agents may mask the signs of bleeding, e.g. pain at the surgical site.)

Sometimes, the only distinguishing features are clinical signs at the site of surgery. For example, there may be progressive abdominal distension or rigidity, associated with raised intra-abdominal pressure with evidence of intra-abdominal compartment syndrome (see p. 174).

Management

As soon as postoperative haemorrhage is suspected, inform the surgical team concerned. In severe cases, contact the senior surgeon involved direct to avoid delays that could compromise the safety of the patient.

The management of postoperative haemorrhage is essentially the same as any other form of haemorrhage. (See Major haemorrhage, p. 251.) The key issues are as follows:

- Resuscitate and stabilize the patient, using an ABC approach.
- Resuscitation strategy will depend upon circumstances, but 'hypotensive resuscitation' as practised in trauma may be beneficial in limiting the extent of the bleeding prior to achieving surgical haemostasis (see p. 309).
- Initial resuscitation may be either with a crystalloid solution (such as Hartmann's solution), colloid or blood where this is available.

Following a major surgical procedure blood will often be available in the intensive care blood fridge or transfusion laboratory. Failing that, the transfusion laboratory may be holding a 'group and save' sample which can be used for urgent cross-match. Otherwise you will need to send an urgent sample for cross-match.

 In all cases of major haemorrhage, contact the transfusion laboratory immediately and advise them of the situation. They will prioritize the patient and provide appropriate timely blood products and support.

- Correct coagulopathy (see p. 258).

In some cases, postoperative bleeding is due to coagulopathy rather than failure of surgical haemostasis. Coagulopathy may result from derangement of clotting factors, and/or be exacerbated by the effects of acidosis, hypocalcaemia and hypothermia. Where possible, correct these factors prior to attempting surgical haemostasis.

- The use of clotting products such as fresh frozen plasma, cryoprecipitate and platelets may be guided either by laboratory tests or point of care testing such as thromboelastography (see p. 259).
- Seek advice on the use of antifibrinolytics, such as tranexamic acid or clotting factor concentrates such as prothrombin complex or activated factor V11a (see p. 261).

In many cases surgical exploration and haemostasis will be required. Therefore, good communication with both the haematology laboratory and the surgical and theatre team is required throughout. Do not forget to arrange for such devices as blood warmers, and in the case of massive haemorrhage, a rapid infusion device (such as the Level-1 infuser) or a cell saver if these are available.

ANAPHYLACTOID REACTIONS

Anaphylactoid is a term which encompasses all life-threatening acute 'allergic' reactions, regardless of their exact pathogenesis. It includes true immune-mediated type 1 or anaphylactic hypersensitivity reactions. These reactions are relatively uncommon and are clearly not confined to the peri-operative period. Common causes include nut allergy and bee stings. In the hospital setting, however, drugs, contrast media, intravenous colloid solutions and latex are common precipitating agents.

Clinical manifestations

The onset of symptoms may occur within 1–2 min of exposure to the precipitating agent or may be delayed up to 1–2 h and may be modified by the effects of general or regional anaesthesia. The clinical manifestations may include:

- cutaneous flushing urticaria, angio-oedema
- abdominal pain, nausea, vomiting and diarrhoea
- laryngeal oedema, bronchospasm, increased airway pressure
- acute pulmonary oedema
- tachycardia, hypotension, cardiac arrest.

Life-saving treatment depends on early recognition and appropriate management. The differential diagnoses are given in Box 14.7.

> **Box 14.7 Differential diagnosis of anaphylactoid reactions**
>
> Vasovagal reaction
> Dysrhythmia
> Myocardial infarction
> Effects of drugs (including illicit drugs)
> Pulmonary embolism
> Bronchospasm
> Pulmonary oedema
> Aspiration
> Hereditary angioneurotic oedema
> Idiopathic urticaria
> Carcinoid tumours

Management

- Stop precipitating drugs.
- Give oxygen. If airway compromised by facial oedema, laryngeal oedema or bronchospasm, secure airway by endotracheal intubation as soon as possible. Ventilate and commence external cardiac massage if necessary.
- Establish i.v. access if not already done, and give rapid fluid load, e.g. 2–4 L crystalloid or colloid (remember that synthetic colloids may be the cause of the reaction!).
- Give adrenaline (epinephrine) 0.5–1.0 mg i.m.

> ⚠ The use of intravenous adrenaline in patients with a spontaneous circulation has been associated with profound hypertension, myocardial infarction and dysrhythmia. Current recommendations are that i.v. adrenaline should only be used in extreme cases and by those with experience in titrating the dose given to an appropriate haemodynamic response. Therefore avoid i.v. adrenaline unless patient is in extremis or cardiac arrest.

- Establish arterial and central venous catheterization when appropriate.
- Take blood (EDTA and serum) for later analysis.
- Measure arterial blood gases. If significant acidosis consider 50–100 mmol sodium bicarbonate. (See Metabolic acidosis, p. 212.)
- If persistent bronchospasm, give nebulized salbutamol 2.5–5 mg.

- Glucocorticoids reduce late sequelae. Give hydrocortisone 200 mg i.m./i.v. followed by 50 mg 6-hourly.
- Antihistamines are of no proven benefit but are often given. Consider chlorpheniramine (chlorphenamine) 10 mg i.m or i.v.

Following resuscitation, these patients should be managed in the ICU. Late reactions can result in clinical deterioration even some hours after initial stabilization. Cancel surgery and/or other interventional procedures unless life-saving. For further advice, see: http://www.aagbi.org/anaphylaxisdatabase.htm.

Evaluation of cause of anaphylactoid reactions

Following an anaphylactoid reaction, it is important to try and establish the cause so that future reactions may be avoided. Take a detailed history of this and other previous allergic reactions. Blood samples taken as soon after the reaction as possible and at regular intervals thereafter can be analysed for immune markers, including antibodies (IGE), complement and mediator levels. Mast cell tryptase peaks within 1–2 h of the event, so should be sampled within this time frame. A negative mast cell tryptase result does not rule out an anaphylactic reaction. Peri-event blood tests may help point toward a diagnosis of an anaphylactic reaction, but do not help identify the causative agent.

Radioallergosorbent tests (RAST) and interval skin-prick testing may determine the causative agent, but this is often inconclusive. Seek advice from laboratory services/immunology department.

It is essential that patients and their relatives are made aware of the reaction. In the case of nut allergy or bee sting anaphylaxis, patients are now given prefilled adrenaline (epinephrine) injectors for emergency use.

MALIGNANT HYPERPYREXIA

Malignant hyperpyrexia (MH) is a rare inherited life-threatening condition in which there is an abnormality of ionic calcium transport in muscles. Following exposure to trigger agents (including volatile anaesthetic agents and suxamethonium) susceptible individuals may develop increased muscle tone, increased metabolic rate and hyperpyrexia. The clinical features are shown in Box 14.8.

Management

- Discontinue trigger agents. Monitor ECG, SaO_2 and core temperature.

Box 14.8 Clinical features of MH

Increased muscle tone

Increased metabolic rate

Hyperthermia (typically increase > 2°C/h)

Rising ETCO$_2$

Falling SaO$_2$

Mixed respiratory/metabolic acidosis

Hyperkalaemia/hypocalcaemia

Myoglobinuria and renal failure

Cardiac failure/dysrhythmia/cardiac arrest

- Intubate if not already.
- Ventilate with 100% oxygen.
- Monitor ETCO$_2$. Manage hypercarbia by hyperventilation.
- Paralyse and ensure adequate sedation and analgesia.
- Institute active cooling measures.
- Give dantrolene 1 mg/kg i.v. over 10 min; repeat as necessary up to 10 mg/kg.
- Monitor blood gases, potassium and calcium. Treat metabolic acidosis, hyperkalaemia and hypocalcaemia as appropriate.
- Measure urine output and myoglobin. Give fluids and consider dopamine to maintain urine output. Mannitol and sodium bicarbonate increase the clearance of myoglobin. (Note: Dantrolene also contains mannitol to improve clearance of myoglobin).

Following stabilization, these patients must be monitored in the ICU. The half-life of dantrolene is approximately 5 h. Hyperpyrexia may recur, requiring further doses of dantrolene. Seek advice from national/regional MH centre.
(See Hyperthermia, p. 224.)

OBSTETRIC PATIENTS

 Obstetric patients admitted to the ICU are by definition young and critically ill, and the management issues are complex. You should always seek senior advice.

Any medical condition can present in pregnancy, and a small number of obstetric patients are admitted to the ICU each year. The principles of management are the same as in the non-pregnant female, although the physiological changes associated with pregnancy and the safety of the fetus in utero are important considerations.

All pregnant women over 20 weeks' gestation must be nursed in the lateral position or with lateral tilt to avoid hypotension and uterine hypoperfusion due to compression of the inferior vena cava by the gravid uterus.

Obstetricians and neonatologists should be involved in decisions regarding the viability of the unborn child and the appropriateness and timing of early termination of the pregnancy/delivery of the child.

There are some specific conditions associated with late pregnancy that may precipitate admission to ICU. In most cases patients will be admitted post-delivery, as the primary management of most specific obstetric problems is urgent delivery of the fetoplacental unit.

PRE-ECLAMPSIA/ECLAMPSIA

Pre-eclampsia is a condition characterized by proteinuria, oedema and hypertension. Eclampsia, which may be preceded by pre-eclampsia or present acutely, is a more severe manifestation of the same disorder in which there are seizures. These conditions usually occur in late pregnancy but may occasionally present immediately post-delivery. The exact pathogenesis of the condition is not known, but urgent delivery of the fetoplacental unit, usually by caesarean section, initiates resolution. Hypertension and seizures may, however, continue for 48 h.

- Give oxygen by face mask. Intubate and ventilate if necessary. Beware of rises in blood pressure and intracranial pressure on laryngoscopy/intubation. Bolus alfentanil 10 μg/kg may modify this. Subsequently ensure adequate sedation.
- Control hypertension. Hypertension results from vasoconstriction and is accompanied by reduced plasma volume. Vasodilatation and restoration of plasma volume should proceed synchronously. Use labetalol/nifedipine/hydralazine to control blood pressure. (See Hypertension, p. 88.)
- Control seizures. Simple measures include benzodiazepines. Consider prophylactic anticonvulsant therapy with phenytoin or magnesium. Magnesium sulphate 4 g (16 mmol) over 20 min followed by infusion of magnesium sulphate 1 g (4 mmol) every hour. Monitor magnesium levels: aim for 2.5–3.5 mmol/L.

- Plasma volume is reduced and oliguria is common. Volume expansion is appropriate but can exacerbate hypertension and lead to pulmonary oedema. Use invasive monitoring to guide fluid challenges (CVP and PA catheter or equivalent).

Complications include DIC, HELLP syndrome, pulmonary oedema, cerebral oedema, cerebral haemorrhage and renal failure. These should be managed as appropriate.

PERIPARTUM HAEMORRHAGE

Peripartum haemorrhage remains a significant cause of mortality in the obstetric patient. Control of the bleeding will usually require delivery of the fetoplacental unit and/or surgical repair. Occasionally packs will be placed in the uterus in an attempt to control bleeding in the hope that hysterectomy can be avoided. These patients are usually then admitted to ICU for continued management. Arterial and CVP monitoring is usually required. Large quantities of blood and blood products are often necessary and DIC is common. Seek senior help. (See Major haemorrhage, p. 251.)

HELLP SYNDROME

HELLP syndrome (haemolysis, elevated liver enzymes, low platelets) is a distinct condition occurring in the peripartum period but frequently accompanies pre-eclampsia/eclampsia. There are abnormalities of the microvascular circulation associated with red cell destruction and increased platelet consumption. The liver is particularly affected, resulting in some cases in hepatic necrosis and rupture. The clinical features are primarily those of abdominal (right upper quadrant) pain and mild jaundice. Thrombocytopenia may result in bleeding. The diagnostic criteria are shown in Table 14.2.

TABLE 14.2 Diagnostic criteria for HELLP syndrome	
Haemolysis	*Abnormal blood film and hyperbilirubinaemia*
Elevated liver enzymes	LDH > 600 units/L AST > 70 units/L
Low platelets	$<100 \times 10^9$/L

Management is largely supportive. Adequate resuscitation, volume loading and epoprostenol (prostacyclin) infusion may improve microvascular circulation. Platelets are generally unnecessary unless there is active bleeding. Plasma exchange may be of value in severe cases. Seek advice.

PREGNANCY-RELATED HEART FAILURE

Pregnancy and delivery are characterized by increased physiological demands on the heart. In patients with pre-existing heart disease or pregnancy-related cardiomyopathy the heart may be unable to meet these demands and heart failure supervenes. Management is supportive, as for other causes of heart failure. Pregnancy-related cardiomyopathy usually improves after delivery. (See Cardiac failure, p. 105.)

CHAPTER 15

PRACTICAL PROCEDURES

General information   370

Arterial cannulation   372

Use of pressure
    transducers   374

Central venous
    cannulation   376

Changing and removing central
    venous catheters   386

Large-bore introducer sheaths/
    dialysis catheters   387

Pulmonary artery
    catheterization   389

Measuring PAOP   393

Measurement of cardiac output
    by thermodilution   394

Pericardial aspiration   395

Defibrillation and DC
    cardioversion   396

Intubation of the trachea   398

Extubation of the trachea   403

Insertion of laryngeal mask
    (supraglottic airways)   403

Percutaneous
    tracheostomy   404

Cricothyroidotomy/
    minitracheostomy   410

Fibreoptic bronchoscopy   412

Bronchoalveolar lavage   415

Insertion of chest drain   416

Passing a nasogastric tube   421

Passing a Sengstaken–
    Blakemore tube   422

Peritoneal tap/drainage of
    ascites   424

Turning a patient prone   425

Transport of critically ill
    patients   426

GENERAL INFORMATION

Critically ill patients require large numbers of practical procedures. The information in this chapter is intended only as a guide. The advice is generalized; you should always read the instructions provided with the equipment that you use, and follow your local hospital guidelines.

 Always seek senior help if you are not familiar with a procedure.

Consent
Formal consent/assent may be appropriate for some procedures, such as tracheostomy, while consent/assent may be implied for minor or life-saving procedures. In any event, always explain to patients, even if apparently 'unconscious', what you intend to do and keep relatives informed. Document your intentions, and what has been said/agreed. (See Consent to treatment, p. 29.)

Local anaesthetic
Paralysed and sedated patients in ICU may still feel pain from invasive procedures. Use local anaesthetic for all potentially painful procedures.

Universal infection control precautions
Contamination with blood or other body fluids imposes significant risk to staff from blood-borne infection, particularly hepatitis and HIV infection. Universal precautions should be adopted for all invasive procedures. These are intended to prevent the spread of infection, to protect you, your patients and colleagues. It is not always possible to know who has an infection; universal infection control precautions apply to everybody, all of the time:

- Wash your hands thoroughly.
- Cuts or grazes on the hands or forearms should be covered with a waterproof dressing while at work. Seek medical advice about any septic or weeping areas.
- Single-use gloves should be worn for direct contact with blood or body fluid, broken skin or mucous membranes.
- Full face visors should be worn to protect against blood or body fluids that may potentially splash the face/eyes.
- Gowns or plastic aprons protect clothing from contamination.
- Place all sharps directly into a sharps bin; do not manually resheath or break needles. Do not overfill sharps bins, and ensure that the bin is securely fastened before disposal.

- Clinical waste should be discarded into colour-coded bags for incineration.
- Blood or body fluid spills should be disinfected immediately according to local policies.

If you do accidentally cut, scrape or puncture your skin, follow the 'accidental inoculation procedure', encourage bleeding, wash with warm soapy water, dry and cover with a waterproof dressing. Report the incident to the senior person in charge and ensure a report is completed. Seek advice from the occupational health department or A&E. In some cases, post-exposure prophylaxis may be required. This is time-critical, so seek immediate advice. It may be appropriate for someone else to complete the practical procedure.

Always follow guidelines and safety information that apply to your department. If you need further information, talk in the first place to a senior member of nursing staff. Where necessary, further advice can be obtained from specialists in microbiology, infection control, occupational health, COSHH (Control of Substances Hazardous to Health), health & safety, etc.

Aseptic technique

ICU patients are generally severely debilitated and at increased risk of infection; therefore, when performing procedures, no matter how minor, good infection control procedures are important. For all invasive procedures strict aseptic technique is required:

- Collect all necessary equipment before starting.
- Ensure assistance is available to open packs, etc.
- Wash hands with disinfectant (generally chlorhexidine or iodine).
- Dry hands on towel provided in gown pack.
- Put on gown.
- Put on gloves using closed technique.
- Prepare the equipment on the trolley.
- Prepare the patient by washing with 2% chlorhexidine solution (see Epic 2: National Evidence-Based Guidelines for Preventing Healthcare-Associated Infections in NHS Hospitals in England. http://www.neli.org.uk/IntegratedCRD.nsf).
- Place sterile towels around the proposed site to make a sterile field.
- Remember to keep hands up to avoid contamination.

ARTERIAL CANNULATION

Arterial cannulation is one of the most commonly performed procedures in the ICU. There is, however, an associated risk of morbidity and the indication for arterial cannulation in the individual patient should be considered carefully.

Indications

- Haemodynamic monitoring: particularly in situations where non-invasive measurements are inadequate, e.g. where changes in arterial blood pressure are likely to be sudden or profound, at extremes of blood pressure and in the presence of arrhythmias.
- Repeated blood sampling. Especially for repeated arterial blood gas sampling. The complications associated with arterial cannulation are outweighed by the morbidity and inconvenience of repeated arterial puncture.

Contraindications

These are relative. Exercise caution in arteriopaths and do not recannulate an artery where previous vascular compromise has occurred. Where possible avoid areas of local sepsis and trauma, limbs with dialysis fistulae and end arteries such as the brachial artery.

Procedure

Arterial cannulation. You will need:
Universal precautions; sterile gloves
Minor dressing pack
Skin disinfectant
Syringe of local anaesthetic/needle
Syringe of heparinized saline flush
Arterial cannulae (usually 20 gauge or 22 gauge)
Extension line and three-way tap
Suture
Dressing

Decide which artery to cannulate. The radial artery of the non-dominant hand is usually preferred in the first instance. Alternatives include the ulnar, dorsalis pedis and posterior tibial arteries. It is pointless, however, to persist with attempts at peripheral arterial cannulation in patients who are hypotensive and 'shut down'. The femoral and brachial arteries are useful during resuscitation of profoundly shocked patients. Ultrasound guidance is potentially useful at all sites to aid arterial cannulation, particularly in hypotensive patients and those whose landmarks are obscured by oedema or obesity.

- Arterial cannulation often results in blood spillage. Universal precautions should be used.
- Clean the puncture site and establish a sterile field.
- Gently palpate the artery and inject local anaesthetic to raise a small intradermal bleb at the puncture site 1 cm distal to the proposed cannulation site.
- A Seldinger technique or a direct cannulation technique may be used.

Seldinger technique
- Advance needle through the puncture site towards the artery at a shallow angle. As the vessel is punctured, a flashback of arterial blood is seen in the hub. Pass the guide wire through the needle into the artery. Withdraw the needle and pass the cannula over the guide wire. The guide wire is then discarded.

Direct cannulation
- Either: advance the cannula and needle through the puncture site towards the artery at a shallow angle. As the vessel is punctured a flashback of arterial blood is seen in the hub. Holding the needle still, advance the cannula over the needle into the artery. This should be a single smooth movement without resistance.
- Or: advance the cannula at a steeper angle and, after observing the flashback, continue through the artery to transfix it. Withdraw the needle slightly from the cannula and then pull the cannula back gently until the tip is in the artery and flashback is again observed. Advance the cannula into the artery.

Following cannulation
- Attach extension tubing and three-way tap.
- Aspirate blood from the line to confirm placement and to remove any air bubbles, then flush line with saline.
- Secure in place and cover with occlusive dressing.
- (If using stitches, do not place stitches too deeply. It is possible inadvertently to damage peripheral arteries.)
- Attach the arterial catheter to a pressure transducer and flushing device.
- Ensure catheter clearly labelled as 'arterial' to prevent inadvertent injection of drugs.

Box 15.1 Complications of arterial cannulation

Immediate	Early	Late
Bleeding	Arterial embolism	Infection
Haematoma	Vasospasm	Ulceration
Arterial damage		Thrombosis
		Arteriovenous fistulae

Sampling from an arterial line

- Clean sample port with alcohol swab and attach syringe.
- Aspirate 3–5 mL blood into the syringe and then discard this syringe.
- Aspirate sample into fresh syringe or vacuum container.
- Samples for blood gases should be drawn into pre-heparinized syringes to prevent damage to the blood gas analyser. Any air in the syringe should be expelled. If not analysed immediately in the ICU, the syringe should be capped and placed on ice.
- Flush the line with saline and place a clean cap on the sampling port.

Complications

Complications of arterial cannulation are shown in Box 15.1.

Vascular compromise may occur at any stage. Inadvertent injection of drugs into an arterial catheter is an important avoidable cause of morbidity and all cannulae and lines should be clearly labelled. Risk of infection increases with time. Any manifestly infected catheter should be removed. After removal press firmly for at least 5 min. Occasionally, persistent bleeding may require a suture (5/0 nylon) to close the skin wound and then further pressure.

USE OF PRESSURE TRANSDUCERS

A transducer converts one type of energy (e.g. arterial pressure) into another (e.g. electrical impulse). There are a number of different types of transducer available but the principle is similar for all:

- The patient's arterial catheter is connected to the transducer by a continuous column of (heparinized) saline. A pressurized flushing device maintains a small forward flow (approximately 2–3 mL/h) to keep the cannula patent.
- Pressure changes in the vessel are transmitted via the saline to a diaphragm. As this diaphragm moves in response to the

pressure changes, its electrical conductivity changes. This results in fluctuations in electrical signal from the diaphragm, which is interpreted by a monitor and displayed as an arterial waveform and blood pressure values. Systolic, diastolic and mean pressures are usually displayed.

In order for the arterial waveform and blood pressure recording to be accurate, the transducer must be used appropriately. Therefore:

- There must be no air bubble in the connection tubing or transducer chamber. This will damp the trace and produce lower blood pressure values. Flush well before connecting the transducer to the patient.
- The transducer should be maintained at the level of the left atrium and appropriately zeroed. (If raised above this level the recorded pressure will be too low, and vice versa.)

Zeroing transducers

- To zero a transducer turn the three-way tap so the transducer is open to air and the patient connection is switched off. The transducer is now connected to atmospheric or zero gauge pressure.
- Zero the monitoring system according to the manufacturer's instructions. (There is usually a single button to press.)
- When zeroing is complete, turn the three-way tap back to reconnect the patient to the transducer. Check that the trace and values obtained are as expected.

COMMON PROBLEMS WITH INVASIVE PRESSURE MONITORING

Invasive and non-invasive pressures disagree

If the blood pressure displayed by the invasive arterial monitoring differs from that obtained by non-invasive methods this is usually the result of either damping or resonance in the invasive monitoring. In most cases the mean arterial pressures are usually in close agreement.

- Check the arterial line is correctly sited and flush the lumen with heparinized saline.
- Check that there are no air bubbles in the connecting tubing or transducer chamber.
- Check zero on invasive monitoring.
- Check that the transducer is at the level of the left atrium.

In some cases, peripheral vasospasm may be a cause of this error. If in doubt, resite the arterial line, or use the non-invasive measurements of blood pressure. In this case, the line can still be retained for arterial blood gas sampling.

CENTRAL VENOUS CANNULATION

 Do not attempt central venous cannulation without supervision until you have been adequately taught to do so. You must be aware of possible complications and how to manage them.

Indications
Central venous access is almost universal in intensive care patients. Indications include:

- monitoring of CVP
- drug administration
- total parenteral nutrition
- fluid resuscitation
- insertion of temporary pacing wires
- insertion of pulmonary artery catheters
- dialysis
- lack of peripheral venous access.

Contraindications
These are relative, but include inability to identify landmarks, limited sites for access, previous difficulties or complications, severe coagulopathy, thrombocytopenia and local sepsis. In addition, if an awake patient is unable to lie flat, central venous cannulation may be impractical.

Ultrasound guidance for vascular access
The use of ultrasound to guide central venous access procedures is recommended in all cases (NICE Guidance. Central venous catheters, ultrasound locating devices, Sept. 2002. www.nice.org. uk/guidance/TA49).

Ultrasound allows for:

- direct visualization of the vessels (artery and vein) and their associated structures
- identification of thrombosis, valve or anatomical abnormalities
- identification of target vessel

- first-pass cannulation in the midline of a vessel directly avoiding other vital structures
- visualization of guide wire and cannula entering vein
- reduction of puncture-related complications.

Use of ultrasound clearly requires understanding of the ultrasound appearances of the anatomy at the various sites of interest. Arteries can be distinguished from veins by their round cross-section, non-compressibility and their pulsatility. Veins, by contrast, show respiratory fluctuation and are easily compressible. When using ultrasound for vascular access you should:

- Ensure you are familiar with the device available.
- Ensure depth settings, gain and other settings are appropriate.
- Place the monitor opposite you at eye level.
- Ensure correct orientation of the probe (vessels should be in the anatomical orientation as it would appear from where you are standing.
- Identify patent target vessel. (To exclude thrombus in a vein ensure it empties completely with pressure.)
- Identify collateral structures to avoid artery, nerves, chest wall and pleura.
- Use sterile ultrasound gel and a sterile sheath to maintain sterility.
- Puncture the vessel of choice using real time guidance to direct the needle into the vein using longitudinal or transverse approaches.
- Verify intravenous placement of the needle, guide wire and catheter with ultrasound.

> **Effective use of ultrasound requires practice. In particular the needle must be visualized as it passes into the vessel. Seek instruction before attempting to use it on a patient.**

Traditional approaches to the central veins are described below.

Internal jugular vein

Right sided internal jugular vein cannulation is associated with a lower incidence of complications and higher incidence of correct line placement than other approaches. It is especially appropriate for patients with coagulopathy or those patients with lung disease in whom pneumothorax may be disastrous. It may be best avoided in those patients with carotid artery disease or those with raised intracranial pressure because of the risks of carotid puncture and of impaired cerebral venous drainage. Internal jugular cannulation is associated with a higher incidence of catheter infection than subclavian cannulation but both have a much lower infection rate than the femoral approach.

The internal jugular vein runs from the jugular foramen at the base of the skull (immediately behind the ear) to its termination behind the posterior border of the sternoclavicular joint, where it combines with the subclavian vein to become the brachiocephalic vein. Throughout its length it lies lateral, first to the internal and then common carotid arteries, within the carotid sheath, behind the sternomastoid muscle (Fig. 15.1A). Ultrasound demonstrates the close proximity of the vein to the carotid artery (Fig. 15.1B). Many approaches to the internal jugular vein have been described. A typical landmark approach is from the apex of the triangle formed by the two heads of the sternomastoid (Fig. 15.1).

- Slightly extend the neck.
- Turn the head slightly to the opposite side.
- Palpate the carotid artery at the level of the cricoid cartilage.
- Look for the internal jugular vein pulsation. If compressed, the internal jugular can usually be seen to empty and refill.
- Introduce the needle from the apex of the triangle at an angle of 30° and aim towards the ipsilateral nipple.
- Often when attempting to puncture the vein it collapses under the pressure of the needle and puncture is not recognized. The vessel may then be located by aspirating as the needle is slowly withdrawn. Blood is aspirated as the needle tip passes back into the vein, which refills once the pressure has been removed.

> It is a common mistake to assume the internal jugular vein is deep. Typically it is <2 cm from the skin. Do not introduce the needle to its full length. There is a danger of puncturing the apex of the lung.

- Typical catheter length required is 15 cm from the right and 20 cm from the left. The right side is preferred because left-sided catheters have to traverse two 'corners' to get to the SVC and are associated with a higher complication rate.

External jugular vein

The external jugular vein lies superficially in the neck, running down from the region of the angle of the jaw, across the sternomastoid before passing deep to drain into the subclavian

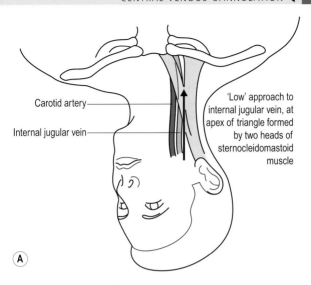

Carotid artery

Internal jugular vein

'Low' approach to internal jugular vein, at apex of triangle formed by two heads of sternocleidomastoid muscle

(A)

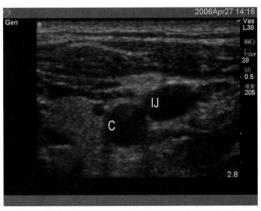

(B)

Fig. 15.1 (A) Approach to the internal jugular vein. **(B)** Ultrasound appearance of internal jugular vein. Right side viewed from the head of the patient. IJ internal jugular vein, C, carotid artery.

vein. It can be used to provide central venous access, particularly in emergency situations when a simple large-bore cannula can be used for the administration of drugs and resuscitation fluids. Longer central venous catheters can be sited via the external jugular but the angle of entry to the subclavian vein often leads to inability to pass guide wires centrally and results in a high failure rate.

Subclavian vein

Subclavian vein cannulation is associated with a higher incidence of complications, particularly pneumothorax, and a higher incidence of incorrect line placement than right internal jugular cannulation. It is, however, more comfortable for the patient long-term and is associated with a lower incidence of line infection than other sites of central venous cannulation.

The subclavian vein is a continuation of the axillary vein. It runs from the apex of the axilla behind the posterior border of the clavicle and across the first rib to join the internal jugular vein, forming the brachiocephalic vein behind the sternoclavicular joint. See Fig. 15.2.

- Position the patient supine (some people advocate placing a sandbag between the patient's shoulder blades, which allows the shoulders to drop back out of the way).
- Identify the junction of medial third and outer two-thirds of the clavicle.
- Introduce the needle just beneath the clavicle at this point, and aim towards the clavicle until contact with bone is made.
- To locate the vein, redirect the needle closely behind the clavicle and towards the suprasternal notch.

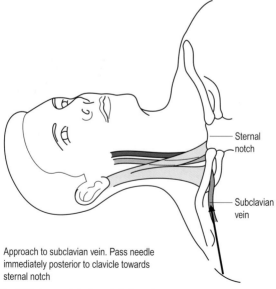

Sternal notch

Subclavian vein

Approach to subclavian vein. Pass needle immediately posterior to clavicle towards sternal notch

Fig. 15.2 Approach to the subclavian vein.

Ultrasound can be used to guide cannulation of the subclavian vein using a more lateral approach. The axillary vein can be identified in the apex of the axilla at a depth of 3–4 cm in the average patient. Cannulation of the axillary vein is relatively straightforward under ultrasound control and minimizes the risk of pneumothorax owing to its position lateral to the pleura and chest wall. Longer catheters (20 cm left and 25 cm right) are required by this approach.

Femoral vein

The femoral vein lies medial to the femoral artery immediately beneath the inguinal ligament. It is particularly useful for obtaining central access in small children and in patients with severe coagulopathy.

● Palpate the femoral artery.
● To locate the vein, introduce the needle 1 cm medial to the femoral artery close to the inguinal ligament. It is a common mistake to go too low where the superficial femoral artery overlies the vein. Long catheters, 24 cm plus, are required to get the tip of the catheter into the IVC, which may be required for good flows (e.g. for dialysis).
● Ultrasound can be used to identify the vessels and ensure that the vein is punctured near the inguinal ligament where the artery and vein lie side by side. See Fig. 15.3.

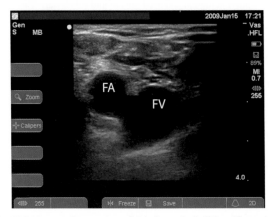

Fig. 15.3 Ultrasound appearances of right femoral vein (FV) and femoral artery (FA), viewed from below, at the level of the inguinal ligament. Below this level the superficial femoral artery partially overlaps the vein and the long saphenous vein and other superficial veins join making access more difficult.

Procedure

Central venous cannulation. You will need:
Universal precautions; sterile gown and gloves
Skin disinfectant
Sterile towels
5-mL syringe of local anaesthetic
CVP line kit
Three-way taps
Heparinized saline to flush line
Suture
Dressing
Ultrasound machine
Ultrasound probe cover and sterile gel
ECG monitoring and defibrillator

- Central venous catheterization is almost universally achieved using a catheter over a guide wire (Seldinger) technique. This is associated with a lower incidence of incorrect line placement and complications than cannula over needle techniques.
- For internal jugular, external jugular and subclavian veins position the patient supine with 10–20° head down tilt. This distends the vein to aid location and helps prevent air embolism.
- Monitor ECG in case of dysrhythmias (a defibrillator should be immediately available).
- Universal precautions.
- Use aseptic technique, sterile gown and gloves.
- Prepare sterile field.
- Prepare all equipment.
- Check wire passes through the needle freely. Attach three-way taps to all open ports of the cannula. Flush the lumens with heparinized saline.
- Inject local anaesthetic to the entry site. Do not forget to anaesthetize suture sites as well.
- Identify the target vessel by ultrasound and/or landmark technique.
- Using a 10-mL syringe and needle enter the central vein by the chosen approach, maintaining suction on the syringe at all times.

If you appear to have missed the vein on the first pass, pull back slowly while maintaining suction on the syringe. You often find you have gone through the vein and can identify it on withdrawal.

- Pass the Seldinger wire through the needle. This should pass freely and without any force into the vein. Watch for dysrhythmias. To reduce the risk of dysrhythmias, avoid introducing the wire further than necessary.
- Never pull the wire back through the needle once it has passed beyond the end of the bevel: it may shear off.
- Use a scalpel blade to make a small nick in the skin. Hold the blade up and cut away from the wire.
- If provided, pass the dilator over the wire into the vein. Then remove it, leaving the wire in situ.
- Pass the cannula over the wire into the vein. Make sure that before you push the cannula forward the wire is visible at the proximal end. Hold on to the wire at all times, to prevent it being lost inside the patient!
- For an average adult patient the central venous cannula does not need to be inserted more than 12–15 cm. Check markings on the cannula. Many are 20 cm long and do not need to be inserted up to the hub.
- Draw back blood, flush all the lumens of the line with heparinized saline and lock off the three-way taps. At this point the patient can be levelled.
- Suture the line into place using the anchorage devices provided and cover with an adhesive sterile dressing.
- Attach a transducer and display the waveform on the monitor.
- Dispose of your sharps and clear away your trolley.
- Obtain a CXR to verify position of the line and check for complications, including pneumothorax and haemothorax.
- Document the procedure in the patient's notes.

Position on chest X-ray

The catheter should lie along the long axis of the vessel and the distal segment and tip should be in the superior vena cava (SVC) or at the junction of the SVC and right atrium but ideally outside the pericardial reflection. Catheters below this level may perforate the heart and cause cardiac tamponade. The pericardial reflection

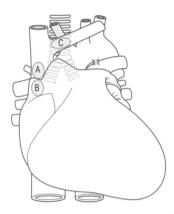

A: Ideal position for tip of all upper body central venous catheters, at or just above the level of carina (outside pericardium)

B: Acceptable position for the tip of right internal jugular catheters (just within pericardial reflection)

C: Acceptable position for tip of left sided central venous catheters that are too short to reach the ideal position A. DO NOT allow the tip of the catheters to abut the wall of the IVC

Fig. 15.4 Optimal position for tip of central catheters on chest X-ray.

lies below the level of the carina and this can therefore be used as a radiological marker. Catheters placed via subclavian veins of left internal jugular vein must not be allowed to lie with the tip abutting the wall of the superior vena cava. This may cause pain, perforation and accelerated thrombus formation. Either advance the catheter to lie in the long axis of the SVC or pull it back to lie in the brachiocephalic vein. See Fig. 15.4.

COMMON PROBLEMS DURING CENTRAL VENOUS ACCESS

Cannot find the vein
Check position (ultrasound and/or landmarks) and try again. If unsuccessful do not persist with repeated passages of the needle in the hope of striking oil! You may have misinterpreted the landmarks, or the vein may be absent or occluded (e.g. with thrombus). Seek help.

Do not proceed immediately to attempt cannulation on the contralateral side: this increases the risk of complications, such as bilateral pneumothorax!

Aspirating blood but cannot pass wire

Check needle position by drawing back on the syringe; good flow is essential. Adjust the angle of incidence of the needle to the vein to improve flow. Tip the patient further head down to further distend the vein. Try rotating the needle through 180° and draw back again. Remember, the wire must pass easily without force. If this doesn't work, re-puncture the vein at a slightly different angle.

Is it arterial?

Occasionally, particularly if using a technique where the wire passes through the barrel of the syringe, it is difficult to know whether you have hit the artery or the vein. In this case it is important to avoid passing a large central venous catheter into the vessel which if arterial could result in vessel damage, stroke or TIA. Consider the following:

- Remove the syringe from the needle and observe for pulsatile flow.
- Connect a transducer directly to the needle in the vessel and look at the waveform.
- Pass the wire into the vessel and remove the needle. Pass an 18-gauge i.v. cannula over the wire into the vessel and remove the wire. Attach a transducer or manometer set directly to the cannula. When venous placement is confirmed, pass the wire back through the i.v. cannula and continue as before.

Arterial puncture

- Needle only, then simply remove and press for 10 min (watch clock!).
- If large-bore cannula, then action depends on circumstances. Usually can remove and press until bleeding stops. If severe coagulopathy, leave in situ and give platelets and FFP before removing. Seek advice and consider the need for surgical exploration and removal under direct vision.

Complications

Complications of central venous cannulation depend in part on the route used but include those in Box 15.2.

Box 15.2 Complications of central venous cannulation

Early	Late
Arrhythmias	Infection
Vascular injury	Thrombosis
Pneumothorax	Embolization
Haemothorax	Erosion/perforation of vessels
Thoracic duct injury (chylothorax)	Cardiac tamponade
Cardiac tamponade	AV fistula
Neural injury	
Embolization (including guide wire)	
AV fistula	

The management of pneumothorax depends upon the size of the pneumothorax and the patient's condition, particularly whether they are ventilated or not. A small pneumothorax in an unventilated patient with good gas exchange may be observed, or aspirated using a small-bore cannula and syringe with three-way tap. Larger pneumothoraces, those that fail to resolve or those that cause any impairment of gas exchange and/or haemodynamics require a formal chest drain. Any significant haemothorax should be formally drained as soon as possible. Once blood has clotted in the chest, drainage is difficult. (See Chest drainage, p. 418.) Seek cardiothoracic/surgical opinion.

Bleeding around the puncture site can occasionally be a persistent problem. If this does not resolve with pressure, use a suture (5/0 nylon) to tie a purse string around the puncture site. This usually stops the bleeding.

Thrombus formation around central venous cannula is common and may lead to deep venous thrombosis and/or pulmonary embolus. Avoid insertion at sites where there is evidence of thrombus on ultrasound scanning. If thrombi are identified around an existing cannula, these should be removed and therapeutic anticoagulation commenced unless contraindicated.

CHANGING AND REMOVING CENTRAL VENOUS CATHETERS

Line colonization with bacteria and fungi is common and there is no evidence that changing lines on a regular basis (e.g. every 5–7 days) is of benefit. (See Catheter-related sepsis, p. 340.)

Changing catheters over a wire

If new central venous catheters are required these should usually be placed at a clean site. Occasionally it may be necessary to change a catheter over a guide wire using an existing site. The technique is similar to that described above for placing any central venous catheter. The main problem is avoiding contamination of the new catheter.

● Cut sutures and remove the dressing from the old line before scrubbing.
● Use universal precautions, aseptic technique, gown and gloves.

 The difficulty with this technique is retaining sterility. Wear two pairs of gloves and discard the top pair when you have removed the old line.

● Clean and prepare area (including old catheter).
● Pass the wire down the central lumen of the old central venous catheter. (Make sure that the new wire is longer than the old CVP line.)
● Remove the old catheter, leaving the wire in place, and send the tip of the old catheter for culture.
● Clean the puncture site with antiseptic solution.
● Use the wire to site the new line as required.

Removing central venous catheters

Removal of central venous catheters can precipitate air embolism, pneumothorax, haemothorax, embolization of thrombus and bacteraemia/sepsis.

Before removing central lines ensure that all drugs and infusions have been stopped or relocated to other lines. Lay the patient down to reduce the risk of air embolism and remove the line smoothly, applying pressure to the puncture site. Apply an occlusive dressing, then sit the patient up. If infection is suspected, send the tip of the line in a dry specimen pot for culture. (See Catheter-related sepsis, p. 340.)

LARGE-BORE INTRODUCER SHEATHS/DIALYSIS CATHETERS

Indications

Introducer sheaths are available in a number of sizes for different applications, including insertion of pulmonary artery catheters and temporary pacing wires. In adults, 7.5 or 8.5 Fr are generally used. They may be used as large-bore access for volume resuscitation. Smaller sheaths may be used for introducing specialized monitoring such as jugular bulb oximetery. Large-bore double lumen dialysis catheters are used for haemodialysis, haemofiltration, plasma exchange and rapid transfusion.

Procedure
See Central venous cannulation above.

All these devices are inserted using a Seldinger technique and a large stiff dilator is used to dilate the initial needle track sufficiently to allow the large-bore catheter to be passed easily into the vessel. These dilators do not pass around tight bends easily and can readily damage or perforate vessels. The left internal jugular vein is best avoided. Introducer sheaths can usually be sited safely at all other sites. Dialysis catheters may be best placed by the right internal jugular or femoral routes. The femoral route may be particularly appropriate in patients with chronic renal failure, to preserve the venous drainage of the arm for subsequent AV fistula formation.

- Universal precautions.
- Aseptic technique, sterile gown and gloves.
- Enter vein with needle, as for central venous line, and pass Seldinger wire.
- Make small nick in the skin with a blade.
- Either: Pass the sheath mounted on the introducer/dilator over the wire into the vein. The dilator is generally longer than needed and does not need to be passed right up to the hub. When the dilator has entered the vein, slide the sheath forward without advancing the dilator any further.
- Or for dialysis catheters, pass the dilator over the wire into the vein then remove dilator and introduce catheter over the wire.

 The dilators provided are often very stiff and can easily kink guide wires and tear vessels if advanced too far or too aggressively. If difficulties are encountered in inserting dilators, abandon the procedure and call for help. If possible avoid left internal jugular routes.

- Remove wire and dilator.
- Draw back and flush catheter with (heparinized) saline. (For dialysis catheters use heparin 1000 units/mL and flush to the volume of the catheter printed on the hub.)

- When in situ and not in use the sheath port should be occluded with an obturator.
- Get CXR to check position and complications.

Haemodialysis catheters

You should ensure that the line used is of an adequate length. It is best if the tip of the line lies freely within a great vein so that the risk of obstruction due to it abutting the vessel wall or being trapped in a 'collapsing' vein is minimized. A line longer than 24 cm is often needed to pass from the femoral vein to the lower IVC.

PULMONARY ARTERY CATHETERIZATION

The place of pulmonary artery catheters has been questioned recently and their use has diminished. In general non-invasive cardiac output monitoring and the ready availability of bedside echocardiography have superseded them. (See Haemodynamic monitoring, p. 74.) They may be of value, however, in conditions where haemodynamic instability or shock is unresponsive to fluid and inotrope therapy guided by conventional CVP measurement, particularly where pulmonary hypertension/right heart failure are thought to contribute to the problem. As insertion of a PA catheter is not without hazard, you should always seek senior guidance. Traditional indications and contraindications are shown in Box 15.3.

Box 15.3 Indications and contraindications for pulmonary artery catheterization

Indications	Relative contraindications
Shock	Severe coagulopathy
Sepsis/SIRS	Unstable ventricular rhythm
ARDS	Heart block
Valvular heart disease*	Temporary transvenous pacemaker (wire dislodgement)
Left ventricular failure	Stenosis tricuspid or pulmonary valve†
Cor pulmonale/pulmonary hypertension	
High-risk surgical patients	

*Relative indication.
†Severe stenosis or mechanical valves absolute contraindication.

Procedure

PA catheterization. You will need:
Universal precautions; sterile gown and gloves
Sterile towels
Skin cleaning solution
5-mL syringe of local anaesthetic
Introducer sheath (see previous section)
Ultrasound/sterile probe cover and gel
Pulmonary artery catheter
Three-way taps
Heparinized saline to flush line
Transducer and monitor
ECG monitoring and defibrillator

 Before attempting to insert a PA catheter, ECG monitoring must be established and a defibrillator must be immediately available because of the risks of dysrhythmia.

- Use universal precautions.
- Full aseptic technique. Sterile gown and gloves.
- Insert introducer sheath as above.
- Position the patient flat before inserting the PA catheter. (This reduces the pulmonary artery pressures and reduces the risk of pulmonary artery rupture.)
- Connect 3-way taps to the open ports, and flush lumens with heparinized saline.
- Connect 1.5 mL syringe to the balloon port and test the balloon. (Check the size of the balloon before starting.)
- Pass protective sleeve over PA catheter.
- Pass the proximal end of the catheter to an assistant who can connect a pressure transducer to the PA port (yellow) and flush the lumen. Then zero the transducer and check the signal on the monitor. Need to display trace on the monitor (scale 0–75 mmHg) continuously.
- Calibrate fibreoptics if using a fibreoptic PA catheter.
- Insert PA catheter into introducer sheath and pass to 20 cm. Note normal CVP trace.
- Inflate balloon and advance catheter gently to right ventricle at approximately 30–40 cm. Advance further until the pulmonary artery is entered at approximately 40–50 cm.

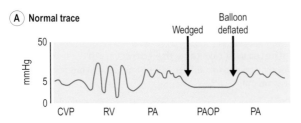

(A) **Normal trace**

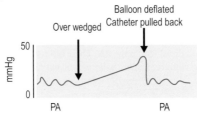

(B) **Over wedged trace**

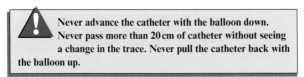

Fig. 15.5 Waveforms during PA catheterization. **(A)** Normal trace. **(B)** Over wedged trace.

- Advance the catheter until pulmonary artery occlusion trace or wedge trace is observed, approx. 20 cm from RV (approximately 50–60 cm total). Deflate the balloon and see return of the PA trace (Fig. 15.5).

> ⚠ Never advance the catheter with the balloon down.
> Never pass more than 20 cm of catheter without seeing a change in the trace. Never pull the catheter back with the balloon up.

- Once the PA catheter is in position, perform a CXR; check the position of the catheter in the proximal pulmonary artery and exclude pneumothorax / haemothorax / knotting of the line.
- While in use, ensure that the PA pressure trace is displayed continuously on the bedside monitor so that inadvertent 'wedging' of the catheter can be recognized and the catheter pulled back to prevent pulmonary infarction.

COMMON PROBLEMS DURING PULMONARY ARTERY CATHETERIZATION

Catheter will not take the correct path

This may be due to a dilated RV or low CO. Do not persist if unsuccessful:

- Remove completely, check direction of curvature of catheter and try again.
- To enter RV place patient head down and left side up.
- To enter PA place patient head up and supine.

Catheter is 'over wedged'

- Always watch the pressure trace when wedging the catheter. If pressure rises, then catheter is 'over wedged' (Fig. 15.4.).
- The catheter is too distal within the PA. There is a risk of pulmonary artery rupture. Deflate balloon, pull catheter back and try again.

Catheter will not wedge

- This may be because the catheter is curled up within the PA. Do not pass more than 20 cm without a change in trace. Pull back and try again.
- In the presence of severe mitral regurgitation or pulmonary hypertension, it may not be possible to obtain a satisfactory wedge trace and attempts may be associated with increased risk of PA rupture. Accept that the catheter will not wedge and use pulmonary diastolic pressure instead of PA occlusion pressure.
- In low CO states, there may be insufficient blood flow in the pulmonary artery to advance the catheter when the balloon is inflated. Do not persist. Use PA diastolic as above.

Complications

PA catheterization is not without risk and is certainly not a therapeutic manoeuvre in its own right! If patients are to benefit then regular collection and interpretation of haemodynamic and oxygen delivery variables, together with the appropriate therapeutic response, is required.

Potential complications of pulmonary artery catheterization are shown in Table 15.1.

TABLE 15.1 Complications of pulmonary artery catheterization

Complication	Comment
Central venous puncture	Any complications of central venous cannulation
Dysrhythmia	Usually on passage through tricuspid valve and RV Especially if hypoxia, acidosis, hypokalaemia: withdraw catheter and reposition Complete heart block may occur
Pulmonary infarction	Check catheter is in proximal PA on chest X-ray Never leave balloon inflated Display PA trace continuously
Pulmonary artery rupture	Pulmonary haemorrhage and blood up the endotracheal tube Avoid overinflation of the balloon Watch trace and never inflate against resistance
Infection	Risk includes endocardial damage and endocarditis Careful aseptic technique and catheter care Remove after 72 h or ASAP
Knotting	Poor insertion technique Do not insert more than 20 cm without a change in trace Do not attempt to pull back. Call for help

MEASURING PAOP

Most monitoring systems have a specific function key for use when measuring PAOP. These generally display the pulmonary artery pressure trace on a larger scale, allowing changes in the trace to be more easily observed and provide a cursor that can be positioned to indicate the PAOP:

● Enter PAOP function on the monitor.
● Inflate the balloon and observe the wedge trace.
● Position cursor over the 'wedge trace' at the point corresponding to end expiration (Fig. 15.5).

MEASUREMENT OF CARDIAC OUTPUT BY THERMODILUTION

Pulmonary artery catheters incorporate a thermistor near the tip to allow thermodilution measurement of cardiac output. A volume of cold 5% dextrose solution (usually 10 mL) is injected through the central venous port of the PA catheter (in SVC or RA) and the temperature change in the PA is detected by the thermistor. The degree and the rate of temperature change is used to calculate cardiac output. (Some catheters incorporate a heated coil and fast reacting thermistor to allow continuous cardiac output measurement.)

- Ensure that the correct cables are connected between the monitor and the PA catheter (one to the distal thermistor and one to measure the temperature of the injectate).
- Enter cardiac output function on monitor.
- Check that the correct computation constant is entered into the monitor. This depends upon the volume and temperature of the injectate and also the type of catheter used. The correct computation constant is found on the packaging information of the PA catheter.
- Enter the patient's height and weight for calculation of body surface area (BSA).
- Set the computer to measure cardiac output, and when prompted inject 10 mL of 5% dextrose into the right atrial (CVP) lumen of the PA catheter. Time the injection at the end of inspiration and inject as rapidly as possible.

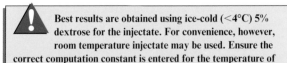

> ⚠ **Best results are obtained using ice-cold (<4°C) 5% dextrose for the injectate. For convenience, however, room temperature injectate may be used. Ensure the correct computation constant is entered for the temperature of injectate used.**

- Repeat the measurement. The individual cardiac output values obtained should not vary more than 5% from each other. Discard any inconsistent value and take the average reading for cardiac output.

Having measured the cardiac output and PA occlusion pressure a range of haemodynamic variables can be calculated. This is generally performed by the monitoring system. Normal values for these variables are given in Chapter 4. (See Optimizing haemodynamic status, p. 78.)

In addition by measuring blood gases on blood drawn simultaneously from the pulmonary artery catheter (mixed venous) and an arterial line, oxygen delivery and consumption variables may be calculated. (See Oxygen delivery and consumption, p. 68.)

PERICARDIAL ASPIRATION

Indications
- Cardiac tamponade.
- Large pericardial effusions.
- To obtain diagnostic pericardial fluid.

Small localized effusions, not causing haemodynamic compromise and without diastolic collapse on echocardiogram, do not require pericardiocentesis. Seek senior advice.
A cardiology opinion should be sought where available. Use ultrasound guidance in all cases where possible to guide safe drainage, avoiding the liver and other structures. (See Cardiac tamponade, p. 108.)

Procedure
- Place patient supine with 20° of head-up tilt.
- Establish i.v. access if not already present and monitor ECG.
- Provide adequate sedation if necessary.
- Full aseptic technique. Sterile gowns and gloves.
- The point of needle insertion is immediately below and to the left of the xiphisternum, between the xiphisternum and the left costal margin. Infiltrate the skin and subcutaneous tissue with local anaesthetic.
- Using a 10-mL syringe, advance the needle at 35° to the patient, beneath the costal margin and towards the left shoulder, aspirating continuously and observing the ECG (Fig. 15.6).
- Fluid (straw-coloured effusion or blood) is generally aspirated at a depth of 6–8 cm. Hold the needle stationary and pass the guide wire through the needle into the pericardial space.
- Remove the needle, leaving the guide wire in situ and then pass the catheter over the wire into the pericardial space. Attach a three-way tap.
- Use a 50-mL syringe to aspirate pericardial effusion or attach to a closed drainage system such as a vacuum bottle. Aspiration should produce immediate haemodynamic improvement.
- Suture the drain in place.

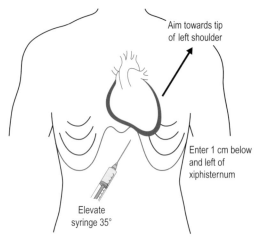

Aim towards tip
of left shoulder

Enter 1 cm below
and left of
xiphisternum

Elevate
syringe 35°

Fig. 15.6 Pericardial aspiration.

> ⚠ **In an emergency situation when aspirating presumed
> cardiac tamponade it is difficult to know whether blood
> aspirated is from the pericardial space or whether the
> ventricle has been punctured. Observe the ECG throughout. If
> the needle touches the ventricle, an injury pattern or arrhythmia
> should be observed.**

Complications

Performed carefully, complications are few. They include
pneumothorax, ventricular tachycardia, myocardial puncture
and damage to the coronary arteries. A repeat CXR and
echocardiogram should be performed after the procedure to confirm
adequate placement and drainage and to identify any problems.

Insertion of a pericardial drain should only be considered a
temporary measure. Seek cardiothoracic surgical advice regarding
repair of the underlying problem and/or creation of a pericardial
window.

DEFIBRILLATION AND DC CARDIOVERSION

Elective cardioversion is beyond the scope of this book. Life-
threatening 'shockable rhythm' should be managed according
to advanced life support protocols. (See pp. 90–98.) For
cardioversion in the emergency situation, i.e. the intensive care

patient with haemodynamic compromise, the following approach is reasonable.

Procedure

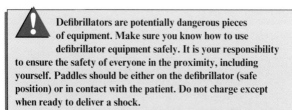

> **Pericardial aspiration. You will need:**
>
> Universal precautions; sterile gown and gloves
>
> Skin cleaning solutions
>
> Sterile towels
>
> 10-mL syringe of local anaesthetic and needle
>
> Pigtail catheter or 14-gauge single lumen central venous catheter (including syringe, needle and guide wire)
>
> Three-way tap
>
> 50-mL syringe or vacuum drainage bottle
>
> Suture
>
> Occlusive dressing

> ⚠ **Defibrillators are potentially dangerous pieces of equipment. Make sure you know how to use defibrillator equipment safely. It is your responsibility to ensure the safety of everyone in the proximity, including yourself. Paddles should be either on the defibrillator (safe position) or in contact with the patient. Do not charge except when ready to deliver a shock.**

- Ensure the patient is adequately sedated/anaesthetized. This may require supplementation of existing sedation/analgesia with a small bolus dose of midazolam, opioid or other similar agent. Conscious patients will require anaesthesia, usually with a cardiostable drug (e.g. etomidate) or volatile agent Seek anaesthetic support.
- Place conducting gel pads over the patient's apex and sternum,
- Select the appropriate mode (asynchronous or synchronous) and select required energy levels (see relevant algorithms) before removing the paddles from the defibrillator.
- Take paddles from the defibrillator and place immediately on to gel pads on the patient. Only charge the paddles once they are in contact with the patient.
- Before charging paddles give an 'all clear' warning to ensure that no-one is touching the patient and check that everyone is clear.
- Before delivering the shock, give a second all clear warning; check that everyone is clear and that any oxygen source is temporarily removed from the patient. Ensure that you yourself are not inadvertently in contact with the patient.

- Deliver shock.
- After delivery of the shock, several seconds may pass before monitors yield an ECG trace. Keep paddles in contact with the patient if you may wish to deliver a further shock, or return them to the safe position on the defibrillator.

If normal rhythm is not restored seek expert help. Consider:

- Higher energy shock.
- Alternative paddle position (e.g. cardiac long axis, anteroposterior).
- Use of antidysrhythmic drug before repeat attempts.
- Many patients on ICU develop atrial fibrillation that does not return to sinus rhythm for more than a very short period after DC cardioversion, until their underlying condition has improved.

INTUBATION OF THE TRACHEA

This is covered at greater length in standard anaesthesia texts; however, there are some aspects of tracheal intubation of particular relevance to patients in intensive care.

 Do not attempt tracheal intubation without senior help if you are not experienced in the technique. In an emergency, ventilate the patient with a bag and mask or via a laryngeal mask and await reinforcements!

Indications

These fall broadly into three groups: relieving airway obstruction, protection of the airway from aspiration and facilitation of artificial ventilation of the lungs. Typical indications are given in Box 15.4.

Patients requiring intubation in ICU frequently have limited physiological reserve and are liable to haemodynamic collapse. Drugs used to facilitate intubation must therefore be used judiciously. In some cases patients may already have a markedly obtunded conscious level and small doses of benzodiazepines (e.g. diazepam 5–10 mg) may be all that is required. In other patients, low doses of i.v. anaesthetic agents may be appropriate (e.g. propofol 1–2 mg/kg or etomidate 0.1–0.2 mg/kg); however, these may be associated with cardiovascular collapse.

Muscle relaxants will usually be required to facilitate intubation. Suxamethonium (1–2 mg/kg) is rapid in onset and relatively short-acting in most patients. It is the drug of choice for

Box 15.4 Indications for tracheal intubation

Airway obstruction	Risks of aspiration	Facilitation of IPPV
Tumours	Obtunded consciousness level	Anaesthesia and surgery
Head and neck trauma	Bulbar palsy	Cardiopulmonary resuscitation
Epiglottitis	Impaired cough reflexes	Respiratory failure
Surgery		Cardiac failure
Airway oedema		Multisystem organ failure
		Major trauma including chest injury
		Brain injury

rapid sequence induction. It has a number of side-effects, however, which limit its use. Atracurium (0.5 mg/kg) is an alternative, but is slower in onset and has a longer duration of action.

 Do not use i.v. anaesthetic agents or muscle relaxants unless you are familiar with them. Seek senior help. (See Sedation and analgesia, p. 34, Muscle relaxants, p. 43 and Contraindications to suxamethonium, p. 43.)

Procedure

Tracheal intubation. You will need:

Skilled assistant

Self-inflating bag (Ambu or similar) and oxygen supply

Face mask

Oral/nasal airways

Suction and suction catheters

Two laryngoscopes (check bulbs)

Selection of endotracheal tubes

Sterile lubricant

Syringe for cuff inflation and tape to tie tube

Gum-elastic bougie, airway exchange catheter or rigid stilette

Laryngeal mask (for use in failed intubation) sizes 3, 4, 5.

Anaesthetic drugs and muscle relaxant

Resuscitation drugs – atropine, adrenaline (epinephrine)

- Preoxygenate the patient. Administer 100% oxygen using a tight-fitting face mask for a period of 3–4 min prior to administering any drugs or attempting intubation, if possible. This will wash out nitrogen and fill the functional residual capacity with oxygen, thereby providing an oxygen reservoir and increasing the safety margin in the event of difficulties.
- Check the head is in the 'sniffing the morning air' position (neck flexed, atlantoaxial joint extended, one firm pillow).
- If the patient might have a full stomach, ask your assistant to apply cricoid pressure; if the neck is supported from behind and the cricoid firmly gripped, downward pressure prevents any passive regurgitation. If possible, avoid inflating the lungs with the face mask and self-inflating bag until the tube is in place, as blowing air into the stomach may increase the risks of regurgitation.
- Give sedative anaesthetic and muscle relaxant as appropriate.
- Hold the laryngoscope in the left hand (size 3 or 4 Macintosh scopes are most commonly used). Slide the scope into the right of the mouth, sweeping the tongue into the groove in the blade, under it and to the left. As you advance the laryngoscope blade over the base of the tongue, the epiglottis pops into sight. With the blade between the epiglottis and the base of the tongue (vallecula), apply traction in the line of the laryngoscope handle, gently drawing the epiglottis forward and exposing the V-shaped glottis behind (Fig. 15.7).
- Pass the endotracheal tube between the vocal cords so that the cuff is just distal to them. There is usually a mark on the endotracheal tube above the cuff, which when placed at the level of the cords indicates the correct position of the tube.
- If you can visualize the vocal cords but are having difficulty passing the endotracheal tube into the larynx, pass a gum elastic bougie or airway exchange catheter into the larynx and then try passing a lubricated endotracheal tube over this.
- Inflate the cuff while ventilating through the endotracheal tube with the self-inflating bag until any gas leak just disappears.

> ⚠️ If immediate intubation proves to be difficult or impracticable, do not persist with fruitless attempts. Ventilate the patient with 100% oxygen using bag and mask or laryngeal mask and call for help.

- Verify correct positioning of the tube by observation of chest movement, auscultation and capnography. Secure it, and attach

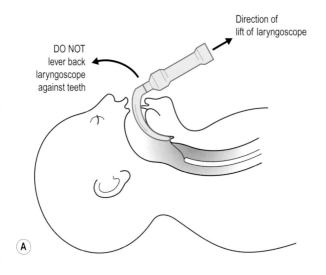

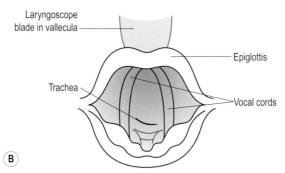

Fig. 15.7 (A) Laryngoscopy. **(B)** View of the larynx.

to the ventilator via a suitable catheter mount. Recheck the tube position and chest movement.
- Check the cuff pressure with a standard pressure gauge to reduce the risks of laryngeal mucosal injury.
- Pass a nasogastric tube if this is not already in situ.
- Obtain a CXR to confirm tube position. Check if the tube is too short, too long (endobronchial?). Check for lobar collapse, pneumothorax, etc.

Use of bougie

The bougie or airway exchange catheter is probably the most useful, simple aid for intubation, In cases of 'poor view' the bougie can be passed through the glottis allowing almost blind passage of the endotracheal tube. (railroad tube over the bougie) .Use of a bougie requires relatively little training and can be a lifesaver. You should familiarize yourself with this device. The bougie can also be used for change of an endotracheal tube. Pass bougie down existing tube, then exchange over the bougie.

Complications

Potential complications of endotracheal intubation are shown in Box 15.5.

The commonest and most immediately life-threatening complication is oesophageal intubation. Always confirm endotracheal intubation by the presence of expired carbon dioxide using a capnograph or end tidal CO_2 detector device (colour change in presence of CO_2). Note that hypoxia is a late sign of oesophageal misplacement particularly following preoxygenation. If you are in any doubt about the position of the tube, remove it, ventilate by facemask, and start again.

Nasal intubation may provoke epistaxis or predispose to mucosal injury (e.g. submucosal positioning of the tube). In the longer term, nasal intubation may occlude the maxillary antrum and give rise to sinusitis. It is nevertheless better tolerated than oral intubation, particularly during weaning from ventilation. Long-term complications include erosion and stenosis of local tissues, particularly of the larynx and trachea. This may present as airway obstruction and stridor after extubation (see p. 138).

Box 15.5 Complications of endotracheal intubation

Immediate	Late
Hypoxia (prolonged attempts)	Accidental extubation or obstruction of airway
Misplacement of tube	Complications associated with mechanical ventilation
Obstruction of airway	Ventilator associated pneumonia
Aspiration	Sinusitis
Trauma to teeth	Injury to vocal cords
Trauma to airway/larynx/ trachea	Tracheal stenosis

EXTUBATION OF THE TRACHEA

Before you consider extubation, the patient should be breathing spontaneously with a satisfactory respiratory pattern and acceptable blood gases. The patient should have an appropriate conscious level and airway reflexes and not be requiring repeated airway suctioning. (See Weaning from artificial ventilation, p. 135.)

- Check a suitable system for providing humidified oxygen by face mask is available, and that you have everything necessary for reintubation.
- Explain to the patient what you are going to do, then aspirate any secretions from the posterior pharynx.
- Insert a wide-bore suction catheter through the endotracheal tube. Deflate the cuff, and simultaneously aspirate through the suction catheter as you withdraw the endotracheal tube. This ensures that any secretions that have collected above the cuff are removed.
- Finally, fit a face mask and encourage the patient to cough out any further secretions.
- Observe the patient closely for signs of respiratory inadequacy or distress developing over the next few hours. Consider the early use of CPAP/BIPAP if the patient has limited respiratory reserve.

INSERTION OF LARYNGEAL MASK (SUPRAGLOTTIC AIRWAYS)

In the event of being unable to intubate a patient, it is vital that oxygenation is maintained. A number of supraglottic airway devices are available to help maintain the airway in this situation. The laryngeal mask is probably the most commonly used. You should however familiarize yourself with the emergency airway equipment available on your unit.

Laryngeal masks are relatively simple to use, provide a clear airway and effectively free the operator's hands. Laryngeal masks come in a range of sizes for all ages. Size 3 is suitable for average adult females and size 4 for average adult males.

- Maintain oxygenation by bag and mask.
- Deflate the cuff of the laryngeal mask.
- Lubricate with aqueous gel.
- Pass into the mouth and push back over the tongue into the oropharynx until the laryngeal mask fits naturally in the posterior pharynx.
- Inflate the cuff with 20–30 mL of air.
- Attach breathing circuit.

- Gently ventilate the patient with 100% oxygen and check for chest movement and end-tidal CO_2.
- Seek senior help to secure airway by endotracheal intubation.

PERCUTANEOUS TRACHEOSTOMY

In recent years tracheostomy has become a common procedure on the ICU. Traditionally, tracheostomy was only performed after patients had been intubated for about 10–14 days because of fear of laryngeal and subglottic injury resulting from continued intubation. The advent of percutaneous techniques has allowed tracheostomy to be performed safely and easily at the bedside without the use of specialized surgical instruments, lighting or diathermy. As a result, many units now perform tracheostomy earlier.

Potential advantages of tracheostomy

- More comfortable than naso-/orotracheal tubes, which allows significant reductions in muscle relaxants, sedative and analgesic drugs. This promotes return of GI tract function.
- Patients easily switched from IPPV/assist modes/CPAP/ T-piece without the need for extubation and reintubation.
- Easier clearance of tracheal secretions by suction.
- Speech is possible with cuff deflation or speaking tube.
- There may be a lower risk of airway problems after prolonged tracheostomy than after prolonged translaryngeal intubation.

Despite these potential advantages, the large UK TracMan study failed to show significant benefit from early tracheostomy.

Indications

- Actual or impending airway obstruction. Tracheostomy should be considered early, before progressive swelling makes reintubation in the event of tube blockage or dislodgement potentially impossible.
- Known difficult intubation.
- The need for prolonged IPPV (see below).
- Aid to weaning (see below).
- Inability of patients to protect or maintain their own airway in the longer term, e.g. severe brain injury, bulbar palsy.

Contraindications

These are relative and include:

- coagulopathy
- distorted or abnormal anatomy
- $FiO_2 > 0.6$
- significant haemodynamic instability.

Percutaneous vs surgical tracheostomy

There remains some debate about the relative benefits of percutaneous versus open surgical tracheostomy. Generally percutaneous techniques are associated with less bleeding complications, a lower risk of surgical site infection and better cosmetic result. Otherwise there is little evidence to suggest one is better than the other. Percutaneous techniques are appropriate for most patients on intensive care. Occasional patients with anatomical problems may benefit from an open surgical approach.

Choice of tracheostomy tube

There is a wide range of tracheostomy tubes commercially available. Check what is available in your unit and seek advice on the appropriate choice for different clinical situations. Soft and flexible tubes provide maximum patient comfort, minimizing trauma to trachea and associated structures. More rigid tubes may be preferred in the longer term as they better maintain stoma patency and are easier to change. Cuffed tubes provide airway protection and facilitate intermittent positive pressure ventilation. Disadvantages include the risk of excessive cuff pressure, difficulty in swallowing and communication. Cuff pressure should not exceed 25 cm H_2O (18 mmHg) to reduce the risk of mucosal damage, and subsequent tracheal stenosis. Conventional length tracheostomy tubes may occasionally be too short and tubes with adjustable length flanges are available.

Procedure

Percutaneous tracheostomy. You will need:

Anaesthetic assistance

Nurse to help (not scrubbed)

Universal precautions; sterile gown and gloves

Skin disinfectant

Local anaesthetic (1% lidocaine (lignocaine) + adrenaline (epinephrine), syringe and needle

10 mL normal saline and syringe

Basic surgical instruments (e.g. venous cut down set)

Percutaneous tracheostomy kit

Appropriate size cuffed tracheostomy tubes (1 size smaller and larger than planned)

Suture and securing tapes

Drugs and equipment for emergency reintubation

Bronchoscope (camera/monitor) and light source

> ⚠️ **This procedure requires a separate anaesthetist to manage the patient and airway and an operator to perform the tracheostomy. On no account should percutaneous tracheostomy be attempted by a single operator.**

Explain to the patient (and relatives) what you are going to do. Get written or verbal consent. Check the patient's coagulation status. Position the patient flat with the head and neck extended over a pillow. The majority of patients are already intubated and ventilated and are given either an intravenous or volatile anaesthetic. This is supplemented by infiltration of the surgical area with 10 mL of local anaesthetic plus adrenaline (epinephrine), which helps reduces skin edge bleeding.

A bronchoscope can be passed into the larynx during the procedure (through the endotracheal tube or laryngeal mask). This allows the anaesthetist to ensure that the endotracheal tube is withdrawn to a safe position and allows the operator to visualize the needle puncture of the trachea and the correct placement of guide wire, dilator and tracheostomy tube. A camera system and monitor make this much easier.

Anaesthetist

- Ensure appropriate monitoring and anaesthetize patient with inhalational or intravenous technique as appropriate. Beware of relying solely on intermittent bolus of propofol, as there is a risk of 'awareness'. A muscle relaxant is usually required.
- Suction trachea and oropharynx.
- Ventilate with 100% oxygen throughout the procedure.
- When the operator is ready, withdraw the endotracheal tube under direct vision using a laryngoscope, until the cuff is visible at the laryngeal inlet. This prevents the endotracheal tube being transfixed by the operator's needle when the trachea is punctured.
- Care must be taken not to lose the airway when the tube is withdrawn. Consider passing a gum elastic bougie or airway exchange catheter down the tube prior to withdrawal, to ensure the tube can be replaced if it is pulled back too far. (Equipment must be available to reintubate the patient in case of difficulty.)
- An alternative approach is to remove the endotracheal tube altogether and to use a laryngeal mask to maintain ventilation and oxygenation.
- If a bronchoscope is to be used, pass this down the endotracheal tube or laryngeal mask and into the larynx so that the operator

has a view of the trachea at the level at which needle puncture
will occur.
● Maintain ventilation until the procedure is complete and
then pass the catheter mount to the operator to attach to the
tracheostomy tube.

Operator

Tracheostomy may be safely performed through the cricothyroid
membrane or in the subcricoid region. In the UK it is recommended
that the tracheostomy stoma should be between the 2nd and 4th
tracheal rings. At higher levels there may be an increased risk
of laryngeal/tracheal stenosis, which may ultimately necessitate
tracheal resection. (Resection may not be possible where the lesion
is very high at the level of the first ring.) At lower levels there is an
increased risk of haemorrhage from major vessels in the thoracic
inlet and subsequent tube changes may be more difficult.

There are a number of different percutaneous tracheostomy
kits available. Most require that the trachea is punctured by a
needle and a guide wire passed through the needle into the lumen
of the trachea. This is then used to guide a tracheal dilator, which
creates the tracheostomy, allowing the insertion of a tracheostomy
tube. The following notes are a guide only; the exact details of the
method of insertion will depend upon the system used.

● Check that all necessary equipment is available and prepared.
● Position patient flat with the neck extended over a pillow.
● Examine the neck and ascertain the position of the trachea.
Look for anatomical abnormalities, large veins or palpable
arterial pulsation. (Ultrasound gives good images of deeper
vessels that may be at risk during the procedure.)
● Clean the skin.
● Palpate the cricothyroid membrane and sternal notch. Infiltrate
the skin with 1% lidocaine (lignocaine) and adrenaline
(epinephrine), midway between the two.
● Make a 2-cm superficial incision horizontally across the midline.
● Use blunt forceps and a finger to dissect the pretracheal tissue until
you can feel the tracheal rings and identify the level. If necessary,
tie off the anterior jugular veins, which occasionally bleed.
● Ask the anaesthetist to withdraw the endotracheal tube until the
tip is just within the larynx.
● Puncture the trachea with the introducer needle below the level
of the first tracheal ring and in the midline. Using a saline-filled
syringe, confirm the position of the needle by aspiration of
air/mucus from the trachea. A bronchoscope passed through
the endotracheal tube can also be used to confirm the correct

position of the needle tip within the tracheal lumen. A green seeker needle may be helpful if difficulties are encountered in cannulating the trachea.

- Pass the guide wire through the needle into the trachea and remove the needle.
- Dilate the trachea according to the manufacturer's instructions supplied with the tracheostomy kit used and insert the tracheostomy tube, again according to instructions.
- Remove the introducer and guide wire.
- Suck out any blood from the trachea. Blood clot in the airway may produce total airway obstruction or act as a ball valve, allowing gas in but not out.
- Inflate the cuff and ventilate the patient through the tracheostomy.
- Correct placement of the tube may be confirmed by bronchoscopy or capnography. (Bronchoscopy has the advantage of being able to confirm the position of the tracheal tube in relation to the carina.)
- Check that chest expansion is symmetrical and that there are bilateral breath sounds, and that oxygen saturations are maintained.
- Tie the tracheostomy tube in place using tracheostomy tapes. In addition, it is advisable to place two stay sutures through the wings of the tracheostomy tube to prevent early accidental decannulation.
- Obtain a chest X-ray to confirm position and exclude any complications.

COMMON PROBLEMS DURING PERCUTANEOUS TRACHEOSTOMY

Bleeding

Heavy bleeding from the wound may sometimes occur, particularly if an anterior jugular vein is damaged. If possible place a clip on the bleeding vessel and tie off. Otherwise pack the wound with gauze, apply pressure and wait. If you are near the end of the procedure insert the tracheostomy tube, as this will often tamponade the bleeding. If bleeding does not stop, consider removing the tracheostomy tube (reintubate the patient via the oral route and pass the endotracheal tube beyond the stoma), pack the wound and seek surgical assistance.

Difficulty ventilating the patient

This usually means that the tracheostomy tube has been misplaced. Do not persist as this may produce a tension

Box 15.6 Complications of tracheostomy	
Early	*Late*
Bleeding (may lead to total airway obstruction)	Tracheal stenosis
Pneumothorax	Tracheo–oesophageal fistula
Tube misplacement or dislodgement	Skin tethering/scarring
Air emphysema	Late haemorrhage from innominate vessels
Mucus plugging/obstruction	
Stomal infection	

pneumothorax! Remove the tracheostomy tube and reintubate the patient by the oral route.

Complications

The potential complications of percutaneous tracheostomy are shown in Box 15.6.

Air emphysema is common but, unless accompanied by a pneumothorax, is usually unimportant and will resolve over time. Pneumothorax is generally the result of attempting to ventilate the patient through a misplaced tube, resulting in air tracking down into the mediastinum and pleural cavities.

Care of the patient with a tracheostomy

Patients with tracheostomy tubes should receive adequate humidification of inspired gases to prevent drying, and regular suction to remove secretions. Spare tracheostomy tubes of the same size and one size smaller should be kept at the bedside, together with a pair of tracheal dilators.

Tracheostomy tubes with changeable inner tubes can remain in place up to 30 days. A disadvantage is that the diameter of the inner lumen will be reduced by 1–2 mm, increasing work of breathing. Fenestrated tubes allow airflow through the vocal cords when the tube is occluded or a speaking valve is attached, but increase the potential for aspiration of gastric contents. They are unsuitable for use in ventilated patients.

Changing tracheostomy tubes

Tracheostomy tubes can be changed at any time if necessary, but it is more difficult if the tract is not well established. Administer 100% oxygen and position as for performing a tracheostomy. Pass a large-bore suction catheter (with the end cut off) or gum elastic bougie through the old tracheostomy tube before removing it and use this as a guide to insert the new tube. Facilities for ventilating the patient with a bag and mask and for reintubation should be available in case of difficulty.

Decannulation

When the patient's condition has improved, the question of when to remove the tracheostomy tube inevitably arises. Consideration should be given to the following:

- respiratory effort
- volume of tracheal secretions and ability to cough effectively
- laryngeal competence and ability to swallow pharyngeal secretions
- general condition and strength (can they hold their head up?)
- conscious level.

The ability to cough sputum forcibly out of the tracheostomy tube is probably the most useful indicator of likely successful decannulation. There is a general tendency to leave tracheostomy tubes in the convalescent patient for too long. There is no difficulty in a trial of decannulation, providing the track is well formed (5–7 days after insertion). If decannulation fails, reinsert the tracheostomy tube.

It is not routine practice to suture stomas: they are usually left to granulate on their own. A simple occlusive dressing should be applied over the stoma. Ideally, patients should be seen in an ICU follow-up clinic. If tracheal stenosis or other problems develop, appropriate referral (ENT or thoracic surgery) should be made.

CRICOTHYROIDOTOMY/MINITRACHEOSTOMY

Cricothyroidotomy is a life-saving procedure used to provide emergency access to the airway (e.g. following obstruction of the upper airway) when measures such as bag and mask ventilation and tracheal intubation have failed. It involves the insertion of a small tube through the cricothyroid membrane, through which oxygen/ventilation can be provided until a definitive airway is obtained.

Minitracheostomy is a term used to describe the insertion of a similar small-bore non-cuffed tube through the cricothyroid membrane (4 mm internal diameter), principally to aid the clearance of secretions. The passage of suction catheters stimulates coughing and allows secretions to be aspirated. As a short-term measure these devices may help to prevent the need for naso-/orotracheal intubation and assisted ventilation. The small size of the tube limits its value and the use of minitracheostomy has declined in recent years.

Both cricothyroidotomy and minitracheostomy kits are commercially available. The technique for the insertion of each is essentially the same.

Procedure

Cricothyroidotomy / minitracheostomy. You will need:

Universal precautions; sterile gown and gloves

Skin disinfectant

Sterile drape

Syringe of local anaesthetic/needle/(10 mL of 2% lidocaine (lignocaine) and adrenaline (epinephrine)

Cricothyroidotomy/minitracheostomy kit (containing needle, guide wire, dilator tube and tape)

Suture

Dressing

Explain to the patient what you are going to do. Get written or verbal consent if appropriate. Check the patient's coagulation status. Position the patient comfortably with the head and neck extended over a pillow. Then:

● Palpate anatomy to identify the cricothyroid membrane.
● Clean the neck with antiseptic solution.
● Infiltrate over the cricothyroid membrane with 2–3 mL of local anaesthetic.
● Warn the patient that you are going to make him or her cough and perform cricothyroid puncture with a green 21-gauge needle. Aspirate air to confirm the tracheal position of the needle and rapidly inject 2 mL of lidocaine (lignocaine). Wait for coughing to subside.
● Perform a superficial skin incision.
● Pass the introducing needle into the trachea and aspirate air.
● Pass the guide wire through the needle and then remove the needle.
● Pass the introducer over the guide wire and then slide the cricothyroidotomy / minitracheostomy tube off the introducer. Remove the introducer and guide wire together, leaving the

cricothyroidotomy/minitracheostomy in place. Suction to remove any blood.
- Confirm correct placement by detection of CO_2.
- Obtain CXR to verify the position.

Complications

The complications of minitracheostomy are the same as for formal tracheostomy. Misplacement and bleeding are particular problems.

FIBREOPTIC BRONCHOSCOPY

Flexible fibreoptic bronchoscopy is a useful diagnostic and therapeutic tool in the ICU. In this situation it is usually performed on patients who have access to their airway via an endotracheal tube or tracheostomy.

Indications
- Fibreoptic intubation.
- Removal of secretions (associated with areas of collapse on CXR).
- Retrieval of sputum samples for microbiology.
- Bronchoalveolar lavage (see below).
- Assessment of airway injury and burns.
- Biopsy of tumours and lung tissue.
- Assessment of endotracheal tube position.
- To guide operator during tracheostomy (see above).

Contraindications

These are relative. Patients with high airway pressures, critical oxygenation, cardiovascular instability or raised intracranial pressure may not tolerate bronchoscopy.

Preparation

The bronchoscope should be leak-tested and sterilized before use. This generally takes about 20 minutes. Most hospitals will have automatic washers for this.

 Use of the bronchoscope clearly requires knowledge of the endoscopic anatomy of the bronchial tree. If you do not know this you should not be performing a bronchoscopy.

Procedure

Bronchoscopy. You will need:

Gown gloves and goggles
Bronchoscope
Light source/battery pack
Bowl of sterile water
Suction
Sputum traps
Sterile saline
Swivel connector with bronchoscopy port

Before commencing the procedure, check that the size of the patient's endotracheal tube is adequate to allow bronchoscopy. Tubes smaller than 8 mm internal diameter may be significantly occluded by the bronchoscope, making ventilation and oxygenation of the patient difficult. There are smaller diameter fibreoptic scopes available specifically to aid fibreoptic intubation that may be useful in this situation.

- Attach the swivel connector to the patient's endotracheal or tracheostomy tube.
- Ventilate the patient on 100% oxygen prior to and during the bronchoscopy.
- Adequately sedate the patient and then give a small dose of muscle relaxant (such as atracurium) to prevent the patient biting or coughing on the bronchoscope. Instil 3–5 mL of local anaesthetic (e.g. 1% lidocaine (lignocaine)) down the trachea. It is sensible to have an assistant to look after patient sedation and ventilation while you perform the bronchoscopy.
- Bronchoscopy should be a clean procedure to avoid contaminating the patient's airway.
- Lubricate the scope with a small amount of lubricant jelly. Avoid getting it over the lens.

 When handling the scope never allow it to bend or fold at an acute angle, as this will break the fibreoptic components.

- Pass the bronchoscope through the bung on the swivel connector and into the endotracheal or tracheostomy tube. Continue forward under direct vision.

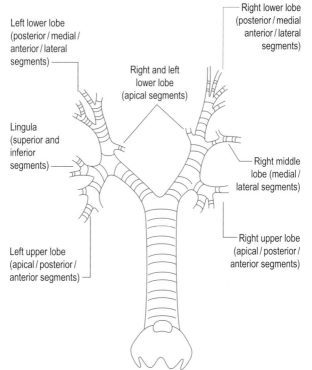

Fig. 15.8 Anatomy of the bronchial tree.

Left lower lobe
(posterior / medial /
anterior / lateral
segments)

Right and left
lower lobe
(apical segments)

Right lower lobe
(posterior / medial
anterior / lateral
segments)

Lingula
(superior and
inferior
segments)

Right middle
lobe (medial /
lateral segments)

Left upper lobe
(apical / posterior /
anterior segments)

Right upper lobe
(apical / posterior /
anterior segments)

- Pass the scope forward to the carina. Then explore each side
  of the bronchial tree in turn. Identify and enter each lobar and
  segmental bronchus (Fig. 15.8). Take note of any abnormal
  anatomy and remove any secretions.
- If there are thick secretions that cannot be sucked up the scope,
  try instilling 10–20 mL of sterile saline down the suction port of
  the bronchoscope. This may help to loosen them. Large plugs
  and blood clots may be dragged out on the end of the scope.
- To obtain microbiology specimens place a sputum trap in
  between the bronchoscope and the wall suction. Use a separate
  trap for each side. Be careful to keep the sputum trap upright
  to prevent the secretions disappearing down the suction tubing.
  Also remove sputum traps before removing the scope from the

patient to prevent specimens being contaminated with upper airway flora.

- Trainees in intensive care should not perform bronchial biopsy. If you see a suspicious lesion that you think is a tumour or something else, leave it. Call for help to ascertain how to diagnose/manage the problem. Note that clotted blood over time becomes white and can mimic tumour appearances to the uninitiated.
- Following bronchoscopy, perform a CXR to exclude pneumothorax and look for improvement in lung expansion where large sputum plugs have been removed.
- Ensure the scope is washed and sterilized according to your hospital policy.

BRONCHOALVEOLAR LAVAGE

Bronchoalveolar lavage (BAL) is a technique for obtaining microbiology specimens from low in the respiratory tree, avoiding contamination of samples with upper respiratory tract flora. It may be performed during bronchoscopy or using specially designed BAL catheters.

Indications

BAL may be used to obtain specimens in any patient with pneumonia. It is of particular value in investigating pneumonia in the immunocompromised patient. In addition to conventional pathogens such as *Streptococcus pneumoniae* and *Haemophilus influenzae*, other likely pathogens in these patients are *Pneumocystis carinii*, either alone or with a co-pathogen, *Mycobacterium* species including tuberculosis, cytomegalovirus and fungi. Discuss the clinical situation with a microbiologist before performing the BAL. He or she will advise on appropriate specimens and tests (see below).

BAL during bronchoscopy

This has the advantage that the operator can be highly selective in the area for lavage in the case of localized disease. It is, however, more invasive and operator-dependent.

- During bronchoscopy advance the bronchoscope into a subsegmental bronchus until it wedges.
- Instil 100 mL of saline down the suction channel.
- Aspirate and collect into a sputum trap.
- Repeat from left/right lung and or different segments as required.

Not all the saline instilled will be aspirated back. This does not matter. If necessary repeat the procedure until an adequate. volume specimen is obtained.

Box 15.7 Investigation following BAL

Microscopy, culture and sensitivity including TB (AAFB)

Differential cell count

Fungi

Viruses

Legionella

Pneumocystis carinii

BAL using catheter

BAL catheters consist of a protective outer sleeve and an inner suction catheter. The suction catheter can be connected via a three-way tap to suction and a syringe for instilling saline. This should be a clean procedure and you should wear apron, gloves and goggles.

● Preoxygenate the patient with 100% oxygen.
● Pass the catheter, with inner tube protected, into the airway, beyond the endotracheal tube.
● Advance the inner protected suction catheter forwards until it meets resistance. Do not use undue force.
● Perform BAL according to local protocol. Generally 80–100 mL of saline are instilled down the suction catheter, and then aspirated into two or three sputum traps. Not all the saline may be aspirated. This does not matter, it will be absorbed.
● Withdraw the inner suction catheter into the protective sleeve before removing from the patient.

Having performed a BAL, telephone the laboratory and then send samples immediately with full diagnostic information and appropriate requests (Box 15.7).

INSERTION OF CHEST DRAIN

The emergency treatment of *life-threatening* tension pneumothorax is large-bore needle decompression. The diagnosis is made on clinical grounds without chest X-ray. (Hyper-resonance, reduced breath sounds, deviated trachea, haemodynamic compromise.) A 14-gauge cannula is inserted into the pleural cavity immediately above the second rib in the midclavicular line to allow air under tension in the pleural space to escape. This should always be followed by placement of a formal chest drain.

> ⚠ **Do not attempt 'blind' needle decompression unless there is clear evidence of life threatening tension pneumothorax. Insertion of a needle in other circumstances is likely to create a problem where one may not have existed before.**

Indications
Chest drains are indicated for the drainage of air (pneumothorax), blood (haemothorax), fluid (pleural effusion), pus (empyema) and lymph (chylothorax) from the pleural cavity. In critically ill patients pleural fluid is a common finding on chest X-rays.

Ultrasound is the best method of assessing pleural effusions at the bedside. Pleural fluid is seen as a black echo-poor medium between the two layers of the pleura. In most cases unless the effusion is large or ventilation is clearly compromised there is no need to drain this fluid. The effusion will resolve as the patient's condition improves. Collections greater than 1–2 cm in depth over a large proportion of the chest, are likely to be significant and may require drainage. Smaller effusions may be tapped/drained for diagnostic purposes, e.g. to identify infection/tumour.

Blood in the pleural cavity should be drained as soon as possible. Once it becomes clotted it will not drain readily and thoracotomy may be required to remove the clot and allow the lung to re-expand.

Type of drain
Chest drains are of two types. Traditionally large-bore tubes, particularly suitable for draining blood or pus, have been placed manually through an incision made in the chest wall directly into the pleural cavity. More recently, Seldinger versions have become available. Seldinger drains should only be used 'blindly' to drain obvious large collections because of the risk that the introducer needle may damage the lung. For smaller collections, Seldinger drains should be placed under ultrasound guidance to reduce the risks of needle damage.

Site of drain
This is partly dictated by the position of the collection clinically and radiographically. In the case of long-standing collections, which may be loculated, ultrasound guidance may be helpful.

In all other cases the drain should be sited in the 5th intercostal space, just anterior to the midaxillary line, and can be directed cephalad for air and caudally for fluid or blood. All drains should be placed immediately above the rib to avoid damage to the neurovascular bundle, which lies underneath.

 Use of the 2nd intercostal space in the midclavicular line (anterior approach) is associated with risk of injury to the internal mammary artery and breast tissue (in the female) and may result in unsightly scarring. Do not use this approach.

Procedure

Chest drainage. You will need:

Universal precautions; sterile gown and gloves

Skin disinfectant

Sterile drape

10-mL syringe, local anaesthetic and needles (lidocaine (lignocaine) 1–2%)

Basic instruments: scalpel, blade, large arterial clamps

Chest drain

Strong silk sutures, adhesive strapping and dressings

Underwater seal, low-pressure vacuum (wall vacuum or pump)

Insertion of drain through thoracostomy

- Explain procedure to the patient.
- Position the patient (supine with arm lifted, a pillow behind back).
- Prepare a sterile field.
- Infiltrate superficial structures down to rib with local anaesthetic.
- Make a 2–4 cm incision.
- Palpate through skin incision and perform blunt dissection down to rib and through pleura.
- Push finger into pleural cavity and sweep around to ensure no viscera are adjacent.
- Insert drain and direct into appropriate position.

 Do not use trocars to insert drains. They are sharp and may cause injury to underlying viscera.

- Connect to underwater drain and confirm position by drainage of collection and respiratory swing.
- Secure drain in position with suture. Purse-string sutures result in very unsightly scarring when chest drains are removed and are best avoided. Use mattress sutures to close the skin edges and a simple tie to hold in the drain.
- Order a chest X-ray.

Insertion of Seldinger drains and pigtail catheters
- Explain procedure to the patient and position as before.
- Ideally determine and mark the optimal position for drain site using ultrasound.
- Prepare a sterile field.
- Infiltrate superficial structures down to rib with local anaesthetic.
- Advance needle through chest until blood/fluid/air aspirated.
- Feed guide wire into pleural space.
- Pass chest drain/pigtail catheter over guide wire.
- For large drains attach underwater seal as above, for pigtail catheters aspirate and/or attach drainage bag.
- Secure in situ and apply dressing.
- Order a CXR.

 DO NOT CLAMP CHEST DRAINS. If moving a patient, simply keep the underwater drain bottle below the level of the chest. Clamping drains may produce a tension pneumothorax.

COMMON PROBLEMS DURING INSERTION OF CHEST DRAINS

Lung will not expand
The stiff non-compliant lung full of secretions and fluid may not re-expand immediately but should do so over time.

- Reassess diagnosis and position of tube.
- Is tube 'swinging' or is it blocked/kinked? Is the effusion loculated?
- Consider low-pressure suction (wall suction or pump 10–20 mmHg).
- Increase tidal volume or add 10 cm of PEEP.
- Consider the need for CT scan and surgical referral (see below).

When assessing a chest drain on X-ray, look at the length of the tube and whether it is kinked or needs to be pulled back or has slipped out. Check the position of the drainage holes – are they within the chest. The limitations of an AP chest X-ray should be appreciated. Tubes may lie within the lung parenchyma and this will only be identified on CT.

Persistent air leak

- Check the drain and reposition if necessary (it may have come out of the chest and be entraining room air). If air leak persists, attempt to minimize airway pressures.
- In trauma patients, consider bronchoscopy to exclude airway rupture.
- Wean patient onto spontaneous breathing modes.
- If ventilated, ensure adequate sedation, analgesia and muscle relaxation.
- Use pressure-controlled ventilation and reduce PEEP.
- Accept a degree of hypercapnia, e.g. $PaCO_2$ 8 kPa.
- Consider high frequency jet ventilation.
- Consider thoracic surgical opinion (see below).

Indications for urgent thoracic surgical opinion

The combination of persistent air leak and non-compliant lungs (e.g. ARDS) may make adequate ventilation and gas exchange impossible. Urgent thoracic surgical opinion may be required (Box 15.8).

Removing chest drains

Chest drains can be removed when they are no longer needed. In practice, this means that if the clinical and CXR findings that required a chest drain have resolved, and the drain is no longer bubbling or draining fluid, it can be removed.

Do not clamp chest drains prior to removal. If a drain is not bubbling or draining, it is not performing any useful function. Remove it and re-site it if necessary.

Box 15.8 Indications for surgical opinion / thoracotomy

Collection not fully drained or lung not fully re-expanded

Massive air leak (bronchopleural fistula / ruptured bronchus)

Continued bleeding

Presence / suspected presence of other intrathoracic injuries

- Clean the site with antiseptic solution.
- Cut the retaining suture, remove the drain and occlude by pressing.
- On removing the drain, ask the patient (if breathing spontaneously) to hold their breath.
- Close the wound with a suture. If this is already in situ it can be tied as the drain is removed to reduce any air entrainment. (Avoid purse strings, as above.)
- Cover with sterile occlusive dressing.
- Obtain a CXR.

PASSING A NASOGASTRIC TUBE

Most patients in the ICU who require ventilation require a nasogastric tube, initially at least, to ensure gastric drainage and early enteral feeding (Box 15.9).

Procedure

Passing a nasogastric tube. You will need:

Gloves and mask

NG tube

Lubricating jelly

Laryngoscope

Magill forceps

- Explain to the patient what you are going to do, even if he or she is apparently unconscious.
- Position the patient supine with head neutral.

Box 15.9 Indications and contraindications for nasogastric tube

Indications	Contraindications
To deflate the stomach after bag mask ventilation	Base of skull fracture (use orogastric tube)
To aspirate gastric contents which might otherwise reflux and soil the airway	Recent gastric or oesophageal surgery (discuss with surgeon)
To provide a route for enteral feeding and drugs	Oesophageal varices (relative contraindication)
	Severe coagulopathy (consider oral route to avoid nose bleed)

- Lubricate the NG tube and, keeping alignment with the long axis of the patient, introduce through the nose. Do not force. If resistance is met, try the other side.
- If the patient is cooperative, ask them to swallow the tip of the tube when they feel it in the back of the throat. In unconscious patients the tube may pass directly into the oesophagus but often coils up in the mouth.
- In this case, use a laryngoscope to examine the pharynx and pass the tube manually into the oesophagus using a pair of Magill forceps. (Be careful not to traumatize the uvula and pharyngeal mucosa.)
- Confirm the position of the NG tube in the stomach by aspiration of gastric contents (turns litmus paper red). Position below the diaphragm should be subsequently verified on chest X-ray.
- Secure the NG tube in position with adhesive tape.

> ⚠ **Beware that the presence of a cuffed endotracheal or tracheostomy tube does necessarily prevent gastric tubes entering the lung. Awake patients can tolerate fine bore tubes within the lung and it should be appreciated that some nasogastric tubes only have a radio-opaque marker on the distal segment, which may be well out in the periphery of the lung.**

Transpyloric feeding tubes

Nasoduodenal/nasojejunal feeding tubes are fine-bore soft tubes designed for long-term use. They are usually provided with the feeding tube mounted on a wire insert, which stiffens the tube during placement and helps X-ray determination of position. This is removed once the tube is in place.

The main difficulty in passing these feeding tubes is getting them to pass through the pylorus. The simplest approach is to pass a reasonable length of tube into the stomach (as for NG tube above) and leave for a few hours before getting an abdominal X-ray. Some tubes will simply migrate into the duodenum/jejunum. Alternatively, transpyloric tubes can be placed using X-ray screening, ultrasound or with endoscopic guidance. Seek advice.

PASSING A SENGSTAKEN–BLAKEMORE TUBE

A number of tubes have been designed to apply pressure to oesophageal varices in order to compress the vessels and reduce bleeding while the patient is resuscitated and definitive treatment carried out. The Sengstaken–Blakemore tube has three lumens. Two are used to inflate balloons, one in the stomach and the other in the oesophagus, while the third is used to aspirate gastric contents.

Procedure

Passing a Sengstaken–Blakemore tube. You will need:

Universal precautions

Suction apparatus

Sengstaken–Blakemore tube (usually kept in a fridge)

500 mL saline

50 mL syringe

Traction (string and 500 mL bag of fluid)

- Read instructions for the specific device you are using.
- Explain to the patient what you are going to do.
- Position the patient comfortably. Left lateral is best if the patient is vomiting.
- Check the patency of the tube lumens and integrity of the balloons.
- Pass the tube orally into the oesophagus and down into the stomach. (Local anaesthetic spray to the pharynx may make this more tolerable in the awake patient.) Insert the tube to at least 35 cm (>55 cm may enter the duodenum).
- Inflate the gastric balloon with 250 mL of saline. You should not feel any resistance.
- Pull the tube backwards gently until resistance is felt as the gastric balloon meets the gastro-oesophageal junction.
- Inflate the oesophageal balloon with air or saline (approximately 100 mL). The pressure in the oesophageal balloon can be measured using a sphygmomanometer and should be 25–35 mmHg. Chest pain, respiratory difficulty and cardiac arrhythmias may occur during inflation of the balloon.
- Apply traction to the tube by tying a piece of string to the end and suspending a 500 mL bag of fluid over a fulcrum. Traction should be released at regular intervals to prevent pressure necrosis of the gastro–oesophageal junction.
- The position of the tube should be checked by CXR. The point where the tube exits the mouth should be marked in order to detect subsequent migration. Check the pressure in the oesophageal balloon regularly.

Removing the tube

After 24 h the traction should be removed and the oesophageal balloon deflated to assess for bleeding. If bleeding recurs, the balloon can be reinflated for a further period of 24 h; however, the need for intervention becomes increasingly likely. If there is no bleeding the tube is usually left in situ (deflated) for 24 h in case bleeding recurs. After this time the tube can be removed. Endoscopy and sclerosis or banding of varices will usually be required.

PERITONEAL TAP/DRAINAGE OF ASCITES

Ascites is common in liver failure, severe right heart failure and some malignancies. Peritoneal tap may be indicated to obtain samples for diagnostic purposes, e.g. microbiological culture/cytology. Drainage of large collections may be indicated where there is raised intra-abdominal pressure, distension and/or respiratory compromise.

Drainage of ascites: You will need:

Universal precautions; sterile gown and gloves

Skin disinfectant

Sterile drape

10-mL syringe, local anaesthetic lidocaine (lignocaine) 1–2% and needles

Pig tail drain

Sutures, adhesive strapping and dressings

Ultrasound

- Before commencing procedure perform ultrasound to demonstrate fluid and verify position for needle puncture away from bowel (Fig. 15.9).
- Clean skin with 2% chlorhexidine in alcohol. Apply drape
- Introduce needle at chosen site (typically low down and lateral to right iliac fosse)
- Aspirate fluid and send for culture.
- Introduce pig tail drain using Seldinger technique if required.
- Suture drain and apply occlusive dressing.

There is debate about how much fluid should be drained and what replacement fluid should be used. Seek local guidance.

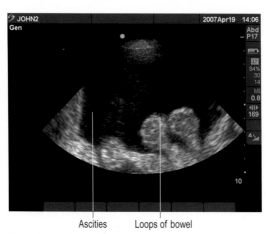

Ascities   Loops of bowel

Fig. 15.9 Ultrasound of the abdomen showing ascites.

TURNING A PATIENT PRONE

Patients may be turned prone when oxygenation is critical despite ventilation and high inspired oxygen concentrations. (See ALI, p. 154.) Turning large adult patients prone can be hazardous both for the staff and the patient. Where possible, hoists or other aids to handling patients should be used. The nursing staff will advise on the best approach. In general terms, whatever approach to physically turning the patient is adopted, there must be adequate numbers of staff available to ensure patient safety, and security of airway, vascular cannulae and drains, etc.

- Temporarily discontinue all non-essential drug and fluid infusions.
- Ensure that all lines and monitoring cables are positioned such that they will not be trapped under the patient when he or she is turned.
- Remove ECG electrodes from the patient's front and replace on the back.
- Designate specific individuals to be responsible for maintaining the security of the endotracheal tube, vascular access and lines. Designate other individuals to turn the patient.
- Position pillows so that they will be under the patient's chest and pelvis when the patient is prone. Alternatively, position

them afterwards. They are to ensure that the abdomen is not compressed, which can impair venous return and CO.
- When everyone is ready, use the commands 'ready, steady, move'. Turn the patient on 'move'.
- Ensure the patient is comfortably positioned and that there is no pressure on the tip of the nose, eyes or any peripheral nerves. The arms should be positioned towards the patient's head (not unduly extended) to ensure there is no tension on the brachial plexus.
- Re-establish any monitoring or drugs and fluid infusions that were previously discontinued.

TRANSPORT OF CRITICALLY ILL PATIENTS

Critically ill patients in intensive care often require transport either within the hospital (for example for investigations or surgery), or between hospitals (for example, for specialist care). You are therefore likely to be involved in transporting a patient at some stage, even if only within your own hospital.

The standards of care during transport, whether intrahospital or interhospital, should be the same as that provided within the ICU. Before moving the patient, it is important that the patient is fully resuscitated and stable. If there is any doubt regarding the adequacy of resuscitation, this should be addressed before transfer. The general principles are as follows:

- Full monitoring should be continued. This should include blood pressure monitoring (preferably invasive), ECG, oxygen saturation, and end-tidal CO_2 for intubated/ventilated patients. If a PA catheter is in situ the pressure trace must be displayed, or the catheter should be pulled back into the SVC to prevent inadvertent pulmonary artery occlusion.
- Ensure that the airway is secure; this usually means endotracheal intubation.
- Ensure adequate supplies of oxygen to complete the transfer. In case the supply fails, an alternative means of ventilating the patient should be available. This should be a self-inflating bag, rather than an anaesthetic breathing circuit.
- Ensure that a portable suction unit is available.
- Ensure adequate intravenous access, usually at least two secure intravenous cannulae.
- Discontinue non-essential drug infusions. Ensure that essential infusions are delivered using syringe pumps with fully charged batteries.

- Ensure any drugs or resuscitation equipment that you are likely to need during the transfer are available.

During the transfer you should be accompanied by an intensive care nurse or an operating department assistant. The transfer should be fully documented, including a record of pulse, blood pressure, ventilation and other vital signs. In the case of inter-hospital transfer, notify the receiving hospital of your departure and expected arrival times in advance to enable suitable preparation to be made.

CHAPTER 16

END OF LIFE ISSUES

Introduction 430

Treatment limitation decisions 430

Managing withdrawal of treatment 431

Confirming death 433

Breaking bad news 434

Issuing a death certificate 434

Post-mortem examinations 435

Reporting deaths to the coroner 436

Brainstem death and organ donation 437

Non-heart beating organ donation 439

Cultural aspects of death and dying 440

Dealing with death at a personal level 443

INTRODUCTION

Mortality rates on ICUs range from 15 to 35%, depending on case mix, and are typically about 20%. In addition, significant numbers of patients die soon after leaving the ICU. The ability to deal with death and the issues surrounding it is therefore an important part of work on an ICU. The dying patient must be afforded respect and allowed to die with dignity, while relatives must also be treated sympathetically. If handled appropriately, relatives will often gain great comfort from the peaceful passing of a loved one and be grateful for all that has been done.

It is particularly important to be honest and to recognize when patients are deteriorating such that death is inevitable. Once recognized, the family can be warned and relatives from further afield given the opportunity to travel to the hospital. Decisions regarding the continuation or withdrawal of treatment should be made in a timely but unhurried manner, avoiding the need for frantic telephone calls in the middle of the night in the event of a cardiac arrest.

TREATMENT LIMITATION DECISIONS

Patients are often admitted to the ICU for a period of stabilization and assessment. Over time, however, it may become clear that the patient has no prospect of meaningful recovery. Under these circumstances, a decision may be made to withdraw treatment or limit further escalation of treatment. In this setting it is important to understand that there is no medico–legal obligation to continue treatment that is futile and, indeed, to do so could be considered as assault on the patient. Treatment limitation may take a number of forms depending on individual circumstances and local practice (see Box 16.1).

Box 16.1 Potential treatment limitation options

Not admitting patient to ICU

Admitting patient to ICU but limiting time for response to treatment (Withdrawal of active treatment if no response)

Limiting range of treatments offered (e.g. not for dialysis/ventilation/inotropes)

Not escalating treatment in face of further deterioration (e.g. ceiling on inotropes)

Not attempting resuscitation in case of cardiac arrest

Withdrawal of active treatment

In general, decisions to limit treatment are made in conjunction with all members of the multidisciplinary team. There should usually be consensus from all clinicians and nursing staff involved with care of the patient that continuation of life-sustaining treatment is inappropriate. If there is any doubt, it is usually better to continue treatment until consensus is reached. The final decision to limit treatment, however, rests with the consultant intensivist and the referring consultant in conjunction with the patient or the patient's representative.

Recent changes in the UK (Mental Capacity Act 2005) have helped clarify the role of the patient's next of kin and independent advocates in decision making in such circumstances.

Independent mental capacity advocates

All decisions regarding the limitation of intensive care treatment should, wherever possible, be made in conjunction with the patient. Intensive care patients are frequently unconscious or sedated, and are therefore rarely competent to be involved in decisions regarding limitation of treatment. In the event that the patient cannot participate, the views of his next of kin should be taken into account. Rarely, neither the patient nor a relation or friend is available to take part in such a discussion. In the United Kingdom, this situation is covered by the Mental Capacity Act 2005, which came into force in 2007. This lays out a framework for the appointment of an independent mental capacity advocate (IMCA). It is the right of all patients lacking capacity to have an advocate to speak up for their interests, whether their next of kin or an IMCA. Individual hospitals have local arrangements for contacting the IMCA service and appointing and IMCA.

Documenting treatment limitation

All treatment limitation decisions and DNR orders must be clearly documented in the notes. Decisions should be reviewed regularly and reversed or revoked if the situation or condition leading to them changes.

MANAGING WITHDRAWAL OF TREATMENT

The best approach to the actual process of withdrawal of treatment will vary from case to case. From a legal point of view, there is no distinction drawn between, for example, the withdrawal of vasoactive drugs and assisted ventilation. Commonly:

● Inotropes and vasopressor agents may be discontinued.
● Artificial ventilation may be withdrawn.

- The endotracheal tube may be removed.
- The inspired oxygen concentration may be reduced.
- The patient should be kept comfortable throughout the process. (See Euthanasia below.)
- Fluids and nutrition are usually continued, as hydration is considered an important aspect of patient comfort.

 Do not use the term 'withdrawal of care'. Care for both the patient and their relatives, continues throughout the process of withdrawal of life-sustaining treatment.

Consideration should be given as to when and where is the best place for withdrawal of treatment to occur. The process is often best managed in the intensive care unit, where staff can support the patient and relatives. Some units have developed so-called 'tender loving care' rooms specifically designed for this purpose. In some circumstances it may be more appropriate to transfer the patient to a general ward. Occasionally, particularly when patients are aware of their surroundings and what is happening, it may be appropriate to transfer the patient somewhere else, such as a hospice, or even home, in order that they may die in peaceful surroundings. Consideration should also be given to the timing of withdrawal of treatment in order that relatives visiting from afar may be present.

Relatives will often ask how long death will take. In general terms, the greater the level of support withdrawn, the more quickly death is likely to occur. In many patients death can be confidently predicted to occur quite quickly, while in others prediction may be more difficult. Rarely patients may even apparently improve temporarily following withdrawal. Unless it is absolutely clear that a patient will die quickly, it is best not to make predictions about the speed of death. Say that you do not know, but will be in a better position to judge once life-sustaining therapy has been withdrawn.

 The withdrawal of life-sustaining therapy such as nasogastric feeding from patients in persistent vegetative state (PVS), who do not otherwise require any form of organ support, is a complex legal issue. This would normally take place outside the ICU and is beyond the scope of this book.

Euthanasia

UK law does not allow the practice of euthanasia. Patients who are dying should not, however, be allowed to suffer needlessly. It is permissible to administer sedative or analgesic drugs to relieve patient distress, accepting that in some cases the administration of these drugs will speed up the process of death. This is known as the 'doctrine of double effect'. Most units would prescribe benzodiazepines or opioids for this purpose and many relatives gain comfort from the fact that the dying patient is not allowed to suffer unnecessarily. It is important in this respect, however, to distinguish between the patient's suffering and the distress of relatives or staff. It is not acceptable to administer drugs that potentially shorten life solely to ease the distress of relatives or carers.

CONFIRMING DEATH

When a patient dies, death must be confirmed by a doctor. Interestingly, there is no legally agreed definition of death in the UK (other than brainstem death); however, it is generally taken to include cessation of breathing and the absence of a heartbeat. Note the following and record findings in the medical records along with the date and time of death:

- Absence of palpable pulse. Absence of heart sounds.
- Absence of respiratory effort (disconnect ventilator). Absence of breath sounds.
- Pupils are fixed and dilated.

> ⚠ **Confirming death in severely hypothermic patients (e.g. following cold water immersion) is very difficult. Remember 'patients should not be declared dead until they are warm and dead'. This may require lengthy attempts at resuscitation and rewarming. If in doubt, seek senior help. (See Hypothermia, p. 224.)**

Who to inform

Once death is confirmed, you must make sure that the relatives have been informed (see below). You should also inform the people listed below, although this can often wait until the next morning if the patient has died out of hours; actions will depend upon the circumstances and, in particular, whether or not the death was expected:

- Referring clinician(s).
- Consultant in charge of intensive care.
- The patient's general practitioner. (This is especially important. It fosters good relations between the hospital and the community and allows the GP an opportunity to offer counselling and support to the relatives.)
- Coroner's officer, if appropriate (see below).

BREAKING BAD NEWS

This is never an easy task, particularly if the death has occurred unexpectedly or if the patient was very young. If the relatives are not present at the time of the death they will generally be called by a senior nurse and asked to come into the hospital. Try to avoid talking on the telephone if at all possible.

When relatives are present or when they arrive, you should speak to them in a quiet side room. It is worth checking that all relevant members of the family are present, as different branches of families may not communicate.

- Follow the basic guidelines on talking to relatives. (See Talking to relatives, p. 28.)
- Be honest but not brutal!
- Avoid euphemisms such as 'he slipped away' as these may not be interpreted in the way you expect. Clearly say that the patient has died.
- Relatives often find it helpful to know that their loved one was not in any pain or distress, if this is true.

The stages of bereavement include denial, anger and gradual acceptance. Any of these emotions may be expressed. It is not uncommon for the initial response to take the form of anger, particularly if relatives believe that things have gone badly for their loved one. Such anger often subsides over time as the realities of the situation become apparent. Sympathetic handling, honesty and compassion with relatives will avoid many later complaints.

Many units now offer relatives the chance to return at a later date to revisit the sequence of events surrounding a patient's death and to ask any questions they may have. This is a valuable part of the grieving process for relatives. Formal grief counselling may benefit some relatives.

ISSUING A DEATH CERTIFICATE

The death certificate asks you to give information about the cause of death. You can issue a death certificate if:

- You have attended to the patient during the last illness, and you have seen the patient alive within 14 days of the death (28 days in Scotland and Northern Ireland).
- You are satisfied that the death was due to natural causes (see below).
- You are reasonably sure of the cause of death.
- There is no specific requirement to inform the coroner.

If you can issue a death certificate, then complete the relevant sections. Once complete, the death certificate is then given to the patient's next of kin so that they can register the death. In many hospitals a bereavement liaison officer will handle these matters. Ensure that you fill in the form as accurately as possible, as it is very distressing for relatives if the registrar of births, marriages and deaths rejects the certificate:

- Write legibly. If your handwriting is difficult to read, it is best to print the details.
- Do not use terms such as heart failure as a sole cause of death. (Strictly this is a mode of death rather than a cause.) If used, these terms must be backed up by an underlying diagnosis, e.g. ischaemic heart disease.
- Print your name next to your signature so that you can be easily identified in case of difficulty.

POST-MORTEM EXAMINATIONS

Where the cause of death is known but information from a post-mortem examination would be of interest, you may ask the family for permission to perform a hospital post-mortem. Where a death occurs after major surgery, most surgeons will request a post-mortem. This may help clarify the events leading up to the death. There is space on the death certificate to record that more information may subsequently be available from a post-mortem. In this case the registrar's office will write to you once the result of the post-mortem is available.

 If you do not know the cause of death, then you cannot ask for a hospital post-mortem. In this instance the death must be reported to the coroner.

Consent to post-mortem examination

Fully informed consent is required from relatives for both post-mortem examination and for the retention of any tissue samples. Consent will often be obtained by the referring clinicians, for example the surgeon, if the patient has died shortly following surgery. If you are required to obtain consent for a post-mortem, you must be aware of what the examination will entail and what samples may be retained. This may require you to discuss the details of the post-mortem with the pathologist. There is an option to request only a limited post-mortem, e.g. a liver biopsy or lung biopsy. This will often provide sufficient information to answer clinical questions and may be more acceptable to the family.

REPORTING DEATHS TO THE CORONER

If you are unable to issue a death certificate, you must report the death to the coroner (Procurator Fiscal in Scotland). The commoner indications for reporting a death to the coroner are given in Box 16.2. If in doubt, ask.

If in any doubt, you should discuss the death with the coroner. You will generally deal with the coroner's officer. There is usually a specially trained policemen with variable degrees of medical

---

Box 16.2 Indications for reporting death to the coroner

Death cannot be certified as due to natural causes

Deceased not seen by a doctor within the last 14 days

Death occurred within 24 h of hospital admission

Death occurred in suspicious circumstances or following an accident or violence

Death occurred during or shortly after imprisonment or while in police custody

Death occurred while deceased was detained under Mental Health Act

Death may have been contributed to by actions of deceased, including self-injury or drug abuse

Death associated with neglect, including self-neglect

Deceased was receiving any form of war pension or industrial disability pension

Death could be in any way related to the deceased's employment

Death associated with abortion, spontaneous or induced

Death occurring during an operation or before full recovery from the effects of an anaesthetic or in any way related to an anaesthetic*

Death was related to a medical procedure or treatment*

Death may be due to lack of medical care*

---

*It is advisable to discuss any death following surgery or other procedure with the coroner. There is no formal time limit laid down for this.

knowledge, but is nevertheless a useful source of advice. When speaking to the coroner's officer, you will need the following information:

- deceased patient's name, date of birth, address
- address and telephone number of next of kin and GP
- brief summary of the patient's last illness, including date of admission, diagnosis, operations, complications, and date and time of death
- reason for reporting death
- suggested cause of death if prepared to offer a death certificate.

If the cause of death is not suspicious, or unnatural, the coroner may give permission for you to issue a death certificate (initial box 'A' on the reverse of the death certificate). In this case, the cause of death cited on the form is agreed with the coroner's officer, who then issues a covering slip to the registrar's office.

If the cause of death is unknown, or is suspicious or unnatural, then the coroner's officer will take over. Generally a coroner's post-mortem will be performed, and if necessary an inquest convened.

Situation in Scotland

In Scotland the situation is slightly different. The Procurator Fiscal investigates deaths reported to him or her. The main concern is to establish evidence of negligence or criminality rather than the cause of death. If satisfied that the death is natural, the Procurator Fiscal may instruct a doctor to examine the body and issue a death certificate. If the cause of death is suspicious, an application must be made to the sheriff for a post-mortem examination. The cause of death is then certified by the pathologist. If there is evidence of negligence or criminality, then the Lord Advocate may order that a fatal accident enquiry be held.

BRAINSTEM DEATH AND ORGAN DONATION

The brainstem is responsible for the maintenance of life-sustaining functions within the body, in particular the maintenance and adequacy of respiration. With the advent of modern intensive care, it is possible for patients in whom brainstem death has occurred to be on a ventilator and still have a heart beat and pulse. These patients are not capable of sustaining life on their own. Brainstem death is therefore now a legally accepted definition of death, the diagnosis of which is governed by strict guidelines and protocols. Patients who are brainstem dead and on a ventilator may be suitable for organ donation. (See Brainstem death, p. 297.)

Consent for organ donation

Patients who are listed on the organ donor register can be considered to have made an advanced directive and their wishes should, where appropriate, be complied with. Keep the relatives informed. If patients are not on the donor register, then consent to the organ donation process can be obtained from the next of kin.

The most appropriate time to approach the subject of organ donation will depend upon the individual circumstances of the case. Relatives will often discuss the subject informally with staff, and it is reasonable to explain about the possibility of donation at any time once the possibility of brainstem death is raised. However, the diagnosis of brainstem death and the request for organ donation are separate issues. You certainly should not make any formal approach until brainstem death has been confirmed. Transplant coordinators are willing to come and speak to relatives about donation if required.

Not all relatives will give consent to organ donation; some religious groups in particular find it difficult. You must accept their wishes, no matter what your own views are. (A code of practice for the diagnosis and confirmation of death. Academy of Medical Royal Colleges 2008. http://www.aomrc.org.uk/aomrc/admin/reports/docs/DofD-final.pdf.)

 You must also seek the coroner's permission for organ donation from those patients whose death would normally require referral to the coroner. (See Reporting deaths to the coroner, p. 436).

Practicalities of donor management

Transplant surgeons are accepting organs (particularly kidneys) from more unstable and elderly patients than in the past, and in addition there is increasing utilization of tissues such as bone, skin and heart valves. If in doubt about what can be used, ask the transplant coordinator. Each region has one or more transplant coordinators who will liaise between the organ retrieval teams and the referring hospital. They will also provide advice on the management of the donor.

The management of a potential brainstem dead organ donor is essentially similar to that of other ICU patients, (particularly those with brain injury). The aim is optimization of physiological parameters, particularly oxygen delivery, and avoidance of secondary physiological insults to organ systems.

Box 16.3 Tests prior to organ donation

Tissue typing
HIV
Hepatitis screening
U&Es
Glucose
LFTs & amylase
ECG
CXR
Height, weight and girth measurements

Problems after brainstem death include:

● Haemodynamic disturbances – with low CO and/or SVR. Oxygen uptake and CO_2, production may be abnormally low. Large volumes of fluid may be required to maintain adequate filling pressures and inotropes/vasopressors are frequently necessary to maintain adequate perfusion pressures. Optimization of the cardiovascular system may require invasive monitoring.

● Poor gas exchange is common (e.g. neurogenic pulmonary oedema), and frequently lungs are unsuitable for transplantation. Ventilation should be optimized.

● Pituitary function is impaired. Diabetes insipidus is common: use DDAVP (0.5–1 μg, i.v.) as necessary to reduce urine output to sensible volumes. (See Diabetes insipidus, p. 286.) There is no evidence that donor organ function is improved by the administration of steroids or thyroid hormone.

● Temperature regulation is lost. Use warmed IV fluids, inspired gases, and warm air blankets to maintain normothermia.

Special investigations

A number of investigations need to be carried out prior to organ donation. These are shown in Box 16.3. There are increasing concerns about the risks of donor transmitted infection and malignancy. The transplant coordinator will give advice, as this is a changing area, particularly in relation to hepatitis serology.

NON-HEART BEATING ORGAN DONATION

The shortage of donor organs from cadaveric, heart beating (brainstem dead) donors has led to renewed interest in the use of non-heart beating (asystolic) donors. Important issues are timing and definition of death, and the time elapsed between death and organ procurement.

TABLE 16.1 Maastricht categories for non-heart beating donors

Category 1	Dead on arrival at hospital
Category 2	Unsuccessful resuscitation (following out of hospital cardiac arrest)
Category 3	Awaiting cardiac arrest
Category 4	Cardiac arrest following confirmed brainstem death
Category 5*	Cardiac arrest in a hospital inpatient

*Maastricht criteria 1995. Category 5 added 2003.

In general, organs may be suitable for organ donation after asystole, if the time interval between death and retrieval is short, so that irretrievable damage to the organs does not occur. Five categories of patients who might be suitable have been described. These are shown in Table 16.1.

Typically patients on ICU are in category 3. The patient does not fulfill criteria for brainstem death, but death is inevitable, withdrawal of treatment is planned, and the family wish their relative to become an organ donor. Following discussion and consent from relatives, there is a planned withdrawal of supportive treatment. Following asystole, there is a 'stand-off' period during which relatives may 'say goodbye' to their loved one, after which the organs are cold perfused in situ by cannulation of the femoral artery and vein before being removed for transplant.

CULTURAL ASPECTS OF DEATH AND DYING

Different groups have different ways of dealing with death. This may clash with your own religious or cultural beliefs. Some groups may have large extended families and publicly display their grief. A number of religious groups are unhappy about post-mortem examinations and some prefer to remove the body from the hospital as soon as possible after death. This can sometimes be arranged. You should respect the views of others.

Table 16.2 gives a brief guide to the beliefs and practices of the more common religious groups. The information has been compiled from a number of sources and every effort has been made to ensure that it accurately reflects religious and cultural beliefs. Any errors or admissions are unintentional and no offence is intended.

- Routine care of the dying and last offices are appropriate unless otherwise stated.
- No religious objection to post-mortem examination or organ donation unless otherwise stated.

TABLE 16.2 Beliefs and practices of common religious groups

Anglicans	May request baptism, eucharist, or anointing
Roman Catholics	May request baptism, holy communion and sacrament of the dying
Members of Christian Free Church	Christians who do not conform to the Anglican or Catholic tradition Generally less emphasis on the sacraments May request a minister for informal prayers
Jehovah's Witnesses	Unrestricted access family and friends and church elders (There are no formal ministers, all Jehovah's Witnesses are ministers). There are no ceremonial rites at death
Christian Scientists	Believe in the power of God's healing and avoid conventional medicine May accept conventional medicine due to family or legal pressure without loss of faith and allow medical care of children No specific ceremonial rites at death Would not wish to consent to post-mortem or organ donation
Afro-Caribbean community	Extended family and church visits More emphasis on prayer than sacraments May prefer body to be handled by staff of same cultural background Older members of the community may believe in the sanctity of the body and not wish to consent to post-mortem or organ donation
Rastafarian	May prefer alternative therapy to conventional medicine. Distinctive hairstyle, may not want hair cut Second-hand clothes are taboo, may be reluctant to wear hospital gowns No specific ceremonial rites at death Unlikely to consent to post-mortem or organ donation
Buddhists	State of mind is important Require peace and quiet for meditation and chanting May request counselling from local Buddhists No specific ceremonial rites at death A Buddhist monk should be informed of the death

Cont'd

TABLE 16.2 Cont'd

Jews	Orthodox Jews will wish to maintain customs of dress, diet, prayer and observe the Sabbath while in hospital
	May object to any intervention which may hasten death (e.g. withdrawal of treatment)
	Relatives may wish to consult a rabbi
	No specific ceremonial rites at death but may recite special prayers
	There is a wish that dying Jews should not be left alone
	Ritual laying out of the body by Jewish burial society with burial arranged ideally within 24 h
	Post-mortem not permitted except where law requires it
	Unlikely to consent to organ donation
Muslims	Muslim women will not want to be seen by male doctors
	Prayer ritual may be continued
	Cleanliness important and running water required for washing
	Friends and family may recite prayer, dying patient may wish to be turned towards Mecca (south-east)
	Body should not be touched by non-Muslims (if necessary wear gloves) and should be prepared according to the wishes of the family or priest
	Funerals should take place within 24 h where possible
	Believe in the sanctity of the body
	Unlikely to consent to post-mortem or organ donation
Hindus	Hindu women prefer female doctors
	Prayer ritual may be continued
	Dying patients may wish to lie on the floor to be close to 'Earth'
	Rites including tying of a holy thread and sprinkling with water from the River Ganges
	Religious tokens should not be removed
	Body should not be touched by non-Hindus (if necessary wear gloves) and should be prepared according to the wishes of the family or priest
	Ideally cremation should be arranged within 24 h, often not practicable
	No specific religious objection to post-mortem or organ donation, although these are not liked

Cont'd

TABLE 16.2 Cont'd	
Sikhs	Sikh women will prefer female doctors
	Sikh men will wish to keep their hair covered at all times
	The five symbols of faith should not be disturbed in life or death
	Running water preferred for washing
	No specific ceremonial rites at death
	Traditionally Sikh families will lay out the body, but no specific objection to others touching the body

DEALING WITH DEATH AT A PERSONAL LEVEL

Working on an ICU can be both very satisfying and very demanding. Doctors and other health care professionals working on the ICU, who frequently deal with dying patients and bereaved relatives, often develop robust coping mechanisms to help them deal with death on a day-to-day basis. There are times, however, when even the most seasoned professional will find it hard to deal with a particular patient's death or a particular set of circumstances. The effects may even be felt some considerable time after the event and staff may even feel guilty about their feelings. It is important at these times to seek support.

If you find yourself affected by anything you come across on intensive care, do not keep it to yourself. Discuss it with friends, colleagues or senior medical or nursing staff, or make use of the support groups and available counselling services.

DRUG INFORMATION

The following drug/prescribing information is for guidance only.
Doses are based on an average 70 kg adult. Requirements will
vary according to patient age, weight and condition. It is the
responsibility of the prescriber to ensure that drugs are prescribed
and used appropriately. For further information refer to ward
pharmacist or see *British National Formulary* (BNF).

Drug	Method of administration	Notes
N-Acetylcysteine	100 mg/kg in 250–1000 mL 5% glucose, continuous infusion over 16–24 h	Acute liver failure
Activated protein C (drotrecogin alfa)	10 mg in 50 mL 0.9% saline. Infuse at 24 μg/kg/h for 96 h	
Adrenaline (epinephrine)	5 mg in 50 mL 5% glucose. 0.1–1 μg/kg/min	Increase concentration and dose according to response
Aminophylline	Loading dose 5 mg/kg in 100 mL 0.9% saline over 20 min. Maintenance 1 g in 1000 mL 0.9% saline 0.5–0.8 mg/kg/h	Omit loading if already receiving theophylline. Increase dose in smokers. Reduce dose if receiving concurrent erythromycin, clarithromycin, or ciprofloxacin. Check levels
Amiodarone	300 mg in 250 mL 5% glucose over 1 h followed 900 mg in 500 mL 5% glucose over 24 h	Half dose after 48 h
Calcium gluconate	10 mL 10% calcium gluconate slow IV bolus, or infusion in 5% glucose	Precipitates with sulphates, bicarbonates and phosphates
Clonidine	600 μg in 60 mL 5% glucose 10–40 μg/h – larger doses have been given (up to 150 μg/h)	For agitation
Digoxin	Loading dose 0.5–1 mg in 50 mL 5% glucose over 30 min. Maintenance 62.5–250 μg over 30 min daily	Check levels

Drug	Method of administration	Notes
Dobutamine	250 mg/50 mL 5% glucose 0–20 µg/kg/min	Increase concentration and dose according to response
Dopamine	200 mg/50 mL 5% glucose 2.5–10 µg/kg/min	Increase concentration and dose according to response
Dopexamine	50 mg/50 mL 5% glucose 0–5 µg/kg/min	Doses above $1 \mu g/kg/min^{-1}$ may produce significant vasodilatation/hypotension
Enoximone	100 mg/40 mL 0.9% saline maintenance 5–20 µg/kg/min	Beware hypotension. Loading dose usually avoided
Glyceryl trinitrate (GTN)	50 mg/50 mL (neat) 0–0.5 µg/kg/min	
Heparin	Use 1000 units/mL solution 5000 units IV loading dose 500–2000 units/h i.v. according to indication	Monitor APTT
Insulin	50 units in 50 mL 0.9% saline, continuous infusion as required to maintain target blood glucose	Monitor blood sugar
Labetalol	100 mg/20 mL (neat) IV bolus 5–20 mg Infusions start at 15 mg/h Double every 30 min to maximum of 160 mg/h according to response	
Noradrenaline (norepinephrine)	4 mg/50 mL 5% glucose 0.1–1.0 µg/kg/min	Increase concentration and dose according to response
Phenylephrine	100 mg in 100 mL 5% glucose 0–10 µg/kg/min	

(Cont'd)

Drug	Method of administration	Notes
Potassium chloride	Intermittent dosing – 10–20 mmol/50 mL 0.9% saline over 30 min Continuous infusion – 50 mmol in 50 mL 0.9% saline at 5–20 mmol/h	Give via central line. Monitor ECG
Phenytoin	Loading 18 mg/kg in 100–250 mL 0.9% saline over 1 h Maintenance 3–5 mg/kg daily by slow i.v. injection in 3 divided doses	Do not exceed infusion rate of 50 mg/min
Prostacycline	250 μg in 50 mL 0.9% saline 5–10 ng/kg/min	
Salbutamol	200–300 μg i.v. bolus repeated if necessary. Infusion 5 mg/50–500 mL 5% glucose 5–20 μg/min	
Vasopressin	20 units in 50 mL glucose 5% 0.01–0.04 units/min	
mg = milligrams, μg = micrograms, ng = nanograms		

DRUG LEVELS

Reference ranges vary according to units of measurement and local guidelines. Confirm with laboratory and/or local pharmacist.

Drug	When to take sample	Desired levels
Ciclosporin	2 h post-dose	800–1200 µg/L Levels vary according to procedure and time post-transplant. Confirm local practice
Digoxin	6–8 h post-dose	0.5–1 µg/L
Gentamicin	Single daily dose regimen TDS regimen	Use Hartford Nomogram. Seek advice Trough < 2 mg/L, peak 5–8 mg/L
Phenytoin	>4 hour post-dose	10–20 mg/L
Tacrolimus	Predose	5–15 µg/L Levels vary according to procedure and time post-transplant. Confirm local practice
Teicoplanin	Predose	10–15 mg/L
Theophylline	Oral route – 2 h post-dose Infusion – any time	10–20 mg/L
Tobramycin	Single daily dose regimen TDS regimen	Use Hartford Nomogram. Seek advice Trough < 2 mg/L, peak 5–8 mg/L
Vancomycin	Pre-dose	5–15 mg/L

If peak level too high, reduce the dose given.
If trough level is too high, omit until level is within desired range.
Give further doses at increased intervals.

USEFUL LINKS

Intensive Care Society	www.ics.ac.uk
Scottish Intensive Care Society	www.scottishintesivecare.org.uk
Intensive Care Society of Ireland	www.icmed.com
ICNARC (Intensive Care National Audit and Research Centre)	www.icnarc.org.uk
European Society of Intensive Care Medicine	www.escism.org
Society of Critical Care Medicine	www.sccm.org
The British Association of Critical Care Nurses	www.baccn.org.uk
The Association of Anaesthetists of Great Britain and Ireland	www.aagbi.org
The Resuscitation Council UK	www.resus.org.uk
The European Resuscitation Council	www.erc.edu
The British Blood Transfusion Society	www.bbts.org.uk
Serious Hazards Of Transfusion (SHOT)	www.shotuk.org
British National Formulary (BNF)	www.bnf.org.uk
The UK Department of Health	www.doh.gov.uk
The National Institute for Health and Clinical Excellence (NICE)	www.nice.org.uk
Toxbase (poisoning/overdose information)	www.toxbase.org

These web sites contain useful information and many have downloadable guidelines. Most also contain links to other related areas of interest.

INDEX

ABCD assessment in trauma, 306–7
  brain injury, 275–7
  see also specific components
abdomen
  compartment syndrome, 174–5, 317
  examination, 24
  imaging, 169
    in renal failure, 187
  injuries, 316–17
  sepsis, 174, 334, 335, 337
ABO incompatibility, 250, 253
  fresh frozen plasma and, 249
abscess
  brain, 296
  lung, 147
absorption
  drug, measures to reduce, 231–3
  enteral feeds, failure, 59
acalculous cholecystitis, 176
ACE inhibitors, cardiac failure, 105
acetylcholinesterase see cholinesterase
N-acetylcysteine, 446
  hepatic failure, 179
  paracetamol overdose, 236
acid/base disturbances, 115–16, 212–15
  in oliguric renal failure, 189
  postoperative, 357
acidifying agents, metabolic alkalosis, 215
acidity, gastric, maintenance in hospital-acquired pneumonia prevention, 144
acidosis
  metabolic see metabolic acidosis
  respiratory, 115–16
  see also ketoacidosis
Acinetobacter, 339
ACTH see adrenocorticotrophic hormone
action plan, formulating, 25–6
activated factor VII, 261–2
activated partial thromboplastin time (APTT), 259
  prolonged, 261
activated protein C, 333, 446
acute coronary syndromes, 101–5

acute lung injury see lung
acute respiratory distress syndrome see respiratory distress syndrome
admission policies, 6–7
adrenal gland
  insufficiency, 221–2
    functional, 222, 332
  secretory tumour, 222–3
adrenaline (epinephrine), 83, 84
  anaphylactoid reactions, 362
  bradycardia, 91
  phaeochromocytoma, 223
  in stress response to surgery and critical illness, 348
  trauma, 307
    brain injury, 283
adrenocorticotrophic hormone (ACTH), in stress response to surgery and critical illness, 348
adrenocorticotrophic hormone (ACTH) analogue (Syncathen) test, 221
adult respiratory distress syndrome see respiratory distress syndrome
advanced directives, 31
advanced life support, algorithm, 110
Advanced Trauma Life Support, 275
Afro-Caribbean beliefs, death and dying, 441
afterload, 72
age
  in APACHE II, 10
  burns assessment, 321
  energy requirements and, 55
  trauma outcome and, 324
    brain, 291
AIDS see HIV
airway
  burns, 321
  obstruction, 138–40
    postoperative, 355
    respiratory failure in, 119
    tracheal intubation in, 139, 399
    tracheostomy in, 139, 404

pressure, high (in ventilated patient), 132–3
damage due to, 130
see also peak airway pressure; pressure-controlled ventilation; pressure-support ventilation
protection in gastric lavage by tracheal intubation, 232
see also respiratory system
airway assessment (A)
for discharge, 14
in trauma, 306
brain injury, 275
airway exchange catheters, 402
albumin, 210–11
administration, 211
low serum levels, 210–11
alcohol *see* ethanol; methanol
alfentanil, 36
alimentary system *see* gastrointestinal system
alkaline diuresis, forced, 232–3
alkalizing solutions in metabolic acidosis, 213
alkalosis
metabolic, 116, 215
respiratory, 116
allergy tests with anaphylactoid reactions, 363
α-blockers, phaeochromocytoma, 223
alveolar–arterial oxygen difference in APACHE II, 11
aminophylline, 446
asthma, 150
chronic obstructive pulmonary disease, 153
amiodarone, 446
atrial fibrillation, 93
supraventricular tachycardia, 93
amitriptyline, 48
amphetamines, 243
anabolic steroids, 243
anaemia, 246
anaesthesia, prolonged, effects, 353
anaesthetic agents
inhaled, as sedatives, 37
local *see* local anaesthetics

anaesthetist, tracheostomy, 406–7
analgesia (and analgesic drugs), 36
postoperative, 349–56, 357
anaphylactoid reactions, 361–3
aneurysm
aortic, repair, 358
cerebral, bleeding, 292
management, 293–4
angina
stable, 100
unstable, 103
angiotensin converting enzyme (ACE) inhibitors, cardiac failure, 105
angiotensin II, 349
anion gap, 212
antacids, pneumonia risk with, 144
anterior cord syndrome, 311
antibiotics, 336, 337, 450
broad-spectrum, pneumonia risk with, 144
empirical use, 336, 337
in immunocompromised patients, 268–9
levels, 450
in pancreatitis (acute), 182
in pneumonia, 147, 148, 337
pseudomembranous colitis associated with use of, 338
in renal failure, pharmacology, 198
in respiratory failure (for underlying condition), 120
in sepsis, 330
anticholinergics, asthma, 150
anticholinesterase drugs, 45
in delayed recovery from neuromuscular block, 353–4
myasthenia gravis, 302, 303
anticoagulants
pulmonary embolism, 108
renal replacement therapy, 193
thrombosis, 266
DVT prophylaxis, 63
anticonvulsants (antiepileptics), 297
in brain injury, 286
in eclampsia, 365
antidepressants, 48
overdose, 237–8

antidiuretic hormone (vasopressin),
    85–6, 448
  excessive secretion, 203
  in sepsis treatment, 332
  in stress response to surgery and
      critical illness, 348
antidotes, 233, 234
antiepileptics see anticonvulsants
antifibrinolytics, Jehovah's
    Witnesses, 255
antifungals, 340
antihypertensive drugs, 89
anti-inflammatory agents, sepsis,
    333
antiretrovirals, 269
antivirals
  cytomegalovirus, 148
  HIV disease/AIDS, 269
anxiety, 48
anxiolytics, 36
aorta
  aneurysm repair, 358
  balloon counterpulsation pumps,
      106, 107
  descending, oesophageal
      Doppler, 77
APACHE II, 8, 8–12
  notes on completing, 10–11
  problems, 11–12
APACHE III, 12
apnoea test, 300
arrhythmias see dysrhythmias
arterial blood gases see blood gases
arterial blood pressure, 374–6
  measurement/monitoring, 374–6
    discrepancy between invasive
        and non-invasive, 375–6
    transducers, 374–5
  systemic see systemic arterial
      blood pressure
  see also pulmonary arteries;
      systemic arterial blood
      pressure
arterial cannulation/catheterization,
    372–4
  accidental (in venous
      cannulation), 385
  pulmonary see pulmonary
      arteries

arterial thrombosis/embolization,
    265–6
ascites, drainage, 424
aseptic technique, 371
aspiration (gastric contents)
  pneumonitis due, 148–9
  tracheal intubation in prevention
      of, 399
aspiration (technique), pericardial,
    395
aspirin
  poisoning, 236–7
  unstable angina/non-ST elevation
      myocardial infarction, 103
assessment, patient, 22–5
  see also primary survey;
      reassessment; secondary
      survey specific systems and
      conditions
assisted spontaneous breathing see
    pressure-support ventilation
asthma, 150–2
asystole, 109
at-risk patients, identification, 4–5
atracurium, 46
  in tracheal intubation, 399
atrial fibrillation (AF), 93, 94
atrial flutter, 95
audit, national databases, 15
autoimmune disease in renal failure,
    187
autonomic neuropathy, 301
autopsy see post-mortem
    examination
autoregulation of cerebral blood
    flow, 273
AVPU assessment in traumatic
    brain injury, 277
awaking from sedation, slow, 40–1

bacterial infections, 336–9
  pneumonia due to, 142
bad news, breaking, 28, 434
barotrauma, 130
barrier nursing, 21
  reverse, 21–2
base deficit/base excess, 115
basic metabolic rate (BMR),
    estimation, 55

bed management issues, 6

benzodiazepines, 237
 antagonists/antidotes, 41, 234, 237
 overdose, 237
 in renal failure, pharmacology, 198
 as sedatives, 35, 37
  combined with opioids, 35
 seizures, 297
  in brain injury, 286

β-agonists
 asthma, 150
 chronic obstructive pulmonary disease, 153

β-blocker
 ischaemic heart disease, 100, 103, 104
  hypertension in the young, avoidance, 90
 sinus tachycardia, avoidance, 91

bicarbonate (HCO_3), serum
 in APACHE II, 11
 loss causing metabolic acidosis, 212
 see also sodium bicarbonate

bile stasis (cholestasis), 176

biochemical tests in acute renal failure
 serum, 185
 urine, 186

biomarkers, acute coronary syndromes, 101–2

biopsy, bronchial, 415

biphasic positive airway pressure (BIPAP), 122–3
 chronic obstructive pulmonary disease, 154

bispectral index, 290

bisphosphonates in hypercalcaemia, 209

bleeding see haemorrhage

blood, pleural cavity see haemothorax

blood flow
 alterations predisposing to thrombosis, 265
 cerebral, 273

blood gases, arterial, 114–16
 sampling, 374

blood group incompatibility, 253
 checking, 250
 fresh frozen plasma and, 249

blood pressure
 arterial see arterial blood pressure
 central venous, 75, 81–2
 see also pulmonary arteries, occlusion pressure

blood samples from arterial line, 372, 374

blood tests, pneumonia, 146

blood transfusion (and blood products) see transfusion

blunt vs penetrating trauma, 309

bones, long, injuries, 317–18
 see also fractures

botulism, 303, 304

bougies, 402

bowel see intestine

brachial artery cannulation, 372–3

bradycardia, 91, 92

brain
 abscess, 296
 injury, 272–92
  catastrophic, 301
  hypoxic see hypoxia
  key concepts, 272–4
  management principles, 272–3
  monitoring, 282, 288–90
  neurosurgical referral, 280–1
  outcome following, 290–2
  patterns and causes, 272
  traumatic see trauma
 see also entries under cerebral

brainstem
 death, 297–301, 437–9
 residual function, 301

breaking bad news, 28, 434

breathing (B)
 discharge criteria, 14
 trauma, 306–7
  brain injury, 275–7

broad complex tachycardia, 95–6, 97

broad-spectrum antibiotics, pneumonia risk with, 144

bronchial biopsy, 415
bronchial tree anatomy, 414
bronchoalveolar lavage (BAL), 415
  indications
    acute lung injury, 157
    infections incl. pneumonia,
      146, 147, 415
bronchoconstriction, asthma, 151
bronchodilators, 120
  asthma, 150, 151
  chronic obstructive pulmonary
    disease, 152, 154
bronchopleural fistula, jet
    ventilation, 134
bronchopneumonia, 141
bronchoscopy (fibreoptic), 412–15
  bronchoalveolar lavage during,
    415
  contraindications, 412
  indications, 412
    tracheostomy, 406, 406–7
  preparation, 412
  procedure, 413–15
Brown–Séquard syndrome, 311
Buddhist beliefs, death and dying,
    441
bumetanide, 188–9
bupivacaine in epidural blockade,
    351
burns, 320–2

calcitonin in hypercalcaemia, 209
calcium, 207–9
  administration (e.g. calcium
    gluconate), 446
    in coagulopathy, 261
    in hepatic failure, 180
    as inotrope, 87
    in septic shock, 332
  disturbances, 208–9
calcium channel blocker,
    myocardial ischaemia, 100
calcium sensitizing agents, 85
calorimetry, indirect, 55–6
cancer, haematological, 269
Candida, 339–40
cannabinoids, 243
cannulation (commonly called
    catheterization)

arterial see arterial cannulation
  sepsis/infection risk, 335, 337,
    340–1
    immunocompromised patients,
      268
    pulmonary artery
      catheterization, 393
  venous see venous catheterization
capacity (mental) to give consent,
    29–30
carbon dioxide (CO_2)
  end tidal ($ETCO_2$), monitoring in
    ventilated patient, 129
  extracorporeal removal, 131,
    132, 151
  tension in arterial blood ($PaCO_2$)
    assessment, 115
    in brainstem death tests, 300
    elevated see hypercapnia
carbon monoxide poisoning, 239
  smoke inhalation and, 322
carboxyhaemoglobin, 239
cardiomyopathy, 302
cardiovascular system, 65–112
  drug overdose affecting, 230
  examination, 24
  invasive monitoring
    in acute lung injury, 156
    in diabetic ketoacidosis, 219
  on patient chart, 23
  postoperative instability, 355–6
  in traumatic brain injury,
    instability, 284–5
  see also circulation; heart
cardioversion, 396–8
care bundles, 34
  sepsis, 329–31
  ventilator, 128
catecholamines
  in phaeochromocytoma
    replacement, 223
    secretion, 223
  in stress response to surgery and
    critical illness, 348
catheters
  airway exchange, 402
  bronchoalveolar lavage, 416
  pigtail (chest drain), 419
  vascular see cannulation

central cord syndrome, 311
central nervous system *see* neurological function
central venous cannulation, 75, 376–89
  accidental, in pulmonary artery cannulation, 393
  changing and removal, 386–7
  complications/common problems, 384–6
  contraindications, 376
  indications, 376
    renal replacement therapy, 193
    transfusion, 252
  procedure, 382–3
  ultrasound-guided *see* ultrasound
  X-ray showing position, 159, 383
central venous pressure (CVP), 75, 81–2
  cerebral perfusion pressure maintenance and, 273–4, 282
cerebral blood flow, 273
cerebral function monitors (CFMs) or analyzing monitors (CFAPs) in brain injury, 285, 290
cerebral haemorrhage, 292, 293
cerebral perfusion pressure (CPP)
  in subarachnoid haemorrhage, 294
  in traumatic brain injury, 273–4, 282–3
  inadequate, 274, 283, 284
cerebrospinal fluid leaks, 288
cerebrovascular accident (stroke), 292
certification of death, 434–5
cervical soft tissue injuries, 310–11
cervical spine control in trauma, airway assessment with, 306
  brain injury, 275
charcoal, activated, 232, 233
chart, patient's, 22–3, 27
chest (thorax)
  trauma, 313–16
  wall abnormalities causing respiratory failure, 119
  X-ray, 158–65
    acute lung injury, 156

of central venous catheter position, 159, 383
    chest drain assessment, 320
    interpretation, 158–65
    mediastinal injury, 314
chest drain, 416–21
children of Jehovah's witnesses, consent issues, 30
chlorhexidine, 371
chlormethiazole, 242
chlorpromazine for acute confusional state, 42
cholangitis, 176
cholecystitis, acalculous, 176
cholestasis, 176
cholinergic agonist, GI dysmotility, 170
cholinergic antagonist, asthma, 150
cholinesterase
  hereditary deficiency, 354–5
  inhibitors *see* anticholinesterase drugs
Christian Free Church beliefs, death and dying, 441
Christian Scientist beliefs, death and dying, 441
chronic health score in APACHE II, 10, 11
chronic obstructive pulmonary disease, 152–4
ciclosporin, 450
circulation (A)
  discharge criteria, 14
  trauma, 307
    brain injury, 277
  see also cardiovascular system
cis-atracurium, 46
clonidine, 446
  for acute confusional state, 42
  for sedation, 38
clopidogrel, unstable angina/non-ST elevation myocardial infarction, 103
Clostridium botulinum and botulism, 303, 304
Clostridium difficile, 171, 338–9
Clostridium tetani and tetanus, 303, 304
clothing, dress code, 20

clotting *see* coagulation
coagulase-negative staphylococci, 338
coagulation (clotting), 255–6
  disorder (coagulopathy), 258–62
    in hepatic failure, 178
    investigations, 259–62
    Jehovah's Witnesses, 255
    in major haemorrhage, 252
    management, 260–1
    disseminated intravascular, 263–4
  see also factors
cocaine, 243
coliforms, 339
colitis, pseudomembranous, 171, 338
collapse (lung - X-ray appearance), 159–60
  entire lung, 160–1
coma, hyperosmolar, 218
  see also Glasgow Coma Scale
communication
  with family/relatives, 28–9
    breaking bad news, 29, 434
  patient difficulties with, 47–8
  team members on patient care, 26
community-acquired pneumonia, 141–3, 337
compartment syndromes
  abdominal, 174–5, 317
  peripheral, 319
compliance (intracranial), 274
compliance (lung)
  acute lung injury scoring, 156
  reduced, 133
    pressure controlled ventilation, 124
compressed spectral array of EEG, 290
computed tomography (CT)
  abdominal, 169
    renal failure, 187
  head injury, 279–80
    neurosurgical referral and, 280, 281
conduction defects, cardiac, 98–9
confidentiality, 27–8

confusion, acute, with sedative withdrawal, 42
congenital heart disease, adults, 111–12
consciousness
  delayed postoperative recovery, 353
  level in traumatic brain injury, 277
  see also unconscious patient
consent, 29–32, 370
  common problems, 30–2
    Jehovah's witnesses and blood transfusion, 30, 254–5
  informed *see* informed consent
  organ donation, 438
  post-mortem examination, 32
consolidation, 159–60
continuous positive airway pressure (CPAP), 121–2
continuous renal replacement therapy, 190–1, 191–3
contractility (myocardial), 72
controlled mandatory ventilation, 123–4
contusions, cardiac, 315–16
convulsions *see* seizures
copper, antidote, 234
core temperature measurement, 224
coronary syndromes, acute, 101–5
coroner
  consent to organ donation, 438
  reporting death to, 436–7
cortical necrosis, acute, 185
corticosteroids (steroids), 221–2
  acute lung injury, 158
  adrenal insufficiency, 221
  asthma, 150
  chronic obstructive pulmonary disease, 153
  hypercalcaemia, 209
  long-term use, 221–2
  in shock states, high-dose, 222
creatine kinase/phosphokinase (CK), 102
  in acute renal failure, 186
  isoenzyme (CM-MB), 102

creatinine in acute renal failure
  clearance, 186
    drug prescribing and, 197
  serum, 185
Creutzfeldt–Jakob disease (vCJD)
    and blood products, 247–8
cricothyroidotomy, 410–12
cryoprecipitate, 249–50
cultural aspects of death and dying,
    440–3
cyanide poisoning, 240
  smoke inhalation and, 322
cyst, pancreatic, 182
cytomegalovirus pneumonitis,
    146, 148

D dimer measurement, 259
daily routine, 19
dantrolene, 225
DC cardioversion, 396–8
dead space ventilation, 118
death (mortality)
  certification, 434–5
  confirming, 433
  cultural aspects, 440–3
  in hypothermia, determination,
    227
  impact on professionals, 443
  rates, 430
    standardized, 8
  reporting to coroner, 436–7
  see also brainstem, death; dying
decontamination
  hand, 20–1
  selective, of digestive tract, 144–5
deep venous thrombosis (DVT), 265
  in diabetic ketoacidosis, 221
  prophylaxis, 63
defibrillation, 396–8
dehydration in diabetic
    ketoacidosis, 219
dental injury, 310
dependency of patient, 48
depolarizing muscle relaxant see
    suxamethonium
dextrose
  in hepatic failure, 179
  in hypoglycaemia, 216–17

diabetes insipidus
  in brain injury, 286–7
  in brainstem death, 439
diabetes mellitus, 217–22
  hyperosmolar non-ketotic states,
    220–1
dialysis catheters, 388
  see also haemodialysis;
    microdialysis; peritoneal
    dialysis
diaphragmatic rupture, 316
diarrhoea, 170–2
  with enteral feeds, 59–60
diastolic dysfunction, 74
diazepam, 37
  in renal failure, pharmacology,
    198
dieticians, 19
  see also nutrition
digestive tract see gastrointestinal
    system
digoxin, 447, 450
  antidote, 234
  atrial fibrillation, 93
  in renal failure, pharmacology,
    198
direct current (DC) cardioversion,
    396–8
disability see neurological
    assessment
discharge from ICU, 6
  policies, 13–15
disseminated intravascular
    coagulation, 263–4
diuresis, forced alkaline, 232–3
diuretics
  in drug overdose, 232, 233
  myocardial ischaemia, 100
  in renal failure, 188–9
  in respiratory failure (for
    underlying condition),
    120
dobutamine, 82, 83, 84, 447
documentation see medical records
dopamine, 83, 83–4, 84, 447
dopexamine, 83, 84, 447
Doppler, oesophageal, descending
    aorta, 77

doxapram in chronic obstructive pulmonary disease, avoidance, 153

drainage
chest, 416–21
peritoneal, 424

dress code, 20

drowning, 323–4

drugs, 19, 446–50
acute lung injury, 157, 158
adrenal insufficiency, 221
anaphylactoid reactions, 362–3
asthma, 150
cardiac failure, 105
right, and pulmonary hypertension, 106
cardiac output optimization, 82–5
cardiogenic shock, 107
chronic obstructive pulmonary disease, 153
GI dysmotility, 170
hypercalcaemia, 208–9
hyperkalaemia, 207
hypertension, 89
information, 446–8
levels, 450
ischaemic heart disease, 100
acute coronary syndromes, 103
stable angina, 100
overdose/poisoning see poisoning
perfusion pressure optimization, 85–6
phaeochromocytoma, 223
postoperative patient in ICU, 357, 358
pulmonary embolism, 108
recreational abuse, 242–4
renal failure, 188–9
prescribing, 196–8
in renal replacement therapy, clearance, 197
respiratory failure (for underlying condition), 120
sepsis, 333
speeding up death, 433
tracheal intubation, 398

traumatic brain injury, 283
specific (types of) drugs

duodenum, enteral feeding directly to, 47, 422

dying patients, 429–43

dysmotility, gastrointestinal, 170

dysrhythmias (arrhythmias), 90–7, 109
in central venous cannulation via Seldinger technique, 383
in electrocution, 322–3
in hyperkalaemia, 206, 207
in hyperthermia, 226
in hypokalaemia, 205
in overdose, 235
in pulmonary artery cannulation, 393

early warning scoring systems, 4–5

ECG see electrocardiogram

echocardiography, 77–8
cardiac contusions, 315–16
cardiogenic shock, 107
infective endocarditis, 341

eclampsia, 365–6

ecstasy, 242, 243

edrophonium test, 303

EEG, compressed spectral array, 290

ejection systolic point, 74

electrocardiogram (ECG)
acute coronary syndromes, 101, 102, 103
atrial fibrillation, 95
atrial flutter, 95
broad complex tachycardia, 96
in hyperkalaemia, 206, 207
in hypokalaemia, 205, 206

electrocution, 322–3

electroencephalogram (EEG), compressed spectral array, 290

electrolytes, 49–53
factors increasing or decreasing requirements, 51
serum measurements
in acute renal failure, 185
frequent, 52

electromechanical dissociation, 109
elimination, drug, measures to
          increase, 231–3
embolism
    fat, 318–19
    thrombotic (=thromboembolism)
        from arterial thrombus,
          265–6
        pulmonary (PE), 107–8, 266
    septic, 335
embolization (technique), cerebral
          aneurysm, 293
emphysema, surgical, X-ray
          appearance, 164
encephalitis, 296
encephalopathy, hepatic, 178, 179
end diastolic volume, 74
end of life issues, 429–43
end systolic point, 74
end tidal CO_2 ($ETCO_2$), monitoring
          in ventilated patient, 129
endocarditis, infective, 334, 341–2
endocrine disturbances, 217–24
endothelial damage, thrombosis
          risk, 265
endotracheal intubation see
          tracheal intubation
energy requirements
    estimation, 54–6
    in parenteral nutrition, 61
enoximone, 84, 447
enteral feeding, 57–60, 421–2
    nasal route see nasal route
    procedure, 421–2
    transpyloric, 47, 422
enterococci, 338
environment, psychological aspects,
          47
epidural analgesia, postoperative,
          350, 351, 352
epileptic seizures see seizures
epinephrine see adrenaline
epoprostenol (prostacyclin), 447
    renal replacement therapy, 193
    right cardiac failure and
          pulmonary hypertension,
          106
erythrocyte see red cells

erythropoietin, 254
Escherichia coli, 339
ethanol (commonly called alcohol),
          241–2
    acute intoxication, 241
    chronic abuse, 241
    in methanol and ethylene glycol
          poisoning, 240–1
    withdrawal, 241–2
ethylene glycol, 240–1
    antidotes, 234, 240–1
etomidate, 37
euthanasia, 432–3
examination
    patient, 23–4
    post-mortem see post-mortem
          examination
exposure, trauma, 308–9
extracorporeal circuits and
          Jehovah's Witnesses, 254
extracorporeal CO_2 removal, 131,
          132, 151
extracorporeal membrane
          oxygenation (ECMO), 131
    in acute lung injury, 158
extubation
    endotracheal tube, 136–7
        stridor following, 140
    tracheostomy tube, 410
eye opening in Glasgow Coma
          Scale, 278

facial injury, 310
factors (clotting)
    concentrates, 254
    factor VII, 255, 256
        activated, 261–2
    factor IX and X, 256
family and relatives
    end of life issues
        brainstem death, 299, 300–1
        consent to organ donation, 438
        treatment withdrawal, 432
    postoperative patient, 358
    talking with see communication
fasciitis, necrotizing, 337, 342
fasciotomy, peripheral compartment
          syndromes, 319

FAST (focused assessment with sonography for trauma), 308–9
fat embolism, 318–19
fear, 48
femoral artery cannulation, 372–3
femoral vein cannulation, 381
fentanyl, 36
fever see pyrexia
fibrinogen, measurement, 259
fibrinolysis, 256, 257
  inhibitors (antifibrinolytics), Jehovah's Witnesses, 255
filling (heart)
  echocardiographic assessment, 78
  optimization of filling status, 80–2
    in cardiac failure, 106
    in hypotension, 88
filling pressure, 81
fistula, bronchopleural, jet ventilation, 134
flaps, free, 358–9
fluid management, 49–53
  anaphylactoid reactions, 362
  CVP and PAOP in optimization of, 81
  diabetic ketoacidosis, 219–20
  drugs overdose, 235
  factors increasing or decreasing fluid requirements, 51
  haemorrhage (major), 252
  postoperative haemorrhage, 360
  pre-eclampsia/eclampsia, 366
  sepsis, 332
  trauma, 307, 309
    blunt vs penetrating, 309
    brain injury, 282
    burns, 321–2
  24-hour monitoring of balance, 52
flumazenil, 41, 237
fluoxetine, 48
focused assessment with sonography for trauma (FAST), 308–9
follow-up clinics, 15
fomepizole, 240, 241

fondaparinux, 266
forced alkaline diuresis, 232–3
fractures
  facial skeleton, 310
    jaw see jaw
  long bone, 318
  rib, 313–14
free tissue transfer (free flap), 358–9
fresh frozen plasma, 249
frusemide see furosemide
fungal infections, 339–40
  pneumonia, 145, 148
furosemide (frusemide)
  hypercalcaemia, 208
  renal failure, 188–9

gamma-hydroxybutyrate (GHB), 243
ganciclovir, cytomegalovirus, 148
gases
  blood see blood gases
  exchange
    in brain injury, 287
    in brainstem death/organ donors, 439
gastric acidity, maintenance in hospital-acquired pneumonia prevention, 144
gastric contents
  aspiration see aspiration
  delayed emptying, 170
gastric lavage, 231–2
gastric pylorus, feeding tube placed through, 47, 422
gastrointestinal system (alimentary/ digestive tract), 167–82
  bleeding see haemorrhage
  drug overdose affecting, 230
  maintaining integrity, 168
  manifestations of failure, 168–9
  motility defect, 170
  in pathophysiology of critical illness, 168
  on patient chart, 23
  selective decontamination, 144–5
gastro(jejuno)stomy, percutaneous endoscopic, 58
gentamicin levels, 450

GHB (gamma-hydroxybutyrate), 243

Glasgow Coma Scale (GCS)
  in APACHE II, 11, 12
  trauma, 307
    brain injury, 278

Glasgow Outcome Scale, 291

glucose, administration see dextrose

glucose, blood
  disturbances see hyperglycaemia; hypoglycaemia
  measurement/monitoring, 216
    in parenteral nutrition, 61

glutamine, 56

glyceryl trinitrate (GTN), 447
  cardiac failure, 105
  cardiogenic shock, 106
  hypertension, 89
  ischaemic heart disease, 100, 103, 104

glycopyrrolate in delayed recovery from neuromuscular block, 354

Goodpasture's syndrome, 187

Gram-negative organisms, 339

Gram-positive organisms, 336–9

great vessel injury, 314

growth hormone in stress response to surgery and critical illness, 348

guidewire
  cannula passed over see Seldinger technique
  in venous cannulation
    changing cannulas over, 387
    inability to pass, 385

Guillain–Barré syndrome, 199, 303

haematological problems, 245–70

haemodiafiltration, continuous venovenous, 193

haemodialysis
  catheters, 389
  continuous, 192
  intermittent, 190
  in overdose, 233

haemodynamic status, 74–80
  brainstem death/organ donors, 439
  monitoring, 74–8, 81–2
    arterial line for, 372
  optimization, 78–80
  traumatic brain injury affecting, 284–5
  ventilation affecting, 130
  weaning from ventilation, 136

haemofiltration, 191
  sepsis, 333

haemoglobin
  carbon monoxide binding to, 239
  optimization, 69

haemolytic uraemia syndrome, 263

haemoperfusion in overdose, 233

haemorrhage/bleeding, 251–2
  central venous cannulation-related, 386
  gastrointestinal, 172–4
    variceal bleeding, 174, 422–4
  intracranial, 272, 292–4
  major, 251–2
  mediastinal, 314
  peripartum, 366
  postoperative patients, 359–61
  tracheostomy-related, 408

haemostasis, normal mechanisms, 255–6

haemothorax (pleural blood), 313
  X-ray appearance, 161–2

haloperidol, 36
  for acute confusional state, 42

hand hygiene, 20–1

Hartmann's solution, 50

head injury
  brain injury in see trauma
  CT scan, 292–3
  neurosurgical referral, 280–1

healthcare staff see multidisciplinary team

heart
  arrest, 109–11
    hypoxic brain injury, 295
  conduction defects (inc. heart block), 98–9
  congenital disease in adults, 111–12
  contusions, 315–16
  failure, 105–6
    pregnancy-related, 367

heart (*Continued*)
  ischaemic disease, 100–5
  output (CO), 70–4
    optimization, 82–5, 88
    thermodilution method of
      measurement, 394–5
    typical adult values, 71
  rate, 71
  rhythm disturbances *see*
    dysrhythmias
  shock related to (cardiogenic),
    67, 106
  tamponade, 108–9
  ultrasound *see* echocardiography
  valvular lesions, 341
  see also cardiomyopathy;
    cardioversion
helium–oxygen mix in airway
    obstruction, 139
HELPP syndrome, 368–9
heparin (incl. low molecular
    weight), 447
  antidote, 234, 261
  deep venous thrombosis
    prophylaxis, 63
  myocardial ischaemia, 100
  pulmonary embolism, 108
  renal replacement therapy, 193
  thrombocytopenia risk with,
    263
  unstable angina/non-ST elevation
    myocardial infarction, 103
hepatic problems *see* liver
high dependency unit (HDU),
    definition, 3
high frequency ventilation, 133–5
highly active antiretroviral therapy
    (HAART), 269
Hindu beliefs, death and dying, 442
histamine H$_2$ blockers and hospital-
    acquired pneumonia, 144
history-taking, 22
  trauma, 308
HIV disease/AIDS, 31, 289–90
  testing for HIV infection, 31–2
hormonal response to surgery and
    critical illness, 348–9
hospital-acquired pneumonia *see*
    pneumonia

human immunodeficiency virus
    see HIV
humidification in ventilation, 129
Hunt and Hess grading scale for
    subarachnoid haemorrhage,
    293
hydralazine, 89
hydrocortisone
  asthma, 150
  chronic obstructive pulmonary
    disease, 153
hydrogen ion (H$^+$) accumulation
    causing metabolic acidosis,
    212
hygiene
  hand, 20–1
  hospital-acquired pneumonia
    prevention, 143–4
hyperbaric oxygen, carbon
    monoxide poisoning,
    239
hypercalcaemia, 208–9
hypercapnia, 120
  chronic obstructive pulmonary
    disease, 152
  management, 120
  raised intracranial pressure and,
    283
  respiratory failure, 117
  in ventilated patients, 131–2
    permissive, 132
hyperchloraemic acidosis, 53,
    214
hyperdynamic shock, 66
hyperglycaemia, 217
  in diabetes, 218
hyperkalaemia, 206–7
  in oliguric renal failure, 189,
    189–90
hypermagnesaemia, 210
hypernatraemia, 204
hyperosmolar (non-ketotic) states,
    218
  in diabetic patients, 220–1
hyperphosphataemia, 209
hyperpyrexia, malignant, 363–4
hypertension
  pulmonary, right heart failure
    and, 105–6

systemic, 88–90
    pre- eclampsia, 365
hyperthermia, 224–5
    drugs overdose, 235
    malignant (=malignant
        hyperpyrexia), 363–4
    traumatic brain injury, 282
hyperthyroidism, 224
hyperventilation, moderate, with
        raised intracranial pressure,
        284
hypoalbuminaemia, 210–11
hypocalcaemia, 208
hypodynamic shock, 66
hypoglycaemia, 216–17
    in diabetic ketoacidosis, 220
    in hepatic failure, 179–80
    in insulin overdose, 238
hypokalaemia, 205–6
hypomagnesaemia, 210
hyponatraemia, 202–4
hypophosphataemia, 209
hypotension, 87–8
    in epidural blockade, 351
hypothermia, 226–7
    after cardiac arrest, 111
    in brainstem death/organ donors,
        439
    drugs overdose, 235
    induced, traumatic brain injury,
        282
hypothyroidism, 224
hypovolaemic shock, 67
hypoxaemia
    acute lung injury scoring, 156
    chronic obstructive pulmonary
        disease, 152
    management, 120
    permissive, in ventilated patients,
        131–2
hypoxia, 117–18
    brain injury in, 272, 294–5
        near drowning, 323–4
    with muscle relaxants, 43
    quantifying degree of, 117–18
    raised intracranial pressure and,
        283
    respiratory failure due to,
        116–17, 117–18

ileus, persistent, 170
imaging
    GI tract, 169
    renal (in acute failure), 187
    sepsis, 334
    spinal trauma, 312
    see also specific modalities
immersion (near drowning), 323–4
immobilization
    pressure-related injuries to, 235
    spine (in trauma), 306, 311, 312
immunocompromized persons,
        266–70
    in APACHE II chronic health
        score, 10
    infection (opportunistic) risk
        and its control, 19–20, 21–2,
        268–9
    pneumonia, 145–7, 148
    see also immunosuppression
immunoglobulin solutions in
        Guillain–Barré syndrome,
        199
immunonutrition, 56
immunosuppression, causes, 267
    transfusion-related, 247
    see also immunocompromized
        persons
independent mental capacity
        advocates, 30, 431
infections, 325–45
    catheter-related *see* cannulation
    control, 19–22
        practical procedures and, 370–1
        source, 336, 338
    diarrhoea due to, 171
    distinguishing, 328–9
    neurological/CNS, 295–6, 335
    opportunistic *see* immuno-
        compromized persons
    predisposing factors in critical
        illness, 326
    problem organisms, 336–40
    respiratory, 141–8
        bronchoalveolar lavage, 146,
        147, 415
    transfusion-associated risks,
        247–8, 253
    see also microbiology; sepsis

inflammatory response (syndrome), systemic (SIRS), 325–6, 326, 327
influenza, pandemic, 143
informed consent, 30
  HIV test, 31
inhalant (solvent) abuse, 243
inhalation, smoke, 322
  see also aspiration
inhaled anaesthetic agents as sedatives, 37
injury, traumatic see trauma
Injury Severity Score (ISS), 324
inotropes, 82–5
  cardiogenic shock, 106
  choice, 84–5
  no response, 86–7
  rational use, 86–7
inspiratory time–expiratory time (I:E) ratio, 125
insulin
  in diabetic ketoacidosis, 220
  in non-diabetic patients, 217
  overdose, 238
intensive care unit
  admission policies, 6–7
  definition, 3
  discharge see discharge
intercostal space, chest drains in 5th vs 2nd, 418
intermittent haemodialysis, 190
intermittent mandatory ventilation, synchronized see synchronized intermittent mandatory ventilation
intermittent positive pressure ventilation (IPPV), 154, 158
  chest trauma incl. rib fractures, 314
  complications, 130, 133
  tracheal intubation in facilitation of, 399
intestine (bowel)
  ischaemia, 172
  pseudo-obstruction, 170
intra-abdominal sepsis, 174, 334, 335, 337
intra-aortic balloon counterpulsation pumps, 106, 107

intracerebral haemorrhage, 292, 293
intracranial compliance, 274
intracranial haemorrhage, 272, 292–4
intracranial pressure (ICP)
  monitoring, 289
  raised, 274, 283–4
    in hepatic failure, 178, 180
    management, 283–4
intrathecal drugs, postoperative, 352
intravenous cannulae/access see venous catheterization
intravenous drug abuse, 243–4
intravenous fluids
  composition, 50
  in raised intracranial pressure, 284
intravenous portosystemic shunt, transvenous, 174
intravenous pyelogram, 187
intravenous route, inadvertent enteral feeding by, 59
introducer sheaths, 387–9
intubation see tracheal intubation
investigations, special, 25
iron, antidote, 234
irritable brain-injured patient, 288
ischaemia
  gastrointestinal, 172
  myocardial, and ischaemic heart disease, 100–5
Islamic (Muslim) beliefs, death and dying, 442
isoflurane, 37
ISS (Injury Severity Score), 324
itracuronium, 46

jaw injuries/fracture (incl. mandible), 310
  postoperative management of patients with wiring, 355
Jehovah's Witnesses
  blood/blood product transfusion, 30, 254–5
  death and dying, 441
jejunum, enteral feeding directly to, 47, 422
jet ventilation, high frequency, 133–4

Jewish beliefs, death and dying, 442
joint(s), infections, 335
joint responsibility for admission, 6
Judaic beliefs, death and dying, 442
jugular bulb oxygen saturation, 289
jugular vein cannulation
    external, 378–9, 382
    internal, 377–8, 382

ketamine, 38
    abuse, 243
ketoacidosis, diabetic, 218–20
kidney see entries under renal
Klebsiella, 339

labetalol, 89, 447
lactate–oxygen index, 289
lactated Ringer's, 50
lactic acidosis, 213–14
laryngeal mask insertion, 403–4
laryngoscope in tracheal intubation,
    400
lead, antidote, 234
Legionella pneumoniae, 142–3
lepirudin, 266
levels of critical care, 3–4
levosimendan, 85
life-sustaining treatment see
    treatment (at end of life)
limbs, examination, 24
limitation of treatment, decisions,
    430–1
liver, 176–81
    in APACHE II chronic health
        score, 10
    drug overdose affecting, 230, 236
    dysfunction, 176
    enzymes, elevated in HELPP
        syndrome, 366
    failure, 176–81
    function tests in parenteral
        nutrition, 61
    ruptured, 316–17
    transplantation see transplantation
living wills (advanced directives), 31
local anaesthetics
    in epidural blockade, 350, 351,
        352
    for invasive procedures, 370

long bone injuries, 317–18
    see also fractures
loop diuretics in drug overdose, 233
lorazepam for acute confusional
    state, 42
LSD, 243
Lund and Browder chart, 321
lung
    abscess, 147
    acute injury (ALI), 154–8
        in major haemorrhage, 253
    in chest drainage, failure to
        expand, 419–20
    chronic obstructive disease,
        152–4
    collapse see collapse
    compliance see compliance
    consolidation, 159–60
    gas exchange see gases
    oedema see oedema
    respiratory failure relating to, 119
lysergic acid diethylamide, 243

Maastricht categories for non-
    beating heart donors, 440
magnesium, disturbances, 210
magnesium (sulphate)
    asthma, 150
    phaeochromocytoma, 223
malabsorption of enteral feeds, 59
malignancy, haematological, 269
malignant hyperpyrexia, 363–4
mandibular fracture see jaw injuries
mannitol, 284
    in drug overdose, 232, 233
MDMA (methylenedioxy-
    metamphetamine), 243
mechanical obstruction see
    obstruction
mediastinum
    air, X-ray appearance, 164
    injury, 314
medical records/documents, 26–7
    treatment limitation, 431
meningitis, 295–6, 337
meningococcal sepsis, 342
mental capacity and consent, 29–30
    see also independent mental
        capacity advocates

metabolic acidosis, 53, 116, 212–15
causes, 212
in hepatic failure, 180
postoperative, 357
see also ketoacidosis
metabolic alkalosis, 116, 215
metabolic status
disturbances, 202–7
in hepatic failure, 179–80
in parenteral nutrition, 61
in stress response (to surgery and critical illness), 349
weaning from ventilation, 136
methanol, 240
antidotes, 234, 240–1
methicillin-resistant S. aureus, 226
methylene blue-treated fresh frozen plasma, 249
methylenedioxymetamphetamine (MDMA), 243
microbiology, airway
bronchoalveolar lavage, 415
sputum specimens, 414–15
microdialysis, brain tissue, 290
micronutrients see trace elements; vitamins
midazolam, 37
in renal failure, pharmacology, 198
milrinone, 84
mineral(s), 56
mineralocorticoids, adrenal insufficiency, 221
minitracheostomy, 410–12
mixed venous oxygen saturation, 70
Mobitz type 1 and 2 heart block, 98
monitoring
transferred patients, 426
in traumatic brain injury, 282, 288–90
see also specific items monitored
morphine, 36
in patient-controlled analgesia, 350
mortality see death
Moslem beliefs, death and dying, 442
motility disorder, gastrointestinal, 170

motor response in Glasgow Coma Scale, 278
Mount Vernon formula, 322
moving between patients, infection control and, 21
MRSA, 226
multidisciplinary team, 18–19
communication with, on patient care, 26
impact of death on members of, 443
joint responsibility for admission, 6
multiple injury (incl. brain), priority injury, 279
multiple organ failure (multiorgan dysfunction syndrome)
in infection, 328
in trauma, 309–10
Munchausen-type syndrome, pseudoseizures, 297
muscle relaxants (neuromuscular blocking agents), 43–6
depolarizing see suxamethonium
in hyperthermia, 225
monitoring, 45
neuromuscular conditions and sensitivity to, 302
non-depolarizing, 44, 45–6
prolonged block (delayed recovery), 353–4
in renal failure, pharmacology, 198
reversal, 45–6
in tracheal intubation, 398–9
in traumatic brain injury, 276
muscle weakness in epidural blockade, 351
muscular dystrophies, 302
Muslim beliefs, death and dying, 442
myasthenia gravis, 302–3
Mycoplasma pneumoniae, 142
myocardium
function
blood transfusion and, 246
contractility, 72
infarction, 103–5
acute (STEMI), 104–5

ECG changes, 101
non-ST segment elevation (NSTEMI), 103
ischaemia, 100
see also cardiomyopathy
myoglobin, urinary, 186, 320

naloxone, 41, 237
narrow complex tachycardia, 93, 94
nasal route
enteral feeding (NG tube), 57, 58, 421–2
pneumonia risk, 144
procedure, 421–2
tracheal intubation
risks, 402
sedation vs, 40
national audit databases, 15
near drowning, 323–4
near infrared spectroscopy, brain tissue oxygenation, 289
neck, soft tissue injuries, 310–11
necrosis
acute cortical, 185
acute tubular (ATN), 185, 186
necrotizing fasciitis, 337, 342
Neisseria meningitis, 342
neoplasms *see* tumours
neostigmine
in delayed recovery from neuromuscular block, 353, 354
GI dysmotility, 170
nephrotoxic drugs, 196–7, 230
neurogenic pulmonary oedema, 287–8
neurological assessment in trauma (=disability; D), 307
brain injury, 277
neurological function (incl. CNS), 271–304
discharge criteria, 14
disorders, 271–304
drug overdose-related, 230
infections, 295–6, 335
in recovery on ICU, 304
on patient chart, 23
neuromuscular blocking agents *see* muscle relaxants

neuromuscular conditions (neuromyopathy), 301–3
muscle relaxants causing, 43
respiratory failure due to, 119
neuromuscular status and weaning from ventilation, 136
neuropathy
autonomic, 301
causing respiratory failure, 119
neurosurgical referral in head injury, 280–1
nifedipine, 89
nitric oxide
acute lung injury, 157
right cardiac failure and pulmonary hypertension, 106
nitrogen, 56
nitrous oxide, 37
non-depolarizing muscle relaxants, 44, 45–6
in renal failure, pharmacology, 198
non-ST segment elevation myocardial infarction (NSTEMI), 103
noradrenaline (norepinephrine), 85, 86, 447
hepatic failure, 179
phaeochromocytoma, 223
nosocomial pneumonia *see* pneumonia
nursing staff, 18
talking to relatives in presence of, 28
nutrition, 53–6
daily requirements, 54
enteral *see* enteral feeding
parenteral, 60–2
see also dietician

obstetric patients, 364–7
obstruction (incl. mechanical causes)
airway *see* airway
shock due to, 67
obstructive pulmonary disease, chronic, 152–4
oedema, pulmonary
acute lung injury, 157
neurogenic (in brain injury), 287–8
X-ray appearance, 164–5

oesophagus
  tracheal tube in, 402
  ultrasound imaging of
      heart and aorta via *see*
          transoesophageal ultrasound
  variceal bleeding, 174, 422–4
oliguria, 186
  postoperative, 356
  renal failure, 189–90
opioids
  abuse, 243, 243–4
  antagonists/antidotes, 41, 234
  in epidural blockade, 350, 351
  in renal failure, pharmacology,
      198
  as sedatives, 35
      combined with
          benzodiazepines, 35
  in traumatic brain injury, 276
organ
  failure, multiple *see* multiple
      organ failure
  transplantation *see*
      transplantation
organizational issues, 1–17
organophosphates, antidotes, 234
oscillation ventilation, high
      frequency, 133
osmolality, urine, 186
outcome prediction/scoring, 7–8
  trauma, 324
      brain, 291
outreach, critical care, 5
overdose *see* poisoning
over-sedation, 38–9
oxygen, 68–70
  administration (therapy)
      in anaphylactoid reactions, 362
      in burns, 321
      in carbon monoxide poisoning,
          239
      in chronic obstructive
          pulmonary disease, 152
      in diabetic ketoacidosis,
          218–19
      in respiratory failure, 120
      in tracheal intubation
          procedure, 400

carriage, blood transfusion and,
    246
consumption (VO_2), 68
  typical adult values, 69
delivery (DO_2), 68
  blood transfusion and, 246
  optimization, 69
  typical adult values, 69
extraction ratio, 68–9
fraction of inspired (FiO_2), 114,
    117–18
  acute lung injury, 157
  in APACHE II score, 11
  chronic obstructive pulmonary
      disease, 152
  increasing, in ventilated
      patients, 131
  saturation, venous *see* venous
      oxygen saturation
  tension
      arterial (PaO_2), assessment,
          114
      brain tissue (PO_2), 290
  see also helium–oxygen mix;
      hypoxaemia; hypoxia
oxygenation
  brain tissue, measurement,
      289–90
  extracorporeal membrane *see*
      extracorporeal membrane
      oxygenation
  poor (in ventilated patients), 131

P waves, atrial flutter, 95
pacemakers, 99
packed red cells, 248
  in major haemorrhage, 252
pain, 48
  drugs relieving *see* analgesia
  response in brainstem death
      tests, 300
pancreatitis, acute, 181–2
pancuronium, 46
paracetamol, 235–6
  antidote, 234, 236
paranasal sinus infections, 335
parenteral nutrition, 60–2
Parkland formula, 322

patient-controlled analgesia, 349–50

peak airway pressure (ventilated patient), 129–30

pelvic infection, 335, 337

pelvic injuries, 317

penetrating vs blunt trauma, 309

percutaneous endoscopic gastro(jejun)ostomy, 58

perfusion pressure
cerebral *see* cerebral perfusion pressure
optimization, 85–6
in hypotension, 88

pericardium
aspiration, 395
echocardiography, 78
effusions, 108–9

peri-operative optimization, 348

peripartum haemorrhage, 366

peripheral compartment syndromes, 319

peripheral venous catheterization
for transfusion, 252
in trauma, 307

peripheral venous thrombosis, 265

peritoneal dialysis, 194–5

peritoneal tap, 424

personal impact of death, 443

personnel *see* multidisciplinary team

phaeochromocytoma, 222–3

pharmacists, 19

phencyclidine, 243

phenylephrine, 85, 86, 448

phenytoin, 297, 447, 450
brain injury, 286

phosphate disturbances, 209

phosphodiesterase (III) inhibitors, 84
cardiogenic shock, 107

physical examination *see* examination

physiological derangement in APACHE II, acute, 9, 12

physiotherapists, 18

physiotherapy in respiratory failure, 120
ventilated patient, 129

pigtail catheter drains, 419

pituitary gland
dysfunction in brainstem death/ organ donors, 439
hormone response to surgery and critical illness, 348

plasma, fresh frozen, 249

plasma exchange (plasmapheresis), 199
Guillain–Barré syndrome, 199, 303

platelets
assessment and normal range, 259
low levels
in HELPP syndrome, 366
transfusion, 250, 261
see also thrombocytopenia

pleural cavity
air leak *see* pneumothorax
blood *see* haemothorax

pleural effusions
in pneumonia, 147
ultrasound, 417
X-ray appearance, 161–2

Pneumocystis carinii pneumonia, 145, 148

pneumomediastinum, X-ray appearance, 164

pneumonia, 141–3, 143–8
atypical, 141–3, 337
community-acquired, 141–3, 337
hospital-acquired, 143–5, 147
antibiotics, 147, 148, 337
immunocompromised persons, 145–7, 148
management, 146–8

pneumonitis, aspiration, 148–9

pneumothorax (air leak into pleural cavity), 313
central venous cannulation- related, 386
persisting with chest drain, 420
tension, life-threatening, 416–17
X-ray appearance, 162–3

poisoning and overdose, 229–42
antidotes, 233, 234
intensive care management, 234–5
investigations, 231
measures to reduce absorption or increase elimination, 231–3
see also specific substances

polymorphic ventricular tachycardia, 96, 98
portosystemic shunt, transhepatic intravenous, 174
positive airway pressure (positive pressure ventilation)
  acute lung injury scoring, 156
  continuous (CPAP), 121–2
  intermittent *see* intermittent positive pressure ventilation
  non-invasive, 122–3
positive end expiratory pressure (PEEP), 126
  asthma, 151
  trauma, 314
post-mortem examination, 435–6
  consent, 32, 435–6
postoperative patients, 348–64
  common problems, 352–6
  haemorrhage, 359–61
  ICU management, 357–9
post-renal failure, 184
potassium, 204–7
  administration (KCl), 205–6, 448
  disturbances *see* hyperkalaemia; hypokalaemia
pre-eclampsia, 365–6
pregnancy, 364–7
preload, 71–2
  optimization in cardiac failure, 105
premature beats, ventricular, 95
prerenal failure, 184, 187
pressure
  airway *see* airway
  blood *see* blood pressure
  immobilized patients, injuries due to, 235
  intra-abdominal, 175
  intracranial *see* intracranial pressure
  perfusion *see* perfusion pressure
pressure-controlled ventilation, 124–5, 127
  settings, 128
pressure-support ventilation (assisted spontaneous breathing), 125–6, 127
  settings, 128

triggering, 126–7
pressure–volume–flow loops (heart), 72–4
primary survey in trauma, 306–7
  brain injury, 275–7
Procurator Fiscal, reporting death to, 437
prone position, turning patient to, 425–6
prone positioning, acute lung injury, 158
propofol, 36, 37
  seizures in brain injury, 286
prostacyclin *see* epoprostenol
protamine, 261
protein, 56
protein C, activated, 333, 446
prothrombin complex concentrate, 261
prothrombin time (PT), 176, 177, 178, 179, 259
  prolonged/raised, 176, 261
proton (hydrogen ion/H$^+$) accumulation causing metabolic acidosis, 212
pseudocyst, pancreatic, 182
pseudohyponatraemia, 204
pseudomembranous colitis, 171, 338
Pseudomonas, 339
pseudo-obstruction, intestinal, 170
pseudoseizures, Munchausen-type syndrome, 297
psychiatric consultation in overdose, 235
psychological care, 47–8
pulmonary arteries
  catheterization, 75, 76, 389–93
    in cardiac output measurement, 394–5
    common problems, 392, 393
    indications and contraindications, 389
    X-ray showing position, 159
  embolism (PE), 107–8, 266
  hypertension, right heart failure and, 105–6
  occlusion pressure (PAOP), 75, 78–9, 393
  procedure, 390–1

pulmonary non-vascular tissue *see* lung
pulse contour analysis, 75–6
pulse power analysis, 76–7
pulseless electrical activity (PEA), as electromechanical dissociation, 109
pupils (size/responses) in traumatic brain injury, 276, 278, 285
purpura, 264
    thrombotic thrombocytopenic, 263
pyelogram, intravenous, 187
pylorus (gastric), feeding tube placed through, 47, 422
pyrexia (fever)
    and raised intracranial pressure, 283
    of unknown origin, 335
    see also malignant hyperpyrexia

radial artery cannulation, 372
radiograph *see* X-ray
radiology *see* imaging *and specific modalities*
ranitidine, 62
rapid screening tests for infection, 329
Rastafarian beliefs, death and dying, 441
reassessment in trauma, 307
    brain injury, 277–8
records *see* medical records
recreational drug abuse, 242–4
red cells (blood product), 248
    packed *see* packed red cells
refeeding disease, 62
regional blockage, 350–2
relatives *see* family and relatives
religious beliefs, death and dying, 440, 441–3
remifentanil, 36
renal failure/dysfunction, 184–90
    acute, 189–95
        investigation, 185–7
        management, 188–95
        outcomes, 195

chronic, 195–6
    and hepatic failure, 179
    high-output, 190
    oliguric, 189–90
    prescribing in, 196–8
renal replacement therapy (RRT), 190–4
    drug clearance in, 197
    indications, 190
        lactic acidosis, 214
    problems/complications, 193–4
renal system, 183–99
    drug overdose affecting, 196–7, 230
    function
        discharge criteria, 14
        examination addressing, 24
        failure *see* renal failure
        on patient chart, 23
renal tubules *see* tubules
respiratory acidosis, 115–16
respiratory alkalosis, 116
respiratory distress syndrome, acute/adult (ARDS), 154, 165
    diagnosis, 155
    in major haemorrhage, 253
    management, 155–8
    outcome, 158
    pathophysiology, 155
    X-ray appearance, 165
respiratory drive, loss, 119
respiratory failure, 116–21
    definitions/types, 116–18
    management, 118–21
respiratory insufficiency, postoperative, 355, 356
respiratory stimulants in chronic obstructive pulmonary disease, avoidance, 153
respiratory system, 113–65
    in APACHE II chronic health score, 10
    drug overdose affecting, 230
    examination, 23–4
    infections *see* infections
    on patient chart, 22
    trauma affecting, 313

resuscitation
  burns, 320–2
  in hypothermia continued to
      normothermia, 227
  postoperative haemorrhage,
      360
  sepsis and septic shock, 330,
      331–2
reverse barrier nursing, 21–2
Revised Trauma Score (RTS), 324
rewarming see warming
rhabdomyolysis, 320
rheology, 247
rheumatoid disease, 187
rib fractures, 313–14
Ringer's lactate, 50
Riyadh Intensive Care Program, 8
rocuronium, 44–5, 46
role of intensive care, 2–3
Roman Catholic beliefs, death and
      dying, 441
RTS (Revised Trauma Score), 324

salbutamol, 447
  asthma, 150
  chronic obstructive pulmonary
      disease, 153
salicylate poisoning, 236–7
  see also aspirin
saline solutions, intravenous, 50, 53
  in raised intracranial pressure, 284
salt solutions see saline solutions
SAPS (Simplified Acute Physiology
      Score), 12
Scotland, reporting death in, 437
screening tests
  for infection, rapid, 329
  vasculitis, 187
secondary survey in trauma, 308–9
  brain injury, 277–8
sedation, 34–43
  choice of agents, 35–8
  common problems, 39–43
    excessive sedation, 38–9
  ideal agents, 34–5
  nosocomial pneumonia
      predisposition, 144
  periods free from, 39

postoperative maintenance, 357
  scoring, 39, 40
seizures/convulsions, 285–6, 296–7
  in brain injury, 285–6
  in drug overdose, 235
  in eclampsia, 365
  raised intracranial pressure and,
      283
Seldinger technique
  arterial cannulation, 373
  central venous cannulation, 383
  chest drains, 419
  introducer sheaths, 388
selective decontamination of
      digestive tract, 144–5
selective serotonin reuptake
      inhibitor overdose, 238
Sengstaken–Blakemore tube, 174,
      422–3
sepsis, 80, 327–8, 329–31
  care bundle, 329–31
  catheter-related see cannulation
  coagulopathy in, 258
  in hepatic failure, 179
  immunocompromised patients,
      268
  intra-abdominal, 174, 334, 335, 337
  meningococcal, 342
  shock, 328, 331–4
  unexplained, 334–5
Septifast, 329
Sequential Organ Failure
      Assessment (SOFA) score, 13
severity of illness scoring systems,
      8, 8–13
sharps and other objects puncturing
      skin, 370, 371
shock, 66–7
  cardiogenic, 67, 106
  high-dose steroids, 222
  septic, 328, 331–4
shunt and shunt fraction, 118
sick euthyroid syndrome, 223–4
Sikh beliefs, death and dying, 443
Simplified Acute Physiology Score
      (SAPS), 12
sinus (paranasal) infections, 335
sinus tachycardia, 90–1

skeletal injuries, 317–18
skin examination (incl. wounds), 24–5
smoke inhalation, 322
sodium, 202–4
  disturbances, 202–4
  loss from body, 202, 203
sodium bicarbonate administration in metabolic acidosis, 213
  in lactic acidosis, 214
sodium thiosulphate in cyanide poisoning, 240
SOFA (Sequential Organ Failure Assessment) score, 13
soft tissues
  cervical, injuries, 310–11
  infection, 335
solvent abuse, 243
solvent/detergent-treated fresh frozen plasma, 249
sonography see ultrasound
spinal cord injuries, 311–13
spine (in trauma)
  cervical see cervical spine control
  imaging, 312
  immobilization, 306, 311, 312
spiritual beliefs, death and dying, 440, 441–3
splenic rupture, 316
sputum specimens for microbiology, 414–15
ST segment changes, 101, 103
  acute myocardial infarction (STEMI), 104–5
staff see multidisciplinary team
standardized mortality rate, 8
staphylococci
  coagulase-negative, 338
  methicillin-resistant S. aureus, 226
status epilepticus, 296–7
steroids see anabolic steroids; corticosteroids; mineralocorticoids
stitches (sutures), chest drain-securing, 419
stomach see entries under gastric

streptokinase
  acute myocardial infarction, 104
  pulmonary embolism, 108
stress response to surgery and critical illness, 348–9
stress ulcer, 172
  prophylaxis, 62, 179
    in traumatic brain injury, 282
stroke, 292
stroke volume, 71–2
subarachnoid haemorrhage, 292, 292–4
subclavian vein cannulation, 380–1, 382
substance abuse, 242–4
sucralfate, 62
sugammadex, 45–6
supraglottic airway, 403–4
supraventricular tachycardia, 91–3
surgery
  prolonged, effects, 353
  stress response, 348–9
  subarachnoid haemorrhage (incl. aneurysm), 293–4
  see also postoperative patients
Surviving Sepsis Campaign guidelines for initial treatment, 330
sutures, chest drain-securing, 419
suxamethonium, 43–5
  in renal failure, pharmacology, 198
  in tracheal intubation, 398–9
  trauma, 312
    brain injury, 276
Syncathen test, 221
synchronized intermittent mandatory ventilation (SIMV), 125, 127
  settings, 128
  triggering, 126–7
syndrome of inappropriate ADH secretion, 203
systemic arterial blood pressure
  abnormal see hypertension; hypotension
  maintenance in right cardiac failure and pulmonary hypertension, 106

systemic inflammatory response
        syndrome (SIRS), 325–6,
        326, 327
systemic lupus erythematosus, 187
systemic vascular resistance,
        shock related to reduction
        alterations in, 67
systole, end systolic point, 74

tachycardia
    broad complex, 95–6, 97
    narrow complex, 93, 94
    polymorphic ventricular, 96, 98
    predisposing factors, 90
    sinus, 90–1
    supraventricular, 91–3
tacrolismus, 450
tamponade, cardiac, 108–9
technicians, 19
teeth, injury, 310
teicoplanin, 450
temperature
    dysregulation, 224–7
        in brainstem death/organ
            donors, 439
        in drugs overdose, 235
        in traumatic brain injury, 282
    measurement, 224
Tensilon test, 303
tension pneumothorax, life-
        threatening, 416–17
terlipressin, 86
terminal care, 429–43
tetanus, 303, 304
theophylline, 450
Therapeutic Intervention Score
        System (TISS), 12
thermal injury, 320–2
thermodilution, cardiac output
        measurement by, 394–5
thermoregulation see temperature
thiopental/thiopentone (in brain
        injury)
    with raised intracranial pressure,
        284
    with seizures, 286
thoracostomy, chest drain insertion
        through, 418–19

thoracotomy, 417, 420
thorax see chest
thrombin time (TT), 259
thrombocytopenia, 262–3
thrombocytopenic purpura,
        thrombotic, 263
thromboelastography, 260
thrombolysis
    acute myocardial infarction, 104
    pulmonary embolism, 108
thrombosis, 264–5
    central venous cannula-induced
        (around cannula), 386
    deep venous see deep venous
        thrombosis
    embolization see embolism
    predisposing factors, 264, 265
    in thrombocytopenia, 262
thrombotic thrombocytopenic
        purpura, 263
thyroid dysfunction, 223–4
thyroxine (T3), 223, 224
TISS (Therapeutic Intervention
        Score System), 12
tissue plasminogen activator,
        acute myocardial infarction,
        104
tooth injury, 310
torsades de pointes, 96, 98
total parenteral nutrition, 60–2
toxicology, 229–44
trace elements, 56
    parenteral nutrition, 61
tracheal intubation, 398–402
    airway obstruction with, 140
    communication difficulties, 47–8
    indications, 398, 399
        airway obstruction, 139, 399
        airway protection in gastric
            lavage, 232
        trauma see subheading below
    nasal see nasal route
    procedure, 399–401
    removal see extubation
    risks/problems/complications,
        130, 132, 133, 402
        pneumonia, 144
        in prolonged intubation, 130

trauma
  brain, 275–7
  facial, 310
  spinal, 312
  tubes, 400–1
    in tracheostomy, 406–7
    X-ray showing position, 159
tracheal suction, ventilated patient, 129
tracheostomy, 404–10
  advantages, 404
  in brain injury, 287
  contraindications, 404
  indications, 404
    airway obstruction, 139, 404
    weaning from ventilation, 137
  percutaneous, 404–10
    procedure, 405–8
    surgical vs, 405
  risks and complications, 408–16
    airway obstruction, 140
    pneumonia, 144
  sedation vs, 40
  tubes, 409
    changing, 409–10
    choice, 405
    misplaced, 402, 408–9
    removal, 410
    see also minitracheostomy
transfer of patients, 426–7
transfusion (blood and blood products), 246–55
  administering products, 251
  indications, 246–7
  recipient identity checks, 250
  refusal (incl. Jehovah's Witnesses), 30, 254–5
  requesting products, 250
  risks and complications, 252–4
    infections, 247–8, 253
  storage of products, 251
  UK available products, 247–51
transhepatic intravenous portosystemic shunt, 174

transoesophageal ultrasound
  Doppler, descending aorta, 77
  valves dysfunction, 341
transplantation, 270, 359
  liver, 180–1
    in paracetamol poisoning, 236
  organ donors for, 437–40
    non-beating heart, 439–40
    register, 31
transport of patients, 426–7
transpyloric feeding tubes, 47, 422
trauma
  brain (from head injury), 272, 274–88
    common problems, 284–8
    ICU management, 281–3
    immediate management, 274–9
    monitoring, 282, 288–90
    multiple (with brain injury), priority injury, 279
  other than brain, 305–25
    ICU management, 309–10
    outcome, 324
    primary survey, 306–7
    reassessment and secondary survey, 308–9
Trauma Score and Injury Severity Score (TRISS), 324
treatment (at end of life)
  limitation decisions, 430–1
  withdrawal, 431–3
tricyclic antidepressant overdose, 237–8
triggering of ventilation, 126–7
TRISS (Trauma Score and Injury Severity Score), 324
troponin, cardiac (troponin I), 101–2
tubules, renal
  acidosis due to dysfunction of, 214–15
  acute necrosis (ATN), 185, 186
tumours (neoplasms)
  adrenal gland, secretory, 222–3
  malignant haematological, 269

ulcers, stress *see* stress ulcer
ultrasound
abdominal, 169
ascites, 425
in renal failure, 187
abdominothoracic, trauma,
308–9
arterial cannulation guidance,
373
central venous cannulation
guidance, 376–7
femoral vein, 381
internal jugular vein, 378
subclavian vein, 381
pleural effusions, 417
see also Doppler;
echocardiography
unconscious patient, spinal cord
injury signs, 312
urea, serum, 186
urethral injury, 317
urinary tract infection, 335, 337
urine
biochemistry in acute renal
failure, 186
myoglobin, 186, 320

valvular (heart) lesions, 341
vancomycin, 450
enterococci resistant to, 338
variceal bleeding, 174, 422–4
vascular access *see* cannulation
vascular endothelial damage,
thrombosis risk, 265
vascular injury, great vessels, 314
vascular resistance, systemic,
shock related to reduction
alterations in, 67
vasculitis screen, 187
vasoactive drugs, 80
vasoconstrictors/vasopressors, 85
no response, 86–7
rational use, 86–7
in traumatic brain injury,
283
vasopressin *see* antidiuretic
hormone
vecuronium, 46

vegetative state following cardiac
arrest (in hypoxic brain
injury), 295
venous catheterization/access
burns patient, 321
central *see* central venous
cannulation
infection risk in
immunocompromised
patients, 268
peripheral *see* peripheral venous
catheterization
venous oxygen saturation
jugular bulb, 289
mixed, 70
venous pressure, central *see* central
venous pressure
venous thrombosis, 265
deep *see* deep venous thrombosis
venovenous haemodiafiltration,
continuous, 193
venovenous haemodialysis,
continuous, 192
venovenous haemofiltration,
continuous, 191
ventilation (artificial), 121–39
common problems/difficulties,
131–3
in tracheostomy, 408–9
complications, 130
in gastric lavage, 232
high frequency, 133–5
hypoxic brain injury, 295
indicated conditions (in
respiratory failure), 121
acute lung injury, 157
asthma, 150–1
chest injury incl. rib fractures,
314
chronic obstructive pulmonary
disease, 154
traumatic brain injury, 275–7
invasive, 123–7
non-invasive, 122–3, 137
patient care, 128–30
strategies and settings, 127, 128
transferred patients, 426
triggering, 126–7

weaning, 135–9
  jet ventilation as aid to, 135
ventilation–perfusion mismatch, 118
ventricles
  fibrillation, 109
    defibrillation, 396–8
  filling of RV, optimization in cardiac failure, 106
  polymorphic tachycardia, 96, 98
  premature beats, 95
  pressure–volume–flow loops in LV, 72, 73
  stroke volume, 71–2
ventricular demand pacemaker, 99
verbal response in Glasgow Coma Scale, 278
viral infections
  pneumonia due to, 142
  transfusion-associated, 247, 253
vitamins (organic micronutrients), 56
  parenteral nutrition, 61
volume-controlled ventilation, 123–4, 127
  settings, 128
volume trauma (in ventilation), 130
volumetric haemodynamic monitoring, 81–2
VVI pacemakers, 99

waking up from sedation, slow, 40–1
warfarin, antidotes, 234

warming/rewarming, 226
  postoperative, 357
water
  daily requirements, 49
  excessive intake, 202
  reduced clearance, 202
websites, 452
wedging of pulmonary artery catheter, problems, 382
weight measurement in fluid management, 52
Wenckebach phenomenon, 98
whole blood, 248
wire *see* guidewire
withdrawal of treatment, 431–3
withdrawal phenomena/symptoms
  alcohol, 241–2
  opioids, 244
  sedatives, 42
World Federation of Neurological Surgeons grading scale for subarachnoid haemorrhage, 293
wounds
  examination, 24–5
  infection, 335, 337

X-ray
  abdominal, 169
    in renal failure, 187
  chest *see* chest
  spine, 312

young hypertensive patients, 89–90